Suicide

an unnecessary death

Suicide

an unnecessary death

SECOND EDITION

Edited by

Danuta Wasserman

National Centre for Suicide Research and Prevention
of Mental Ill-Health (NASP)
Karolinska Institute
Stockholm, Sweden

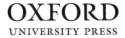

In 1882, Jules Michelet wrote the following existential reflection on Vincent van Gogh's drawing Sorrow: 'Comment se fait-il qu'il y ait sur la terre une femme seule – . . . ' This reflection brings to the fore the role of solitude and loneliness.

Suicide is a predominantly male phenomenon. Millions of mothers, wives, sisters and daughters are left alone in indescribable grief. Along with the male relatives, they are survivors tormented by sorrow and pain.

However, suicide is also becoming a female phenomenon. Our contemporary world, with its fascinating opportunities for development, has a shadowy side that most of us seek to avoid. An increasing number of girls and women, hurt in their loneliness and abandonment, and in their sense of exclusion from human fellowship, can no longer cope with life. In some countries, for some age groups, female suicide outnumbers male suicide.

The words of grief kill none.
Dumb silence is what kills.
Speaking, we live;
Speechless, we die.
Listen, then, to my voice–
a paltry flame that lights up
the walls of our cave.
'There is no one here,
there is nothing to fear
as long as the world exists
and the flame is lit.'

Olof Lagercrantz
(Swedish poet, 1911–2002)

Front cover illustration: *Sorrow*, Vincent Van Gogh, 1882.
Reproduced with the kind permission of
The New Art Gallery   Walsall, Garman Ryan Collection, UK.

OXFORD
UNIVERSITY PRESS

Great Clarendon Street, Oxford, OX2 6DP,
United Kingdom

Oxford University Press is a department of the University of Oxford.
It furthers the University's objective of excellence in research, scholarship,
and education by publishing worldwide. Oxford is a registered trade mark of
Oxford University Press in the UK and in certain other countries

© Oxford University Press 2016

First Edition published by Martin Dunitz/Informa in 2001
Second Edition published by Oxford University Press in 2016
Impression: 1

Published in the United States of America by Oxford University Press
198 Madison Avenue, New York, NY 10016, United States of America

British Library Cataloguing in Publication Data
Data available

Library of Congress Control Number: 2015938211

ISBN 978–0–19–871739–3

Printed and bound by
CPI Group (UK) Ltd, Croydon, CR0 4YY

Contents

VIIB *Public health perspective*

About the editor

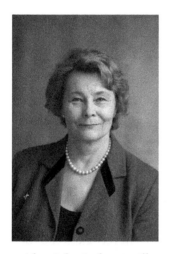

Danuta Wasserman, MD, PhD, is Professor of Psychiatry and Suicidology at Karolinska Institute (KI) in Stockholm, Sweden and Head of the National Centre for Suicide Research and Prevention of Mental Ill-Health (NASP) at KI. She is Director of the WHO Collaborating Centre for Research, Methods Development and Training in Suicide Prevention. NASP, which Professor Wasserman founded in 1993, is active in four main areas: research and development of new suicide-preventive methods, epidemiological surveillance, information, and teaching. The Centre's researchers collaborate in many international preventive projects.

Professor Wasserman's research activities comprise epidemiological, psychodynamic, psychiatric, and genetic studies of suicidal behaviours. She also has experience of clinical practice with depressive and suicidal patients. The study of suicidal communication and responses of the closest family members and the care-givers, as well as psychological problems arising in patients and in the staff in the treatment process, are of particular interest to Professor Wasserman's research. High priority is also given to randomized controlled trials (RCTs) designed to promote new suicide-preventive measures aimed at young people. Professor Wasserman is the Principal Investigator for the Saving and Empowering Young Lives in Europe (SEYLE), Working in Europe to Stop Truancy Among Youth (WE-Stay), and Suicide Prevention by Internet and Media-Based Mental Health Promotion (SUPREME) projects, which are school-based suicide-preventive intervention studies conducted in several European countries and funded by the European Union. She is Principal Investigator for the Genetic Study of Suicidal Behaviours

(GISS), which is focusing on the interplay between genes and environment in families of suicide attempters. GISS comprises the biggest collection in the world of both parents and their suicidal offspring. She received the honour from the Nobel Assembly at Karolinska Institute (KI) to organize the Nobel conference on the role of genetics in promoting suicide prevention and mental health of the population. Professor Wasserman has written and co-authored several hundred publications and book chapters. She is editor of the Oxford Textbook of Suicidology and Suicide Prevention: A Global Perspective.

Professor Wasserman was President of the International Academy of Suicide Research (IASR), the President of the European Psychiatric Association (EPA), and Chairman of the Section on Suicide Prevention of the World Psychiatric Association (WPA) and EPA. She served as Chairman of the Department of Public Health Sciences at Karolinska Institute. She has won numerous national and international honours and awards, including, the Stengel Research Award from the International Association for Suicide Prevention (IASP) in recognition of her outstanding contributions in the field of suicide research and suicide prevention, the Distinguished Research Award from the American Foundation for Suicide Research (AFSP), the Hans-Rost-Prize from the German Association for Suicide Prevention, and the Book of Science Award from the British Medical Association for her book Depression: the facts published by the Oxford University Press. The Nordic Council of Ministers of Health awarded Prof Wasserman for her outstanding contributions to public health research and prevention. She is an honorary fellow of the Royal College of Psychiatrists in the UK, and an honorary member of several other European Psychiatric Associations, including memberships to various Executive Committees and Working Groups on suicide research in both national and international scientific organizations.

About the contributors

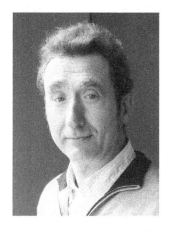

Karl Andriessen

Karl Andriessen, MSuicidology (Griffith University, Brisbane, Australia) is an Anika Foundation PhD student at the School of Psychiatry, University of New South Wales, Australia. Before moving to Australia, he has been working in suicide prevention and postvention nationally and internationally for 25 years. He is an affiliated researcher with the Faculty of Psychology and Educational Sciences, University of Leuven, Belgium, and has published many peer-reviewed articles and book chapters in English, Dutch and French. He is a Co-Chair of the Special Interest Group on Suicide Bereavement of the International Association for Suicide Prevention (IASP), and received the 2005 IASP Farberow Award for outstanding contributions in the field of bereavement and survivors after suicide.

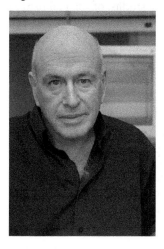

Alan Apter

Alan Apter, MD, PhD, is a Professor in Child and Adolescent Psychiatry and graduated in medicine from the University of Witwatersrand. He then emigrated to Israel and was a Battalion Medical Officer in the Israel Defense Force. He completed his training in adult psychiatry at the Sackler School of Medicine at the University of Tel-Aviv and his training in child and adolescent psychiatry at Children's National Medical Center in Washington DC, US. His fellowship in biological psychiatry was at Albert Einstein College of Medicine in New York. He served as Chairman of the Department of Psychiatry at Sackler School of Medicine and is Director of the Feinberg Child Study Center at Schneider's Children's Medical Center of Israel.

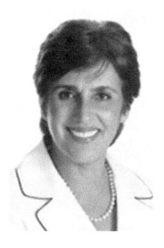

Victoria Arango

Victoria Arango is the Associate Director of the Division of Molecular Imaging and Neuropathology at the New York State Psychiatric Institute and a Professor of Neurobiology in the Department of Psychiatry at Columbia University. She is an internationally renowned expert in the biology of completed suicide. Her research focuses on the examination of monoamine systems in individuals who die by suicide and in structural and morphometric abnormalities in the same subjects.

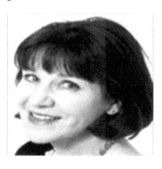

Annette L Beautrais

Professor Annette L Beautrais works and teaches in suicide research and prevention at University of Canterbury, Christchurch, New Zealand. Her work includes: suicide-related presentations to emergency departments; geospatial mapping of suicide clusters; psychological autopsy studies of suicidal behaviour; postvention support for people bereaved and impacted by suicide; text-messaging interventions to reduce suicide-related presentations to the emergency department; and longitudinal studies of suicidal behaviour.

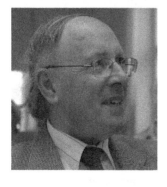

Per Bech

Per Bech, MD, Dr Sci, FRCPsych, is Professor of Psychiatry and Clinical Psychometrics at the Psychiatric Research Unit, Mental Health Centre North Zealand Hillerød, University of Copenhagen, Denmark. He became an honorary member of the European Psychiatric Association (EPA) in 2000 and of the Danish Psychiatric Association in 2014. He was awarded the Anna Monika Prize for studies on the use of rating scales in 1983 as well as the Strömgren Award in 2009 and the CINP Pioneers in Psychopharmacology Award in 2010.

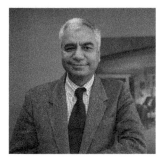

Dinesh Bhugra

Dinesh Bhugra, CBE, is a Professor and the President of the World Psychiatric Association (2014–2017). In 2008–2011, he was President of the Royal College of Psychiatrists in the UK. He was Chair of the UK's Mental Health Foundation in 2011–2014, and is its President. His research interests are in cultural psychiatry, sexual dysfunction, and service development. He has authored/co-authored more than 350 scientific papers and 30 books. He is the Editor of *International Journal of Social Psychiatry, International Review of Psychiatry*, and *International Journal of Culture and Mental Health.*

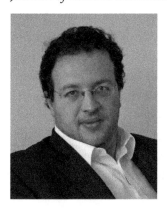

Vladimir Carli

Dr Vladimir Carli, MD, PhD, is Senior Lecturer in Prevention of Suicide and Mental Ill-Health at the National Centre for Suicide Research and Prevention (NASP), at Karolinska Institute (KI). He is Co-Director of the WHO Collaborating Centre for Research, Training and Methods Development in Suicide Prevention. He is Vice President of the International Association for Suicide Prevention, Chair of the Suicidology Section of the World Psychiatric Association (WPA), as well as the Secretary General of the Network on Suicide Prevention of the European College of Neuropsychopharmacology (ECNP) and the Section of Suicidology and Suicide Prevention of the European Psychiatric Association (EPA). He is co-author of more than 60 scientific publications.

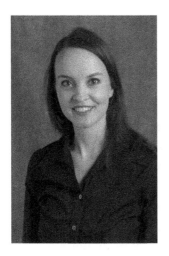

Megan Chesin

Dr Megan Chesin is an Assistant Professor at William Paterson University and a Research Scientist at the New York State Psychiatric Institute. Her research interests include developing and testing mindfulness-based interventions to prevent suicide attempt. She also studies biopsychological factors associated with suicide attempt.

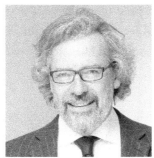

Diego De Leo

Diego De Leo, MD, PhD, is Past President of both IASP and IASR. He has successfully established and managed high-level international collaborations. Director of the Australian Institute for Suicide Research and Prevention (AISRAP) at Griffith University, he is also the Editor-in-Chief of the journal CRISIS, he is the newly appointed Chair of the College of Presidents of IASP, and serves as a board member of the Australian Suicide Prevention Advisory Council. Professor De Leo is the winner of several national and international awards. In 2013, he was appointed as an Officer in the General Division of the Order of Australia, awarded for 'distinguished service to medicine in the field of psychiatry as a researcher and through the creation of national and international strategies for suicide prevention'. Professor De Leo's research expertise includes definitional issues, old-age suicide, international trends, and suicide-prevention programmes.

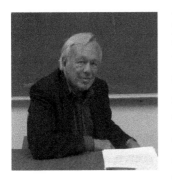

Jan Fawcett

Dr Jan Fawcett graduated from Yale University Medical School, and received psychiatric training at the Langley Porter Neuropsychiatric Institute in San Francisco and the University of Rochester. His research career in the areas of depression and suicide began as research fellow at the Clinical Center of the National Institute for Mental Health in Bethesda, Maryland. He then created an inpatient research unit for the treatment of suicidal patients at the Illinois State Psychiatric Institute in Chicago with the University of Illinois. In 1972, he became the Stanley Harris Jr Chair of Psychiatry at Rush University Medical Center. He then became Principal Investigator of the Rush Site of the NIMH Collaborative Depression Study. He continued his studies of depression and suicide receiving awards from the Anna Monica Foundation, the American Foundation for the Prevention of Suicide, the American Suicide Association, the American College of Physicians, and NARSAD, now known as the Brain and Behavior Research Foundation, for his studies in depression and suicide. In 2002, he retired from his chair to become Professor of Psychiatry at the University of New Mexico School of Medicine, where he continues to teach, and do clinical research and practice with an emphasis on treatment refractory depression.

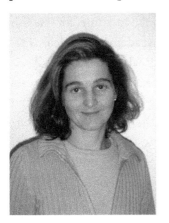

Alexandra Fleischmann

Alexandra Fleischmann is a clinical and health psychologist, who obtained her Doctor of Psychological Science degree at the University of Vienna, Austria, in 1997. She held positions at the University Clinic of Medical Psychology and Psychotherapy, Graz, Austria and at the University Institute of Psychology, Zurich, Switzerland. For the past 15 years she has been working at the World Health Organization, Geneva, Switzerland in the Department of Mental Health and Substance Abuse, particularly on the prevention of suicide.

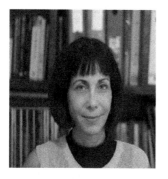

Yari Gvion

Yari Gvion, PhD, is a supervising clinical psychologist who has worked for many years in a psychiatric hospital with adolescents and in private clinic. She is a staff member at Bar-ILan University and Tel Aviv—Yafo College. Her main fields of research include risk factors for suicide attempts, severity of suicide attempts, and self-destruction in adolescent psychiatric patients.

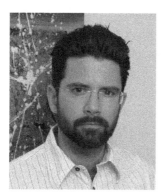

Gergö Hadlaczky

Gergö Hadlaczky, PhD, is a researcher and lecturer at the National Swedish Prevention of Suicide and Mental Ill-Health (NASP) at Karolinska Institute, Stockholm, Sweden. He specializes in experimental psychology and his main research interest areas include decision-making in suicidal individuals and the prevention of suicide through new technologies.

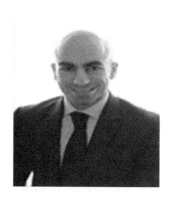

Ahmed Hankir

Ahmed Hankir, MBChB, is a doctor at the National Institute for Health Research and Academic Clinical Fellow in Psychiatry with Manchester University. Dr Hankir's research interests are wide-ranging and he has published extensively on the public understanding of psychiatry, the mental health of health-care professionals, and the policy and provision of mental health services in conflict zones. Dr Hankir has also presented his research findings in international conferences all over the world and is the recipient of numerous prestigious prizes, most notably the 2013 Royal College of Psychiatrists Foundation Doctor of the Year. Dr Hankir conducts research under the auspices of the Ministry of Defence on military mental health with Professor Sir Simon Wessely, President of the Royal College of Psychiatrists.

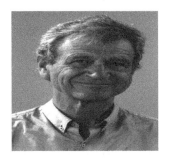

Göran Högberg

Göran Högberg MD, PhD, is active at the Department of Women's and Children's Health, Child and Adolescent Psychiatric Unit, Astrid Lindgren Children's Hospital, Karolinska Institute, Stockholm, Sweden.

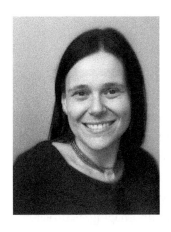

Karolina Krysinska

Karolina Krysinska, PhD, is a Project Coordinator working at the Centre of Research Excellence in Suicide Prevention, Black Dog Institute, Sydney, Australia, and is affiliated as a research fellow at the Faculty of Psychology and Educational Sciences, KUL --University of Leuven, Belgium. Her research interests include risk and protective factors in suicide, suicide prevention, thanatology, psychology of trauma, and psychology of religion. She is an author and co-author of book chapters and peer-reviewed articles on various aspects of suicide, trauma, and bereavement.

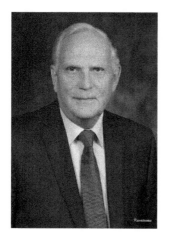

Jouko Lönnqvist

Jouko Lönnqvist, MD, PhD, served as Professor of Psychiatry (University of Helsinki) and as a research professor and director at the National Institute of Health and Welfare in Finland. His main professional and research interests have been mental health, self-destructive behaviour, and psychoses. He has published more than 500 research articles in international journals. Professor Lönnqvist was the President of the International Academy of Suicide Research (IASR) 2008–2009. He received the Stengel Award in 1981, the Award for Scientific Achievement (American Foundation for Suicide Prevention) in 2004, and the Nordic Public Health Prize in 2011.

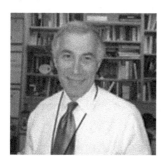

J John Mann

J John Mann, MD, is Director of the Division of Molecular Imaging and Neuropathology at the New York State Psychiatric Institute and is the Paul Janssen Professor of Translational Neuroscience in Psychiatry and Radiology at Columbia University College of Physicians and Surgeons. Professor Mann's research employs functional brain imaging, neurochemistry, and molecular genetics to probe the causes of depression and suicide. He is Head of the NIMH-funded Conte Translation Neuroscience Research Center for the Study of Suicidal Behavior at Columbia University. Professor Mann has edited ten books on suicide and psychiatric disorders.

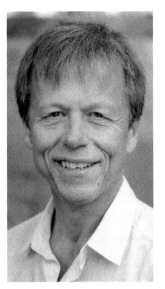

Lars Mehlum

Lars Mehlum, MD, PhD, is Professor of Psychiatry and Suicidology at the University of Oslo and the founding head of the Norwegian National Suicide Research and Prevention Centre. Dr Mehlum has published widely on his research on suicidal behaviour in the young, patients with personality disorders and schizophrenia, and treatment outcome studies on suicide attempters, among them research on dialectical behaviour therapy. He is a policy adviser for suicide prevention, a past president of the International Association for Suicide Prevention, and President of the European Society for the Study of Personality Disorders.

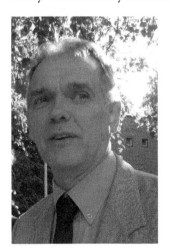

Ilkka Henrik Mäkinen

Ilkka Henrik Mäkinen, PhD, LLM, is Professor of Sociology at Uppsala University. He has published several works on different aspects of suicide as a social/societal phenomenon. His research interests include the epidemiology and sociology of suicide, as well as attitudes, laws, and the history related to this form of death.

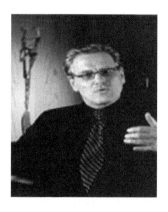

Hans-Jürgen Möller

Hans-Jürgen Möller, MD, served as Professor of Psychiatry and Chairman of the Psychiatric Department at the Ludwig-Maximilians-University in Munich, Germany, where he acts as professor emeritus. Professor Möller has been working in the field of psychiatry for more than 40 years. After obtaining his Doctor of Medical Science in 1972 from the University Germany, he then specialized in psychiatry and completed postgraduate training at the Max Planck Institute of Psychiatry in Munich. From 1980 to 1988, he was Professor of Psychiatry at Munich Technical University, and from 1988 to 1994 Professor of Psychiatry and Chairman of the Psychiatric Department at the University of Bonn in Germany. Professor Möller's main scientific contributions include clinical and neurobiological research into psychiatry, schizophrenia and depression, and clinical psychopharmacology. Professor Möller has written and co-authored more than 1,000 publications and several books. He is co-editor of *European Archives of Psychiatry and Clinical Neuroscience*, and co-editor of *Psychopharmakotherapie*. He is founding editor and former chief editor of the *World Journal of Biological Psychiatry*. He also holds positions on the editorial boards of numerous national and international psychiatric journals. He has been a member of the executive committees of several national and international psychiatric societies. He was President of the World Federation of Society of Biological Psychiatry (WFSBP), President of the European Psychiatric Association (EPA), and Chairman of the Section on Pharmacopsychiatry of the World Psychiatric Association (WPA). He is Past-President of the Collegium Internationale Neuro-Psychopharmacologicum (CINP). He received numerous awards, among others the Jean Delay Price of the WPA and the Long-term Achievement Award of the WFSBP.

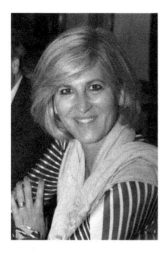

Véronique Narboni

Doctor Véronique Narboni studied medicine in Montpellier, France and graduated in 1991 as a general practitioner. She was a guest researcher at the Karolinska Institute in Stockholm from 1999 to 2000, at the National Swedish and Stockholm County Centre for Suicide Prevention founded in 1993 by Professor Danuta Wasserman. During this period, she collaborated in the development of the WHO project SUPRE, and on the guidance paper 'Preventing suicide: a resource for school teachers and other school staff'. After having worked on the impact of educational programmes on the attitudes and behaviour of general practitioners, with regard to suicide prevention, based in Paris she is now sharing her time between a GP practice and a brain-health project: "Sustainable Brain Health Institute".

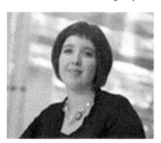

Siobhan T O'Dwyer

Siobhan T O'Dwyer is a research fellow with a joint appointment between the Centre for Health Practice Innovation and the Australian Institute for Suicide Research and Prevention (both at Griffith University, Australia). Siobhan is a gerontologist with a background in psychology and public health. She led the world's first research on suicide risk in family carers. Her other research interests include social robotics and non-pharmacological approaches to dementia care.

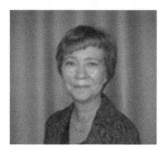

Lis R Olsen

Lis R Olsen, MD, PhD, is a child and adolescent psychiatrist and Head of the Outpatient Clinic for Adolescent Psychiatry, Mental Health Services, Capital Region of Denmark, Child and Adolescent Mental Health Center, Denmark. Her main research interests are psychometrics, depression, and child and adolescent psychiatry.

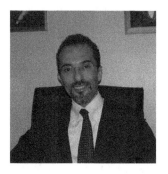

Maurizio Pompili

Maurizio Pompili, MD, PhD, is Professor of Suicidology at the Sapienza University of Rome, Italy. He is Director of the Suicide Prevention Center at Sant'Andrea Hospital in Rome. He is the recipient of the American Association of Suicidology's 2008 Shneidman Award for 'Outstanding contributions in research in suicidology'.

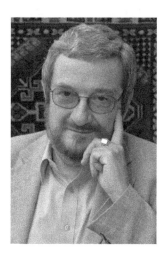

Zoltán Rihmer

Zoltán Rihmer, MD, PhD, DSc, is Professor of Psychiatry at the Department of Clinical and Theoretical Mental Health and Department of Psychiatry and Psychotherapy, Semmelweis University, and Director of the Laboratory of Suicide Research and Prevention, National Institute of Psychiatry and Addictions, Budapest, Hungary. As a full-time clinician, his special interest is the clinical and biological/genetic aspects of mood and anxiety disorders, with particular regards to prediction of treatment response and prediction and prevention of suicide, and the interface between mood disorders and cardiology. Professor Rihmer is a board member of several Hungarian and international organizations and editorial boards. Dr Rihmer has published more than 460 scientific articles/book chapters and five books. He has received several national and international awards and he is a member of several national and international scientific organizations and editorial boards, including *Journal of Affective Disorders, Suicidology Online, World Journal of Biological Psychiatry, International Journal of Psychiatry in Clinical Practice, Psychiatria Hungarica*, and *Neuripsychopharmacologia Hungarica*.

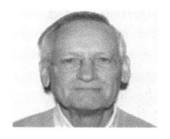

Alec Roy

Alec Roy, MD, is Professor of Psychiatry at the New Jersey Medical School. His main area of research is suicidology, especially risk factors, genetics, alcohol and substance dependence, schizophrenia, depression, and prevention. He received the Louis Dublin Award of the American Association of Suicidology and the Stengel Research Award of the International Association for Suicide Prevention in 1999.

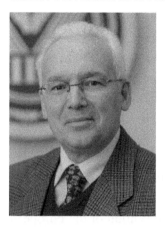

Vsevolod A Rozanov

Vsevolod Rozanov, MD, PhD is a Professor of Suicidology and the Chair of Clinical Psychology at the Institute of Post-Diploma Education, Odessa Mechnikov University. He started his career in clinical neurochemistry and then shifted towards behavioural genetics and suicide prevention. He has been involved in GISS (genetic project on suicidal behaviour) in collaboration with Karolinska Institute. He combines research with suicide prevention and mental health promotion, including initiatives in the armed forces, as well as among GPs and schoolteachers. He is an active member of IASP, EPA, and WPA, where he re-established the section of military psychiatry and serves as the chair of the section.

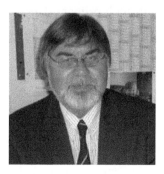

Wolfgang Rutz

Wolfgang Rutz holds an MD from the University of Wurzburg, Germany and a PhD from the University of Linkoping, Sweden. He was director of mental health services on Gotland for many years and has been intensively engaged in the development of mental health services in

Sweden and the Nordic and Baltic countries. Over the last decade his research has focused on the prevention and monitoring of depressive conditions and suicidality. From 1998 to 2005 Dr Rutz was Regional Adviser for Mental Health at the WHO Regional Office for Europe in Copenhagen, and from 2005 to 2009 he headed the Department of Public Mental Health at the Academic University Clinic in Uppsala, Sweden. He is Professor of Social Psychiatry at the University for Applied Sciences in Coburg, Germany and is affiliated as Senior Consultant for Public Mental Health to the Karolinska Institute, Stockholm and the Theological Faculty at Uppsala University, Sweden.

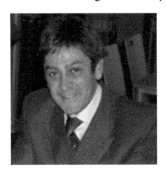

Marco Sarchiapone

Marco Sarchiapone is Associated Professor of Psychiatry at the University of Molise and Psychiatrist at the National Institute for Health, Migration and Poverty (NIHMP). He has been involved in research in the field of suicidology for more than 20 years in an interdisciplinary perspective, ranging from biological aspects to social and psychological correlates. He is the Chairman of the Section of Suicidology and Suicide Prevention of the European Psychiatric Association (www.suicidology.net/epa) and Italian representative at the WHO/Euro Network for Suicide Prevention. He is the editor of the open-access journal Suicidology Online (www.suicidology-online.com). He is the Scientific Coordinator of the "EUDOR-A Multi-centre Research Program - A Naturalistic, European Multi-centre Clinical Study of EDOR Test in adult patients with primary depression" and UNICEF Consultant for the implementation of a programme aimed at preventing suicide among high school adolescents and juvenile offenders in Kazakhstan. He was deputy coordinator of SEYLE (Saving and Empowering Young Lives in Europe) and WE-STAY (Working in Europe to Stop Truancy Among Youth), two research projects funded under the EU 7th Framework Programme and aimed at preventing suicide and risk behaviors among adolescents. He was also site leader of SUPREME (Suicide Prevention by Internet and Media

Based Mental Health Promotion), funded by the European Agency for Health and Consumers, and of the MONSUE project (Monitoring Suicide in Europe). He was President of the 13th European Symposium on Suicide and Suicidal Behaviour and of the 1st Roman Forum on Suicide. In Italy, he has been responsible for a large research project on psychological and genetic factors associated to violence and self-harm behaviour in prisoners.

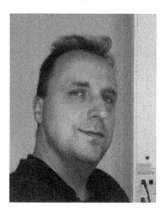

Marcus Sokolowski

Marcus Sokolowski, PhD, is Associate Professor in Public Health Science and Genetics at the National Centre for Suicide Research and Prevention of Mental Ill-Health (NASP), located at the Karolinska Institute in Stockholm, Sweden. Coming from a background of PhD and post-doc in molecular biology and virology, he joined NASP at KI in the 2005 and has since then conducted genetic investigations of suicidal behaviours in Professor Danuta Wasserman's research group. He teaches on the subject and supervises Master and PhD students. He helped Professor Wasserman and Professor Lars Terenius to organize the 2009 Nobel Conference on 'The Role of Genetics in Promoting Suicide Prevention and the Mental Health of the Population'. Dr Sokolowski received the 2010 Andrej Marusic Award at the ESSSB13 conference for his contributions to biological suicidology, in addition to previous awards and stipends.

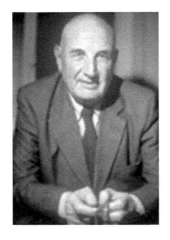

Jean-Pierre Soubrier

Jean-Pierre Soubrier, MD, is professor emeritus at the Collège de Médecine des Hôpitaux de Paris, France, and honorary chief psychiatrist at University Hospital Paris (AP-HP). His suicidology research career began in 1965 as a Fulbright Research Fellow at the Suicide Prevention Center, Los Angeles, US. He was Founding President of the Groupement d'Etudes et de Prévention du Suicide (GEPS), France (1969), Past President of the International Association for Suicide Prevention (IASP), WHO Advisory Board Member International Committee on Suicide Prevention, and First Chairman of the World Psychiatric Association (WPA) Section on Suicidology (2002). His awards include Silver Medal, Faculty of Medicine, Paris (1965); Best Film Medical Festival 'Suicide prevention: myth or reality?', Paris (1974); Stengel Award, IASP (1981); Annual Award, Académie Nationale de Médecine, France (1985); and Best Scientific Poster: 'Print media and suicide', European Congress of Suicidology (ESSSB), Rome, Italy (2010). He is Consulting Editor of the journal *Suicide and Life Threatening Behavior* (US) and is a member of the Scientific Committee National Strategy on Suicide Prevention (France). He was Chairman of the Taskforce Suicide Prevention in old age (2009–2011) and opened a resource centre on suicidology, Centre Ressource En Suicidologie (CRES) in Paris, France in 2012.

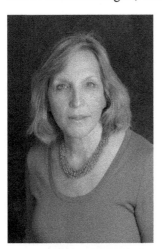

Barbara Stanley

Dr Barbara Stanley is Professor of Medical Psychology in the Department of Psychiatry at Columbia University. She is the Director of Suicide Prevention Training, Implementation and Evaluation in the Center for Practice Innovations at the New York State Psychiatric Institute. She is also a Research Scientist in the Division of Molecular Imaging and Neuropathology at the Institute. She conducts a broad range of research on suicidal behaviour and non-suicidal self-injury, including intervention studies and examination of neurobiological, biobehavioural, and clinical risk factors.

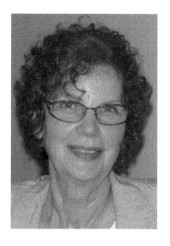

Airi Värnik

Airi Värnik, MD, PhD, is a Professor in Mental Health at Tallinn University and Visiting Professor in Psychiatry at Tartu University. Her doctoral theses are from the Leningrad Behterev Institute and from the Karolinska Institute, National Centre for Suicide Research and Prevention of Mental Ill-Health (NASP). Dr Värnik is a founder and director of the Estonian–Swedish Institute of Suicidology in Tallinn, she is a full member of the IASR, board member of Archives of Suicide Research and of numerous international projects on suicide, a reviewer of scientific journals, and author of 78 scientific articles and book chapters.

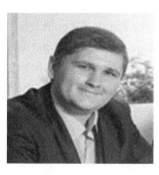

Andriy Yur'yev

Dr Andriy Yur'yev is currently doing post-graduate training in psychiatry at Harlem Hospital Center, Columbia University (US). He obtained his medical degree from Dnepropetrovsk State Medical Academy (Ukraine) and completed his PhD at Tallinn University (Estonia). For several years he worked as a researcher at the Estonian–Swedish Mental Health and Suicidology Institute. His research interests include exploring social and psychological risk factors for suicide.

Foreword

When I first started my research in suicide prevention more than 50 years ago, the taboo surrounding suicide was recognized early as a major hurdle blocking our efforts at suicide prevention—impeding identification, assessment, and treatment. It was also clear that overcoming this hurdle could be accomplished only by much targeted education and information. It is astounding how much in a mere half century the field of suicide has sprung to life and burgeoned, with what is now a vast number of related publications, research and clinical centres, plays, and films. All of these have helped to overcome the general unwillingness to openly discuss and examine the subject.

Though difficult to measure or to quantify, there is no doubt in my mind that the taboo surrounding suicide has diminished. Nevertheless, cultural and religious precepts in many countries continue to play an important role in attitudes towards suicide, and often still keep it from being mentioned even when it occurs within the family. Of course, we do not want to erase all the taboos around suicide—which often act as a deterrent in a moment of overwhelming stress—rather alter perceptions just enough to allow suicidal people to ask for help, now so much more available than when we first started. This at least allows significant others to hear, listen, and prevent what Professor Wasserman has so aptly used to title this welcome publication—an unnecessary death.

Suicide: an unnecessary death is a delight to read—it is as simple and direct as possible, yet includes all the major areas of current concern and interest in the field. Professor Wasserman has written for an important audience that until now has been virtually ignored. This book is not directed at the professional suicidologist/researcher/clinician (although they would also profit greatly from reading it); rather, it is directed at the 'busy clinician' who is dealing with the patient in many different everyday circumstances. *Suicide: an unnecessary death* will also be welcomed by groups such as the police, probation officers, and teachers, who will benefit from a facilitated introduction to the entire field of suicide prevention.

I predict that this book will be of much use and interest to others, as it already has been to me.

Professor Norman L Farberow
Los Angeles, CA, US
Foreword to First Edition, 2001

Foreword

Every suicide is a tragedy. More than 800,000 people die due to suicide every year and there are indications that for each individual who died of suicide there may have been more than 20 others attempting suicide. Notably, suicide is the second leading cause of death in 15–29-year-olds; for young girls, 15–19 years old, it is the first leading cause of death globally. Suicide and suicide attempts affect millions of relatives and loved ones, as well as communities around the world.

Suicide is a serious public health problem in both developed and low- and middle-income countries. In fact, 75% of suicides occur in low- and middle-income countries where resources and services, if they do exist, are often scarce and limited for early intervention, treatment, and support of people in need. Many suicides happen impulsively and, in such circumstances, easy access to the means of suicide, such as pesticides or firearms, can make the difference as to whether a person lives or dies.

The stigma attached to mental disorders and suicide means that many people feel unable to seek help. Despite the evidence that many deaths are preventable, suicide is too often a low priority for governments and policymakers. Therefore, the awareness of suicide as a public health issue needs to be raised and suicide prevention has to be prioritized on the global public health and public policy agendas.

In the WHO Mental Health Action Plan 2013–2020, WHO Member States have committed themselves to work towards the global target of reducing the suicide rate in countries by 10% by the year 2020. In 2014, the first-ever WHO report on suicide prevention, 'Preventing suicide: a global imperative', was published. Practical guidance on strategic actions that countries can take, on the basis of their resources and existing suicide-prevention activities, is given and there are evidence-based and low-cost interventions that are effective, even in resource-poor settings.

Though we know a lot about preventing suicides, there are gaps in knowledge which need further research and systematic evaluation of strategies and programmes in different cultures and settings. A systematic review of existing findings and identification of the most urgent questions to answer for researchers and students can be very helpful to take the agenda forward.

Within this perspective, the revision of this already well-established and authoritative international book, published for the first time in 2001, is very timely. I wish to thank the editor and authors, of whom many belong to the WHO network of experts in suicidology, for contributing to this book. Their efforts will hopefully lead to the strengthening of understanding and actions towards the prevention of suicide.

Dr Shekhar Saxena
Director
Department of Mental Health and Substance Abuse
World Health Organization
Geneva, Switzerland

Preface

More than 800,000 people worldwide commit suicide every year, and at least ten times as many attempt suicide. A considerable number of these are in contact with the health-care and public mental health sectors. Encounters with suicidal individuals are therefore common in the everyday work of health-care staff, and of public mental health professionals.

A massive expansion is under way in psychiatric and public health research. This applies to every field, including suicidology. There has, therefore, been a constant increase in the number of articles and books reporting research findings about suicide and attempted suicide.

The abundance of new literature makes it difficult for busy clinicians, GPs, counsellors, volunteers, and other staff whose clinical practice involves daily contact with suicidal patients to devote sufficient time to penetrating this literature and, accordingly, apply new findings in their clinical practice. Moreover, health-care and public health services in almost every country have undergone restructuring and various cost-cutting measures that, in turn, have reduced the time available to health-care staff for their own education. This is the background to this book as a summary of the latest findings that may be useful to practitioners.

The aim of this book is to convey to the reader the vast experience of research and clinical work gained by leading experts in the field of suicidology and suicide prevention who joined me in this effort. For didactic reasons, all chapters are written in discursive, textbook style, rather than in the style of a scientific paper. Consequently, the number of references carefully selected by the authors, is limited. Each chapter is also of limited length to provide a rapid overview for those who are under heavy time and emotional pressure when assessing suicidal persons and recommending treatment and daily care.

The book is directed at clinical psychiatrists and other physicians, as well as other staff who work with psychiatric patients, but who have no implicit knowledge of the field of suicidology.

Several chapters in this book describe suicide preventive public health measures. If professionals in the health-care sector remain aware of the public health aspects, it will make the clinical practice more effective and synergetic.

The book is also aimed to increase awareness about suicide preventive methods for the general public and professionals in the public mental health sector, as well as for families, friends, colleagues, and workmates of suicidal persons.

The latest developments in suicidology and suicide-prevention research and vast experience of a wide range of international experts are conveyed in this book.

I wish to acknowledge the enthusiastic and considerable support I have received, in the course of preparing this book, from all the contributors and their administrative staff. I would also like to thank my husband Professor Jerzy Wasserman, who read all the manuscripts, and was an unfailing and inspiring discussion partner throughout.

Danuta Wasserman
Professor of Psychiatry and Suicidology at Karolinska
Institute (KI), Stockholm, Sweden
Head of the National Centre for Suicide Research and Prevention
of Mental Ill-Health (NASP) at KI
Director for the WHO Collaborating Centre for Research, Methods
Development and Training in Suicide Prevention
Stockholm, Sweden 2016

Section I

Epidemiology

Chapter 1

Suicide in the world

Alexandra Fleischmann

Epidemiology

Globally, more than 800,000 people died by suicide in 2012, according to World Health Organization (WHO) Global Health Estimates.[1,2] This corresponds to a global age-standardized suicide rate of 11.4 per 100,000 population; 15.0 and 8.0 per 100,000 for males and females respectively. Comparing country-level data, the difference in age-standardized suicide rates ranges from 0.4 to 44.2 per 100,000 (Map 1.1). There are indications that for each adult who died of suicide there were likely to be more than 20 others attempting suicide.[2] Taking into consideration the family members, friends, work colleagues, and communities who experience suicide bereavement,[3] there are many millions of people every year who are affected by both suicide deaths and attempts. According to WHO projections, there will be 1,007,000 deaths from suicide by 2030, with suicide remaining the 15th leading cause of death and contributing 1.4% of all deaths worldwide.[1]

Estimated age-standardized rates by country are presented in Table 1.1.

Among the young (15–29 years old), suicide was the second leading cause of death globally in 2012, and it was the first leading cause of death for young girls aged 15–19 years.[4] Despite preconceptions that suicide is more prevalent in high-income countries (HICs), in reality 75% of global suicides occurred in low- and middle-income countries (LMICs) in 2012 (Fig. 1.1).

Ranking of the top-ten countries for the estimated total number of suicides and total age-standardized suicide rates is presented in Table 1.2.

In general, suicide rates are lowest in people under 15 years old and highest among those 70 years and older. In some regions and countries, suicide rates increase steadily with age, while in others there is a peak

Age-Standardized suicide rates (per 100, 000 population), both sexes, 2012

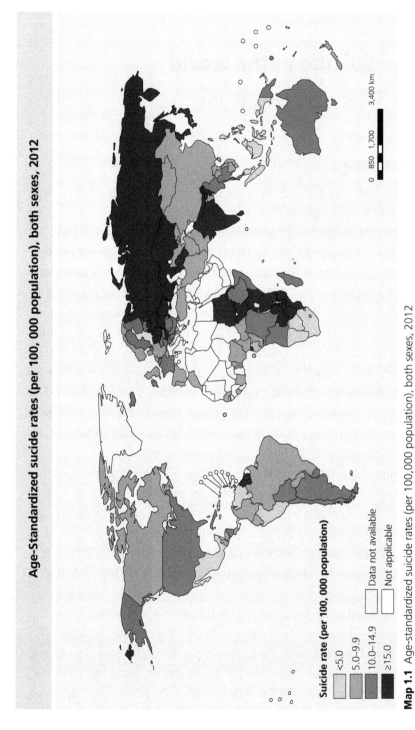

Suicide rate (per 100, 000 population)

- <5.0
- 5.0–9.9
- 10.0–14.9
- ≥15.0
- Data not available
- Not applicable

0 850 1,700   3,400 km

Map 1.1 Age-standardized suicide rates (per 100,000 population), both sexes, 2012

Reproduced from Map Production: Health Statistics and Information Systems (HSI) with permission from the World Health Organization, <http://gamapserver.who.int/mapLibrary/Files/Maps/Global_AS_suicide_rates_bothsexes_2012.png>

Table 1.1 Estimated age-standardized suicide rates by country (per 100,000 population) for 2012*

Country	Men	Women
Afghanistan	6.2	5.3
Albania	6.6	5.2
Algeria	2.3	1.5
Angola	20.7	7.3
Argentina	17.2	4.1
Armenia	5.0	0.9
Australia	16.1	5.2
Austria	18.2	5.4
Azerbaijan	2.4	1.0
Bahamas	3.6	1.3
Bahrain	11.6	2.9
Bangladesh	6.8	8.7
Barbados	4.1	0.6
Belarus	32.7	6.4
Belgium	21.0	7.7
Belize	4.9	0.5
Benin	8.8	3.1
Bhutan	23.1	11.2
Bolivia	16.2	8.5
Bosnia and Herzegovina	18.0	4.1
Botswana	5.7	2.0
Brazil	9.4	2.5
Brunei Darussalam	7.7	5.2
Bulgaria	16.6	5.3
Burkina Faso	7.3	2.8
Burundi	34.1	12.5
Cambodia	12.6	6.5
Cameroon	10.9	3.4
Canada	14.9	4.8
Cape Verde	9.1	1.6
Central African Republic	14.1	5.3
Chad	7.4	2.3

(*Continued*)

Table 1.1 (continued) Estimated age-standardized suicide rates by country (per 100,000 population) for 2012*

Country	Men	Women
Chile	19.0	5.8
China	7.1	8.7
Colombia	9.1	1.9
Comoros	24.0	10.3
Congo	14.7	4.6
Costa Rica	11.2	2.2
Côte d'Ivoire	10.6	4.1
Croatia	19.8	4.5
Cuba	18.5	4.5
Cyprus	7.7	1.5
Czech Republic	21.5	3.9
Democratic Republic of the Congo	15.8	4.8
Denmark	13.6	4.1
Djibouti	20.9	9.5
Dominican Republic	6.1	2.1
Ecuador	13.2	5.3
Egypt	2.4	1.2
El Salvador	23.5	5.7
Equatorial Guinea	24.1	8.6
Eritrea	25.8	8.7
Estonia	24.9	3.8
Ethiopia	16.5	6.7
Fiji	10.6	4.1
Finland	22.2	7.5
France	19.3	6.0
Gabon	12.1	4.5
Gambia	7.6	2.6
Georgia	5.7	1.0
Germany	14.5	4.1
Ghana	4.2	2.2
Greece	6.3	1.3
Guatemala	13.7	4.3

(*Continued*)

Table 1.1 (continued) Estimated age-standardized suicide rates by country (per 100,000 population) for 2012*

Country	Men	Women
Guinea	7.1	2.4
Guinea-Bissau	7.2	2.4
Guyana	70.8	22.1
Haiti	3.3	2.4
Honduras	8.3	2.8
Hungary	32.4	7.4
Iceland	21.0	6.7
India	25.8	16.4
Indonesia	3.7	4.9
Iran (Islamic Republic of)	6.7	3.6
Iraq	1.2	2.1
Ireland	16.9	5.2
Israel	9.8	2.3
Italy	7.6	1.9
Jamaica	1.8	0.7
Japan	26.9	10.1
Jordan	2.2	1.9
Kazakhstan	40.6	9.3
Kenya	24.4	8.4
Kuwait	1.0	0.8
Kyrgyzstan	14.2	4.5
Lao People's Democratic Republic	11.2	6.6
Latvia	30.7	4.3
Lebanon	1.2	0.6
Lesotho	9.2	3.4
Liberia	6.8	2.0
Libya	2.2	1.4
Lithuania	51.0	8.4
Luxembourg	13.0	4.4
Madagascar	15.2	6.9
Malawi	23.9	8.9
Malaysia	4.7	1.5

(Continued)

Table 1.1 (continued) Estimated age-standardized suicide rates by country (per 100,000 population) for 2012*

Country	Men	Women
Maldives	7.8	4.9
Mali	7.2	2.7
Malta	11.1	0.7
Mauritania	4.5	1.5
Mauritius	13.2	2.9
Mexico	7.1	1.7
Mongolia	16.3	3.7
Montenegro	24.7	6.4
Morocco	9.9	1.2
Mozambique	34.2	21.1
Myanmar	16.5	10.3
Namibia	4.4	1.4
Nepal	30.1	20.0
Netherlands	11.7	4.8
New Zealand	14.4	5.0
Nicaragua	15.4	4.9
Niger	5.3	1.9
Nigeria	10.3	2.9
Norway	13.0	5.2
Oman	1.2	0.6
Pakistan	9.1	9.6
Panama	8.1	1.3
Papua New Guinea	15.9	9.1
Paraguay	9.1	3.2
Peru	4.4	2.1
Philippines	4.8	1.2
Poland	30.5	3.8
Portugal	13.6	3.5
Qatar	5.7	1.2
Republic of Korea	41.7	18.0
Republic of Moldova	24.1	4.8
Romania	18.4	2.9

Table 1.1 (continued) Estimated age-standardized suicide rates by country (per 100,000 population) for 2012*

Country	Men	Women
Russian Federation	35.1	6.2
Rwanda	17.1	7.2
Saudi Arabia	0.6	0.2
Senegal	8.6	2.8
Serbia	19.9	5.8
Sierra Leone	11.0	4.5
Singapore	9.8	5.3
Slovakia	18.5	2.5
Slovenia	20.8	4.4
Solomon Islands	13.9	7.2
Somalia	18.1	6.8
South Africa	5.5	1.1
South Sudan	27.1	12.8
Spain	8.2	2.2
Sri Lanka	46.4	12.8
Sudan	23.0	11.5
Suriname	44.5	11.9
Swaziland	8.6	4.1
Sweden	16.2	6.1
Switzerland	13.6	5.1
Syrian Arab Republic	0.7	0.2
Tajikistan	5.7	2.8
Thailand	19.1	4.5
The former Yugoslav Republic of Macedonia	7.3	3.2
Timor-Leste	10.2	5.8
Togo	8.5	2.8
Trinidad and Tobago	20.4	6.2
Tunisia	3.4	1.4
Turkey	11.8	4.2
Turkmenistan	32.5	7.5
Uganda	26.9	12.3
Ukraine	30.3	5.3

(*Continued*)

Table 1.1 (continued) Estimated age-standardized suicide rates by country (per 100,000 population) for 2012*

Country	Men	Women
United Arab Emirates	3.9	1.7
United Kingdom	9.8	2.6
United Republic of Tanzania	31.6	18.3
United States of America	19.4	5.2
Uruguay	20.0	5.2
Uzbekistan	13.2	4.1
Venezuela (Bolivarian Republic of)	4.3	1.0
Viet Nam	8.0	2.4
Yemen	4.3	3.0
Zambia	20.8	10.8
Zimbabwe	27.2	9.7

*In 171 WHO Member States with populations of 300,000 or more. These estimates represent the best estimates of WHO, computed using standard categories, definitions, and methods to ensure cross-country comparability, and may not be the same as official national estimates. The estimates are rounded to the appropriate number of significant figures. Standardized to the WHO World Standard Population.

Adapted from World Health Organization, Preventing suicide: a global imperative, Annex 1, Copyright 2014 with permission from the World Health Organization, <http://apps.who.int/iris/bitstream/10665/131056/1/9789241564779_eng.pdf>

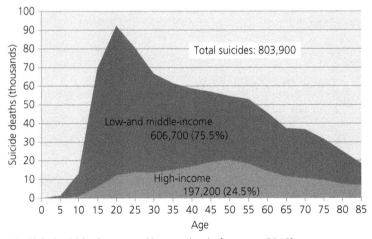

Fig. 1.1 Global suicides by age and income level of country, 2012*

Table 1.2 Ranking of the top 10 countries for the estimated total number of suicides and total age-standardized suicide rates for 2012*

Rank by number of suicides	Country	Number of suicides	Age—standardized suicide rate (per 100,000)	Rank by suicide rate	Country	Age—standardized suicide rate (per 100,000)	Number of suicides
1	India	258,075	21.1	1	Guyana	44.2	277
2	China	120,730	7.8	2	Republic of Korea	28.9	17,908
3	United States of America	43,361	12.1	3	Sri Lanka	28.8	6,170
4	Russian Federation	31,997	19.5	4	Lithuania	28.2	1,007
5	Japan	29,442	18.5	5	Suriname	27.8	145
6	Republic of Korea	17,908	28.9	6	Mozambique	27.4	4,360
7	Pakistan	13,377	9.3	7	Nepal	24.9	5,572
8	Brazil	11,821	5.8	8	United Republic of Tanzania	24.9	7,228
9	Germany	10,745	9.2	9	Kazakhstan	23.8	3,912
10	Bangladesh	10,167	7.8	10	Burundi	23.1	1,617

Adapted from World Health Organization, Preventing suicide: a global imperative, Annex 1, Copyright (2014), with permission from the World Health Organization http://apps.who.int/iris/bitstream/10665/131056/1/9789241564779_eng.pdf

*In 171 WHO Member States with populations of 300,000 or more. These estimates represent the best estimates of WHO, computed using standard categories, definitions, and methods to ensure cross-country comparability, and may not be the same as official national estimates. The estimates are rounded to the appropriate number of significant figures. Standardized to the WHO World Standard Population.

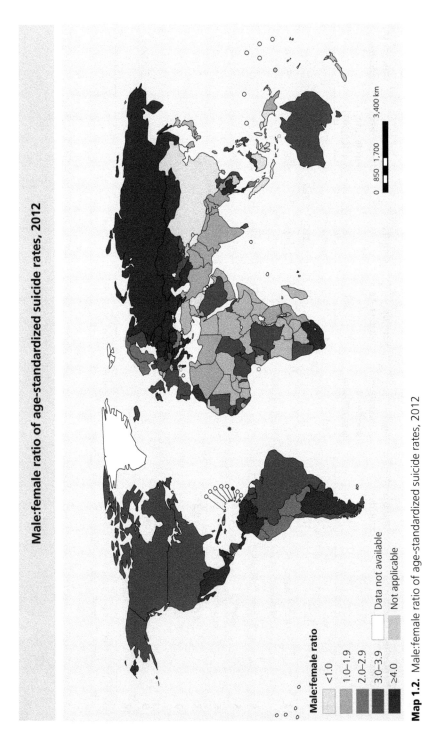

Map 1.2. Male:female ratio of age-standardized suicide rates, 2012

Reproduced from Map Production: Health Statistics and Information Systems (HSI) with permission from the World Health Organization, <http://www.who.int/gho/mental_health/suicide_rates/en/>

in suicide rates in the young that subsides in middle age. Comparing HICs and LMICs, rates are higher in middle-aged men in HICs than in LMICs, and rates are higher in LMICs in the young and in elderly women than in HICs.

The high male-to-female ratio of age-standardized suicide rates is primarily a phenomenon in HICs where it was 3.5 in 2012. It was a much lower 1.6 in LMICs, and globally it was 1.9. This means that there are more men than women who die by suicide globally, with the exception of very few countries where there are more deaths by suicide among women (Map 1.2). Comparing country-level data, the male-to-female ratio of age-standardized suicide rates ranged from 0.5 to 12.5 in 2012.

Suicide has an important contribution to all intentional deaths (i.e., violent deaths), which include deaths from interpersonal violence (i.e., homicide essentially), armed conflict (i.e., war essentially), and suicide. Globally, suicides account for 56% of all violent deaths; 50% among males and 71% among females. In HICs, suicides account for 81% of violent deaths in both males and females, while in LMICs 44% of violent deaths in males and 70% of violent deaths in females are due to suicide.

Methods of suicide

One of the key methods of suicide in LMICs, particularly in countries with a high proportion of rural residents engaged in small-scale agriculture, is pesticide self-poisoning. A systematic review of world data for 1990–2007[5] estimated that around 30% of global suicides are due to pesticide self-poisoning, most of which occur in LMICs around the world. Based on this estimate, pesticide ingestion is among the most common methods of suicide globally.

In HICs, hanging accounts for 50% of the suicides, and firearms are the second most common method, accounting for 18% of suicides. The relatively high proportion of suicides by firearms in HICs is primarily driven by HICs in the Americas where firearms account for 46% of all suicides. In particular settings, e.g., in highly urbanized areas where a majority of the population live in high-rise buildings, jumping from high places is a common method of suicide.

Data quality

Of the 172 countries with populations of 300,000 or greater for which WHO Global Health Estimates were made,[6] only 60 have good-quality vital registration data that can be used directly to estimate suicide rates (Map 1.3). The estimated suicide rates in the other 112 WHO Member States, which account for about 71% of global suicides, are necessarily based on modelling methods. Good-quality vital registration systems are much more likely to be available in HICs. The 39 HICs with good vital registration data account for 95% of all estimated suicides in HICs, but the 21 LMICs with good vital registration data account for only 8% of all estimated suicides in LMICs.

This problem of poor-quality mortality data is not unique to suicide, but given the sensitivity of suicide—and the illegality of suicidal behaviour in some countries—it is likely that under-reporting and misclassification are greater problems for suicide than for most other causes of death. Suicide registration is a complicated, multilevel procedure that includes medical and legal concerns and involves several responsible authorities that can vary from country to country. Suicides are most commonly found misclassified according to the codes of the 10th edition of the International Classification of Diseases and Related Health Conditions (ICD-10) as 'deaths of undetermined intent' (ICD-10 codes Y10–Y34), and also as 'accidents' (codes V01–X59), 'homicides' (codes X85–Y09), and 'unknown cause' (codes R95–R99).[7–9]

National-level data on the methods used in suicide are very limited. The ICD-10 includes X-codes that record the external causes of death, including the method of suicide, but many countries do not collect this information. Between 2005 and 2011, only 76 of the 194 WHO Member States reported data on methods of suicide in the WHO mortality database. These countries account for about 28% of all global suicides, so the methods used in 72% of global suicides are unclear. The coverage for suicide methods data is much better for HICs than for LMICs.

Suicide attempts

The two primary methods for obtaining information about national or regional rates of suicide attempts are from self-reports of suicidal behaviour in surveys of representative samples of community

Quality of suicide mortality data, 2012

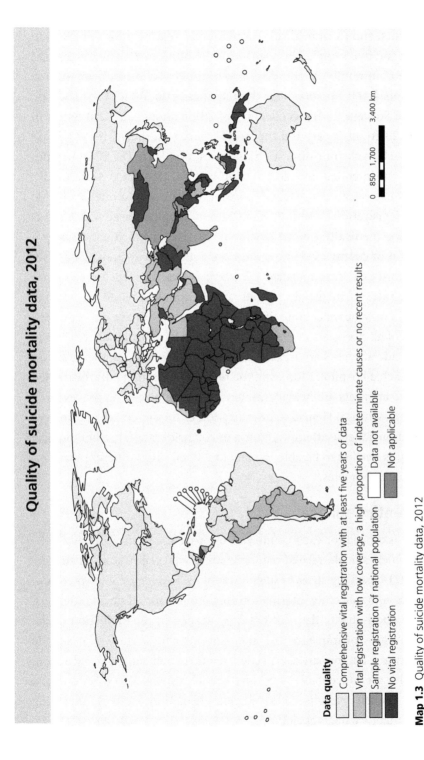

Data quality

☐ Comprehensive vital registration with at least five years of data

☐ Vital registration with low coverage, a high proportion of indeterminate causes or no recent results

☐ Sample registration of national population

☐ No vital registration

☐ Data not available

☐ Not applicable

Map 1.3 Quality of suicide mortality data, 2012

Reproduced from Map Production: Health Statistics and Information Systems (HSI) with permission from the World Health Organization, <http://www.who.int/mental_health/suicide-prevention/mortality_data_quality/en/>

residents, and from medical records about treatment for self-harm in representative samples of health-care institutions (usually hospitals) in the community. WHO does not routinely collect data on suicide attempts, but it has supported the activities of the WHO World Mental Health Surveys[10] which collect information about suicide attempts in some 20 countries around the world. Moreover, the WHO STEPwise approach to chronic disease risk factor surveillance (STEPS) includes questions intended to collect data on suicide attempts.[11] Additionally, WHO has released a resource booklet, in addition to one on suicide case registration,[12] about establishing hospital-based case registries for medically treated suicide attempts.[13] Unfortunately, only a handful of countries is known to have national or regional data from hospital-based case registries. Caution is needed, because estimates of the rates of medically treated suicide attempts based on hospital reports may be inaccurate, if the selected hospitals are not representative of all hospitals in the community or, if a substantial proportion of suicide attempts are treated only by local clinics and, therefore, do not reach a hospital. Moreover, the reported rates of medically treated suicide attempts are heavily influenced by the recording processes in hospital settings. Hence, standardization of the collection of information about suicide attempts, taking into consideration methodological issues, is needed to be able to compare rates across different jurisdictions and countries.[2]

Preventing suicide

There is a need for each country to improve the quality and availability of their suicide-related data, including vital registration of suicide, hospital-based registries of suicide attempts, and nationally representative surveys collecting information about self-reported suicide attempts. These good-quality data are not only needed in the evaluation of the effectiveness of implemented interventions and strategies for suicide prevention, but they are also needed to inform policymaking and action. Suicides are preventable and, for national responses to be effective, a comprehensive multisectoral suicide-prevention strategy, including good-quality data, is essential.[2]

References

1 **World Health Organization (WHO).** Global Health Estimates (website). Geneva: World Health Organization (<http://www.who.int/healthinfo/global_burden_disease/projections>, accessed 15 September 2014).

2 **World Health Organization (WHO).** Preventing suicide: a global imperative. Geneva: World Health Organization, 2014.

3 **Pitman A, Osborn D, King M, Erlangsen A.** Effects of suicide bereavement on mental health and suicide risk. Lancet Psychiatry. 2014;**1**(1):86–94.

4 **World Health Organization (WHO).** Health for the world's adolescents. Geneva: World Health Organization, 2014.

5 **Gunnell D, Eddleston M, Phillips MR, Konradsen F.** The global distribution of fatal pesticide self-poisoning: systematic review. BMC Public Health. 2007;**7**:357.

6 **World Health Organization (WHO).** WHO methods and data sources for global causes of death 2000–2012. Global Health Estimates Technical Paper WHO/HIS/HSI/GHE/2014.7. Geneva: World Health Organization, 2014.

7 **Värnik P, Sisask M, Värnik A, Yur'Yev A, Kõlves K, . . . Wasserman D.** Massive increase in injury deaths of undetermined intent in ex-USSR Baltic and Slavic countries: hidden suicides? Scand J Public Health. 2010;**38**(4):395–403.

8 **Värnik P, Sisask M, Värnik A, Arensman E, Van Audenhove C, . . . Hegerl U.** Validity of suicide statistics in Europe in relation to undetermined deaths: developing the 2–20 benchmark. Inj Prev. 2012;**18**(5):321–325.

9 **Höfer P, Rockett IR, Värnik P, Etzersdorfer E, Kapusta ND.** Forty years of increasing suicide mortality in Poland: undercounting amidst a hanging epidemic? BMC Public Health. 2012;**11**(12):644.

10 **Kessler RC, Ustun TB, editors.** The WHO World Mental Health Surveys. New York (NY): Cambridge University Press; 2008.

11 **World Health Organization (WHO).** STEPS optional module: mental health/suicide. Geneva: World Health Organization, 2014 (<http://www.who.int/chp/steps/riskfactor/modules/en/>, accessed 15 September 2014).

12 **World Health Organization (WHO).** Preventing suicide: a resource for suicide case registration. Geneva: World Health Organization, 2011 (<http://whqlibdoc.who.int/publications/2011/9789241502665_eng.pdf?ua=1>, accessed 15 September 2014).

13 **World Health Organization (WHO).** Preventing suicide: a resource for nonfatal suicidal behaviour case registration. Geneva: World Health Organization; 2014 (<http://apps.who.int/iris/bitstream/10665/112852/1/9789241506717_eng.pdf?ua=1>, accessed 15 September 2014).

Theoretical models of suicide behaviour

Chapter 2

Stress-vulnerability model of suicidal behaviours

Danuta Wasserman and Marcus Sokolowski

Stress-vulnerability model

The causes of suicide are complex and multifactorial, and it is today clear that no simple explanations are to be found. Given the complexity, a variety of study-models to explain the origins of suicidal behaviours have been presented which tend to focus on particular explanatory domains e.g., psychiatric, psychological, or social. In those models, one particular component has often been regarded as dominant for aetiology; for example, that given enough stressful life events almost anyone would develop psychopathology or suicidality. But nowadays, a more comprehensive stress-vulnerability model is mainly used and accepted, introduced by Mann and Arango[1] into suicidology. Here, one instead also takes into account the fact that a current acute stressor ('state')—for example, an ongoing psychiatric illness or recent traumatic life experience—is neither sufficient nor necessary for suicide to occur. For example, although most suicides happen in the context of depression, only a few per cent of depressed are suicidal. This is also valid for exposure to stressful life events such as loss of a loved one, which affects people differently in the same manner. It is instead reasoned that a trait-like characteristic ('stress-vulnerability') must also be present, which pushes certain individuals to engage in suicidal behaviours in situations when most others do not. Such a constitutional predisposition (a 'trait' or 'diathesis') for suicide is thought to be formed (or 'developed') due to the influence of inborn genetic risks which combine with stressful life experiences, trauma, illnesses, or even drugs during childhood and adolescence. The challenge lies in understanding how such a trait-like 'suicidal brain' is formed and how it might manifest itself in adulthood prior to suicide.

Current research combines sociological, psychological, and neurobiological (including genetic) study perspectives into increasingly refined formulations of the stress-vulnerability model,[2-5] and this also makes prevention of, or intervention against, suicidal behaviours relevant across the entire life span and not only during acute suicidal crises.

The role of biology in a suicidal diathesis

The diathesis (or 'trait') in the stress-vulnerability model is mainly understood as a biological trait which is formed and expressed in balance with the inborn genetics of the individual,[1-6] and related to higher-level psychological characteristics such as personality traits (high neuroticism or impulsivity)[7,8] or cognitive functions (deficits in attention, memory, learning, and decision-making).[9] General family and twin studies have consistently shown that suicidality is influenced genetically by 30–50%, an inheritance which is currently understood to be polygenetic and complex.[10] Therefore, any genetic influences will always act in balance with the presence of different protective and risk factors in the environment throughout life, from the level of personal experiences, the family situation to the broader social and cultural situation. While the comprehensive environmental life history of the individual (that is during the early life, when diathesis is formed) is usually difficult to find out, technological advances allow for biological changes and genetic set-up to be assayed with constantly increasing accuracy and completeness in adult persons. Any biological changes observed in a suicidal adult then reflect the sum of all genetic and environmental contributions throughout life. By comparing suicidal with non-suicidal people, but with both having the same current stressor or 'state' (e.g., depression), one can then disentangle what is specifically related to the suicidal 'trait' or diathesis in itself.

Many such biological changes specific to suicidality have been observed, by analysing either blood or cerebral spinal fluid samples of suicide attempters, or by investigating brain tissues in post-mortem autopsies. The most historic and also most studied biological changes relate to various deficiencies in the monoaminergic (serotonin, dopamine, and noradrenaline) neurotransmitter systems. Concerning the role of serotonin, it is also supported by that selective serotonin receptor inhibitors (SSRIs), antidepressants which act to restore serotonin levels in the brain, also reduce the risk of suicidal behaviours among depressed adults. However, it is also increasingly clear that the monoamines are only a part of the explanation, due to the polygenetic and complex aetiology of suicide. For example, there are treatments which do not primarily act on the serotonin system, which are nevertheless useful against suicidalilty.[11] Biological changes which more directly point to the major influences of stress in the diathesis have gained increasing interest, ultimately suggesting permanent changes in a person's responses to stress at different levels of functioning, including serotonergic. As suicidality might be viewed as the outmost consequence of repeated stress-reactions, it seems one may follow the path from stress to the biological and psychological changes that are produced in the person. The nature of such externally influenced changes would then depend on the individual genetic set-up and the cumulative effect of past experiences. Such a perspective integrates excellently with the stress-vulnerability model, which suggests the presence of a step-wise acquired suicidal trait throughout life by stress as a key influence at each step, with subsequent deficient stress-responses during an acute suicidal crisis later in life, as well as the possibilities for rescue from suicidal crises by intervening on the current stress, the stress-vulnerability trait, or both.

Stress-biology and the diathesis

From a biological point of view, one might say that a person's stress is defined by the activity of those neurosystems which are engaged during a stress-response.[2] Psychological stress occurs when there are *perceived* changes in the environment which require some kind of adaptation, ranging from objective events such as physical abuse to subjectively perceived threats such as social cues.[12]

Stress can affect emotions, learning, memory, and decision-making, all being relevant in the suicide diathesis. Acute psychological stress, that is encountering an immediate threat (lasting seconds to minutes), results in a first-wave biological response ('flight-or-fight'): a massive reaction which puts muscles, heart, and brain on high alert. This response, preferentially mediated by monoamines (serotonin, noradrenaline) and neuropeptides, is necessary for our survival and does not affect the brain in any long-lasting way, as the biological 'alarm' is quite easily turned off when the threat has passed. In contrast, chronic psychological stress, such as being in a repeatedly hostile life-situation (lasting hours, days, or longer), involves more long-term actions mediated by the stress hormone cortisol and other neurosteroids.

Chronic stress produces progressive changes in gene expression by, for example, 'epigenetics'[13] and this can have consequences for the structure and function of larger brain circuits—changes which have been observed in adult suicidal subjects. Indeed, chronic stress produces life-long changes in emotions, learning, memory, decision-making, and also how one will respond to stress in the future.

The actions of cortisol, which is produced through the so-called hypothalamic-pituitary-adrenal (HPA) axis, can also induce changes in all monoaminergic systems, including serotonin. It has been shown that cortisol (response) is altered in certain suicidal subjects and that it may be useful for predicting the risk of future suicidal behaviours. The long-lasting changes in the brain by chronic psychological stress depend also on when in life the stress occurs, as different parts of the brain are 'stress-sensitive' during different stages of life. For stress encountered during sensitive periods during early childhood, such as traumatic parent separation, dysfunctional parent–child interactions, or physical and sexual abuses, the hippocampus is the most sensitive with consequences for memory and learning abilities. In adolescents, the prefrontal cortex is instead the most sensitive, affecting mainly decision-making and impulse control. The amygdala implicated in emotions and emotional control of, for example, fear and anxiety, is sensitive throughout childhood to early adulthood. Pre-adult life experiences can generate long-term changes in the HPA axis which contribute to different suicide-related psychology, and can further combine with inherited genetic changes in the HPA axis[2] and beyond, resulting in a stress-vulnerability diathesis for suicide in the adulthood.

Offsetting the diathesis and building resilience to stress

Even though stress-vulnerability is regarded as an inherited 'trait', it is also important to remember that no one is ever predestined to suicidal behaviour.

Nowadays, it is known that brain structures and functions are not static, but that they continue to change throughout the entire life.[14] In fact, this capability of the brain to continuously change its circuits and chemistry in an adaptive manner—its 'neuroplasticity'—is what actually also characterizes the maintenance of mental health.[13] Even more, neuroplasticity is of key importance for a person's maintenance of mental health in the presence of harmful stress, the 'resilience', as well as for recovery from psychopathology during treatment. It has further also been shown that suicidal subjects have less neuroplasticity, which would explain well why they are unable to find coping strategies to their current stressed state, manifested by cognitive disabilities in attention, learning, memory, decision-making, and a general feeling of hopelessness. Furthermore, antidepressants such as SSRIs and even regular physical activity not only act by increasing serotonergic function, but also by promoting the brain to make new neurons and brain-circuit reconnections, that is to increase neuroplasticity. One well-studied molecular player of importance in neuroplasticity is the brain-derived neurotropic factor (BDNF), and BDNF is also one of the most consistent biomarkers found to be reduced in suicidal subjects irrespective of their psychiatric diagnosis. The BDNF-related brain circuits are, in turn, also deactivated by chronic stress, fitting well with the effects of stress-biology discussed above.[15] It is increasingly clear that psychological treatments might require a boost of the suicidal person's neuroplasticity, to have success. To further understand how we can maintain and promote neuroplasticity also in everyday life by, for example, 'healthy lifestyles' is also a research area of great promise for reducing and treating suicidal behaviours, as well as for improving mental health in general.

References

1 Mann JJ, Arango V. Integration of neurobiology and psychopathology in a unified model of suicidal behaviour. J Clin Psychopharmacol 1992;**12**(2 Suppl):2S–7S.

2 Wasserman D, Wasserman J, Sokolowski M. Genetics of HPA-axis, depression and suicidality. Eur Psychiatry 2010;**25**(5):278–280.

3 Turecki G. The molecular bases of the suicidal brain. Nat Rev Neurosci. 2014;**15**(12):802–816.

4 Sokolowski M, Wasserman J, Wasserman D. Genome-wide association studies of suicidal behaviors: a review . Eur Neuropsychopharm 2014;**24**(10):1567–1577.

5 Sokolowski M, Wasserman J, Wasserman D. An overview of the neurobiology of suicidal behaviours as one meta-system. Mol Psychiatry 2014, epub 2 September: 1–16.

6 Ben-Efraim YJ, Wasserman D, Wasserman J, Sokolowski M. Family-based study of HTR2A in suicide attempts: observed gene, gene × environment and parent-of-origin associations. Mol Psychiatry 2013;**18**(7):758–766.

7 Calati R, Giegling I, Balestri M, Antypa N, Friedl M, Konte B, et al. Influence of differentially expressed genes from suicide post-mortem study on personality traits as endophenotypes on healthy subjects and suicide attempters. Eur Arch Psychiatry Clin Neurosci 2014;**264**(5):423–432.

8 Voracek M. Big five personality factors and suicide rates in the United States: a state-level analysis. Perceptual and motor skills 2009;**109**(1):208–212.

9 Richard-Devantoy S, Berlim MT, Jollant F. A meta-analysis of neuropsychological markers of vulnerability to suicidal behaviour in mood disorders. Psychol Med 2014;**44**(8):1663–1673.

10 Voracek M, Loibl LM. Genetics of suicide: a systematic review of twin studies. Wien Klin Wochenschr 2007;**119**(15–16):463–475.

11 Griffiths JJ, Zarate CA, Jr., Rasimas JJ. Existing and novel biological therapeutics in suicide prevention. Am J Prev Med 2014;**47**(3 Suppl 2):S195–203.

12 Brodsky BS, Stanley B. Adverse childhood experiences and suicidal behaviour. Psychiatr Clin North Am 2008;**31**(2):223–235.

13 Turecki G. Epigenetics and suicidal behaviour research pathways. Am J Prev Med 2014;**47**(3 Suppl 2):S144–151.

14 Lupien SJ, McEwen BS, Gunnar MR, Heim C. Effects of stress throughout the lifespan on the brain, behaviour and cognition. Nat Rev Neurosci 2009;**10**(6):434–445.

15 Rothman SM, Mattson MP. Activity-dependent, stress-responsive BDNF signaling and the quest for optimal brain health and resilience throughout the lifespan. Neuroscience 2013;**239**:228–240.

Chapter 3

The suicidal process

Danuta Wasserman

Classification of suicidal behaviour

Suicide is, by definition, a deliberate act. But unconscious psychological components play an important part. If there is no farewell letter, it is sometimes difficult to know the reasons for a suicide and whether it was a deliberate step or accidental or the result of taking prescription drugs, alcohol, or an overdose of narcotics without the intention of dying. Behind many suicides there is probably no real intention to die.

If the person survives, it is recorded as a suicide attempt. People who attempt suicide are, in many cases, different from those who actually take their own lives, and the practice of describing them as two separate but overlapping populations persists. From an epidemiological perspective these two populations differ, although they may not differ so much from the psychological point of view. There are many suicide attempters who resemble people who commit suicide.

Studies on lifetime prevalence of suicidal thoughts show variation ranging from 9% to 25% and on lifetime prevalence of attempted suicide from 3% to 5%.[1–3]

Pokorny[4] introduced the concept of suicidal behaviour to cover suicidal thoughts (suicidal ideation), attempted suicide, and suicide. At the same time, Paykel et al.[5] introduced in addition to suicidal ideation and suicide attempts such concepts as weariness of life and death wishes. These could be regarded as phenomena distinct from, or forerunners to, suicidal thoughts. With these notions, the foundation was laid for the model of the suicidal process.

Beskow[6] took these concepts to the fore and used this model in retrospective studies of completed suicides.

The model of the suicidal process indicates that suicidal behaviour has a previous history and that the current process is a continuum of gradually increasing seriousness in suicidal behaviour, from weariness of life to death wishes, suicidal thoughts, suicide attempts, and suicide (Fig. 3.1).

Studies of the suicidal process in suicide attempters[7] show that most suicidal acts are preceded by a process, of varying length, in which the dynamics are highly individual. The suicidal process usually stretches over months, but for some people it lasts more than a year; for patients with chronic depression, schizophrenics, or substance abusers it can be lifelong. For young people with adjustment disorders, its duration may be only a few days or weeks. Propensity for suicide may be acute, chronic, or latent. For long periods, thoughts of suicide may be entirely absent, only to return in response to new strains.

The suicidal process in the context of the stress-vulnerability model

The stress vulnerability (diathesis) model, described in Chapter 2, can be supplemented with the model of development of the suicidal process in order to provide a better understanding of the dynamics in the inter-action between suicidal people and those around them, and to be able to study the 'suicidal communication' between the suicidal individual and his/her family and other key persons, as well as interplay between inherited and acquired conditions (Fig. 3.1). The factors that are taken into account in this model include:

- the role of the suicidal person's cognitive style and personality;
- the role of environmental factors;
- the way in which stress contributes to the vulnerability (diathesis) becoming manifest;
- how other people's reactions and psychosocial and cultural support can contribute to the outcome; and
- in which circumstances a person's vulnerability is held back (protective factors) and in which circumstances it is expressed in suicide or attempted suicide (risk factors).

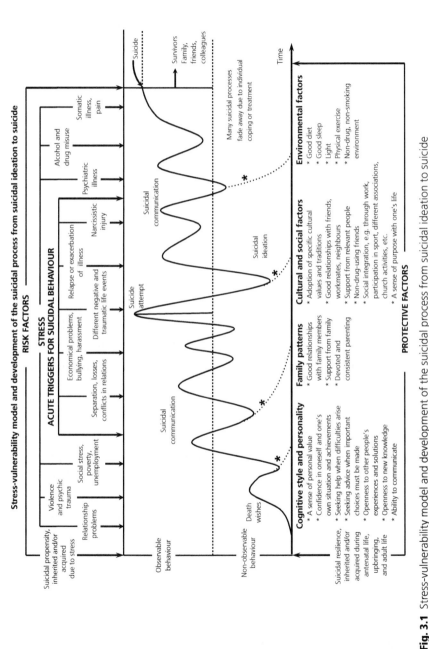

Fig. 3.1 Stress-vulnerability model and development of the suicidal process from suicidal ideation to suicide

Adapted from Wasserman D., Suicide: An unnecessary death, Figure 2.1, Copyright (2001), with permission from Martin Dunitz/Informa

In the model of the suicidal process, the boundaries between suicidal thoughts and suicide attempts are not distinct but fluid. The outcome is affected by the presence of risk and the absence of protective factors in interaction with the diathesis. Suicide is regarded as an act stemming from the interplay between cognitive, affective, and communicative aspects.

The suicidal process can be interrupted due to treatment but it may also abate spontaneously. The fact that the suicidal process is affected by numerous different factors is also suggested by various epidemiological surveys and individual psychological investigations. It is also vital to study the suicidal process not only at the individual level but also at the interpersonal (communicative) level, and in relation to other external factors at the community level (in terms of social integration) as well as in relation to the cultural and the physical environment.

In this book, the term 'suicidal' is used to describe a person who has intense and serious thoughts about committing suicide. The term also covers people who have less intensive or vague suicidal thoughts but are in the risk zone for suicide owing to various factors or who have attempted to take their own lives in the past year. These risk factors include mental illness, personality disorder, and negative life events (see chapters 4 to 13). Risk is particularly high when one or more factors that normally afford a degree of protection disappear.

Suicidal communication

The manner in which other people respond to a person's suicidal communication may afford some protection against suicidal behaviour.[8–11] Unfortunately, however, it may also be an obvious risk factor that adds to the chaos and self-hate experienced by the suicidal person, accelerating the suicidal process in a negative direction. Whether the suicidal process is curtailed or proceeds to a suicide attempt or completed suicide depends on:

- the person's capacity to ask for and receive help; and
- the capacity of other people (including health-care staff) in the suicidal person's surroundings to recognize and take seriously their suicidal communication and intervene.

Poor communication by suicidal people

Through dialogue, and by using friendly words, one can help suicidal people to verbalize their elusive experiences and to convert them into words, which are the foundation of interpersonal communication and contact. To prevent suicidal people from resorting to suicide, it is important to take their every reference to suicide seriously.

The popular belief that people who talk about suicide do not commit it is a myth. However, there are some people on the verge of suicide who do not communicate their intentions. Although they may have partners, they are emotional loners and do not share their reflections with anyone. After a suicide, the family may often express such thoughts as, 'I don't know who I was living with'. Men who live by the principle that strength lies in being alone and who neither wish nor dare to reveal their emotional needs and thoughts are well-known poor communicators. Young people, too, may have marked communication difficulties. People who communicate poorly may, on the surface, behave normally or almost normally while brooding intensely about suicide and planning the act.

Conversation as a means to reduce anxiety and chaos

Suicidal communication (i.e., references to thoughts about the act and plans to commit it) may vary sharply in intensity both over a day and in a longer perspective. By dialogue, a person may be diverted from thoughts of suicide and provided with some scope for alternative ways of solving conflicts. Other options suggested by the helper may perhaps be rejected at first but eventually absorbed and, possibly, applied. Conversation and communication reduce confusion, anxiety, and panic. A sensitive interlocutor—one who does not exacerbate the suicidal patient's feelings of shame or guilt or give offence and who is prepared to provide practical assistance by, for example, telephoning the hospital or helping with something that has been neglected during the chaotic period—is needed. Helpers can arrest the mental paralysis that suicidal people may experience in the face of the slightest commitment. It is possible, by means of dialogue and practical support, to broaden a suicidal person's tunnel vision and loosen his or her cognitive constriction.

Types of suicidal communication

Suicidal communication may be classified as verbal and non-verbal. Both these types of communication can be further divided into direct and indirect communication.[7]

Direct verbal communication

In direct verbal suicidal communication, people directly express their intention to take their own lives or, less clearly, the feeling that everything is hopeless and the only right thing to do is to put an end to it all. This form of communication is sometimes expressed in quarrels, along with accusations directed at significant others—that they have caused difficulties, and, by implication, the suicidal situation.

Indirect verbal communication

Indirect verbal suicidal communication is sometimes less intelligible, since such utterances as, 'I can't go on like this', 'I don't see any point in living', 'Perhaps we won't see each other again', and 'It's hardly surprising that lots of people want to kill themselves, the way society is' are often difficult to interpret. To be comprehensible, such messages need to be put in context. Some are easy to interpret; others can be understood only with hindsight.

Direct non-verbal communication

Examples of direct non-verbal suicidal communication may be the acquisition of a weapon or the collecting of drug prescriptions or medicines.

Indirect non-verbal communication

Writing a will, giving away keepsakes, paying debts, and arranging insurance may be examples of indirect non-verbal suicidal communication. Intensive efforts to get in touch with loved ones or health-care services or to seek solitude and isolation may be other expressions of suicidal intent.

Response of significant others

Empathy of surrounding people

Direct suicidal communication is easier to interpret, but it is often mistrusted by the recipients, who doubt whether the person genuinely intends to take his or her own life. The indirect forms of suicidal communication are more difficult to understand for outsiders, but members of the immediate family often see how the person has changed and instinctively understand the communication. At best, those in proximity to the suicidal person can then become aware of the situation and, besides showing empathy, provide support and ensure that adequate care and professional help are obtained.

Ambivalence of surrounding people

Some people may react with concern, anxiety, and silence. Ambivalence towards suicidal people, with the simultaneous wish to stay with them and to leave them, to seek help for them and to wait, may be present. In extreme cases, people may show direct or indirect aggression towards the suicidal person in various ways. There can be a paradoxical interplay between the hypersensitive suicidal person, who is desperate, chaotic, irritable, sometimes aggressive, or paralysed in terms of coping strategies, and the surrounding people, who tend to be silent, cautious, withdrawn, or show turning-away reactions.

The reactions which significant others display have a crucial bearing on whether the development of the suicidal process is curtailed or accelerated. The silence affords no help to a person who is suicidal. If significant others are ambivalent, the suicidal person's ambivalence may be reinforced and a vicious circle may arise. Suicidal individuals, owing to their disturbed perception, look mainly on the dark side of everything, disparage themselves, and magnify their own difficulties. They often perceive only the negative pole of significant family members' or other peoples' ambivalence and they interpret these expressions as lack of love and interest and as rejection. They have difficulty in perceiving the positive pole of the significant others' ambivalence and often do not see the concern, attention, and wishes to help.

Aggression of surrounding people

If the relatives or significant others of a suicidal person become extremely frustrated and turn their backs or show aggression in verbal or non-verbal ways, the suicidal person is left alone with his or her own aggression, which can then be turned inwards. In some cases the suicidal person can be killed by the indifference or aggression of others.

The life-saving actions of surrounding people

Other people's reactions have a particularly decisive impact when a suicidal person has only one relationship. The reactions of health-care personnel are equally important. Relatives and others who are close to those who are suicidal need (and deserve) a great deal of support and, sometimes, professional help, since their ambivalent and aggressive reactions stem from their own mental conflicts being brought to the fore when they find themselves in a situation of extreme duress.

Menninger,[12] like Freud before him, saw suicide as a reflected murder, or 'inverted homicide'. Menninger believed that anger was turned inwards, instead of being expressed outwardly towards the person who evoked the feeling of anger.

In-depth studies

The model of the suicidal process also provides scope for studying a suicidal person's fantasies, wishes and thoughts, intentions, plans, impulses, and decisions to commit suicide. The stages of the suicidal process may be seen as attempts to resolve various internal psychic and external conflicts, to find new means of adjustment to an untenable life situation, or to communicate a 'cry for help'.[8]

The idea of suicide may at first be fleeting. It may be rejected, then return, only to be rejected once more . . . and so on until, eventually, it may appear to be the only option.

Immediately before the suicidal act (whether suicide attempt or suicide), the intensity of the suicidal process rises and feelings of hopelessness, helplessness, anxiety, anger, and desperation are usually mixed with the symptoms of different psychiatric disorders. Similarly, the personality traits are accentuated. Inappropriate strategies for dealing with the life situation come to the fore when a person loses the capacity for taking an overall view, owing to drastically curtailed cognitive ability and 'blinkered vision'. Anxiety fuels the suicidal process and the mind revolves around thoughts of how and where death will come. All this is communicated frequently to others in various ways.

When a person takes the definite decision to die, all this chaos may be replaced by a phase of tranquillity that often misleads others. However, when protective factors are present, the outcome is often that the act is never committed.

Protective factors

The presence of risk factors, but also the absence of the protective factors, determines whether people lose control over their life situation and the outcome is a suicide, an attempted suicide, or merely suicidal thoughts. Suicidal ideation is situation-dependent, and suicidal acts occur only when risk factors are present and acting in concert and protective factors have disappeared.

Consequently, what makes the difference between life and death is not only the presence of risk factors, but also access to protective factors that strengthen the suicidal person's coping strategies.

Protective factors may be connected with sources of pleasure that are not currently available but may return or, similarly, rewarding contacts, employment, or interesting occupations. Other examples are rediscovering ties with the family—parents, siblings, children, or grandchildren— and neighbours, and rejoining a religious, political, or other group. Finding a responsive person who is prepared to listen, and therapy and medication that may help to make accessible the coping strategies that a person has used successfully in the past, are other ways of strengthening suicide-preventive factors.

Protective factors are contained in both the minds of suicidal people and their surroundings. Nowadays, research focuses on finding the long-term lifestyles that protect people against any suicidal behaviour. Cognitive flexibility, collecting information about the problem, finding alternative solutions, minimizing rather than exaggerating the significance of one's negative life situation, hopefulness, and the propensity of the suicidal person and his or her family to seek help are protective factors. On the other hand, blame, guilt, and avoidance of problems are correlated with suicide risk.[13]

A protective lifestyle is the product of growing up in a secure setting, with continuity in terms of adequate parent figures who are emotionally responsive to the child's needs, values, and norms and who care for the child from birth to adulthood.[14] This security is supplemented in due course by firm friendships, other adult networks, marriage, and a new family. A social, cultural, or religious context with the experience of meaning for the family and the individual's life is another protective factor.

Protective factors are essential for building sufficiently strong defences against suicidal impulses. Such protective factors also include treatment of any mental disorder that is present. The physical environment also plays a part in mental well-being, and a balanced diet and adequate sleep and light (all of which affect neurotransmitter function, and thus mental health), along with other environmental psychosocial factors, are other key protective factors. Risk factors and risk situations for suicidal behaviours are described in detail in chapters 6–19.

References

1 Bertolote J, Fleischmann A, De Leo D, Wasserman D. Suicidal thoughts, suicide plans and attempts in the general population on different continents. In: Wasserman D, Wasserman C, editors. Oxford textbook of suicidology and suicide prevention: a global perspective. Oxford: Oxford University Press; 2009: 99–104.

2 Nock MK, Borges G, Bromet EJ, Alonso J, Angermeyer M, Beautrais A, et al. Cross-national prevalence and risk factors for suicidal ideation, plans and attempts. Br J Psychiatry 2008;**192**(2):98–105.

3 Borges G, Nock MK, Abad JMH, Hwang I, Sampson NA, Alonso J, et al. Twelve-month prevalence of and risk factors for suicide attempts in the WHO World Mental Health Surveys. J Clin Psychiat 2010;**71**(12):1617.

4 Pokorny, AD. A scheme for classifying suicidal behaviors. In: Beck AT, Resnick HLP, Lettieri DJ (eds). The prediction of suicide. Bowie, Maryland, USA: Charles Press; 1974: 29–44.

5 Paykel ES, Myers JJ, Lindenthal JJ, Tanner J. Suicidal feelings in the general population: a prevalence study. Br J Psychiatry 1974;**124**:460–469.

6 Beskow J. Suicide and mental disorder in Swedish men. Acta Psychiatr Scand 1979;Suppl277:1–138.

7 Wolk-Wasserman D. Suicidal communication of persons attempting suicide and responses of significant others. Acta Psychiatr Scand 1986;**73**:481–499.

8 Farberow NL, Shneidman ES. The cry for help. New York, NY: McGraw-Hill; 1961.

9 **Wasserman D, Thanh TTH, Minh PTD, Goldstein M, Nordenskiöld A, Wasserman C**. Suicidal process, suicidal communication and psychosocial situation of young suicide attempters in a rural Vietnamese community. World Psychiatry 2008;7(1):47–53.

10 **Owen G, Belam J, Lambert H, Donovan J, Rapport F, Owens C**. Suicide communication events: lay interpretation of the communication of suicidal ideation and intent. Soc Sci Med2012;75(2):419–428.

11 **Zhou XM, Jia SH**. Suicidal communication signifies suicidal intent in Chinese completed suicides. Soc Psychiatry Psychiatr Epidemiol. 2012;47(11):1845–1854.

12 **Menninger KA**. Man against himself. New York, NY: Harcourt, Brace and World; 1938.

13 **Horesh N, Rolnick T, Iancu I, et al**. Coping styles and suicide risk. Acta Psychiatr Scand 1996;93:489–493.

14 **Rutter M**. Resilience in the face of adversity. Protective factors and resistance to psychiatric disorder. Br J Psychiatry 1985;147:598–611.

Chapter 4

Neurobiology of suicide and attempted suicide

J John Mann and Victoria Arango

Introduction

Suicide is a complication of psychiatric disorders in vulnerable individuals. Psychological autopsies have shown that generally about 90% of people who die by suicide have a diagnosable major psychiatric disorder.[1] However, the majority of people with psychiatric disorders never attempt suicide. Mood disorders account for most suicides and are associated with approximately 60% of all cases. Bipolar disorder requiring hospitalization has a lifetime rate of suicide of 20%, and 15% of people with unipolar or major depressive disorder commit suicide. Despite the high lifetime rate of suicide in depressed individuals, most people with mood disorders never attempt suicide. This raises the question as to why some people with psychiatric disorders are at risk of suicide and others are not. We have proposed that there is a diathesis, or predisposition, to suicidal behaviour. In discussing the biology of suicidal behaviour, it is important to distinguish the biological correlates of this diathesis for suicidal behaviour from the biological correlates of the stressors for suicidal behaviour such as the primary psychiatric disorder.[1] Each of these two domains has different biological correlates.

There is a lot of evidence that the most common stressor or trigger of suicide, major depression, is associated with impaired serotonergic function that involves different brain regions and thus is independent of the serotonergic abnormality associated with the vulnerability or diathesis for suicidal behaviour. In major depression there are fewer platelet serotonin transporters,[2] lower levels of 5-hydroxylindoleacetic acid (5-HIAA) in the cerebrospinal fluid (CSF),[3] and a blunted prolactin response to oral fenfluramine[4] and to intravenous L-tryptophan.[5]

The antidepressant efficacy of selective serotonin reuptake inhibitors also suggests that there is a deficiency in serotonergic function. The abnormality in serotonergic function in major depression may be a biochemical trait because it is present even when the patient is clinically better.[6,7]

Evidence that there are familial and genetic factors that contribute to the risk of suicidal behaviour

Suicidal behaviour is influenced by familial and genetic factors.[8–10] The rate of suicide and suicide attempts is higher in the families of suicide attempters than in families of psychiatric controls (patients with the same psychiatric illness or history). Monozygotic (identical) twins have a higher rate of concordance for suicide compared with dizygotic (non-identical) twins.[11] Roy also found a higher rate of concordance for non-fatal suicide attempts in monozygotic twins than in dizygotic twins who survived the co-twin's suicide.

The largest published twin study found that the concordance rate for a serious suicide attempt in monozygotic twins (23.1%) was more than 17-fold greater than the risk in the total sample. The rate of concordance for attempted suicide was comparable or higher than for completed suicide, indicating that both attempted and completed suicide are heritable. Adoption studies have shown that the risk of suicide is transmitted from the biological family to the adoptees at birth, independent of the transmission of mood or psychotic disorders, which is powerful evidence for genetic transmission. Familial studies have shown that the transmission of suicidal behaviour is independent of the transmission of psychopathology associated with suicidal behaviour. In other words, the familial transmission of the stressors, such as psychiatric illnesses, is independent of the familial transmission of the diathesis for suicidal behaviour.[12]

This cumulative body of evidence indicates that there are familial, and almost certainly genetic, factors related to the diathesis for suicidal behaviour. The consequence of such genetic factors must be a biological abnormality or phenotype.

Biological correlates of attempted suicide

One of the strongest findings in biological psychiatry is the observation that low levels of the main metabolite of serotonin (5-HIAA) in the cerebrospinal fluid (CSF) are associated with a history of serious suicide attempts in patients with mood disorders, schizophrenia, or personality disorders.[13] Moreover, it has been shown that low levels of 5-HIAA in the CSF can predict future suicide and suicide attempts.[14]

Studies of CSF 5-HIAA levels in humans and non-human primates indicate that this index of serotonergic activity in the brain is a biochemical trait that is under significant genetic control. As a biochemical trait under genetic control, it may be one mechanism by which genes can influence behaviour, and specifically by which genes can influence the risk for suicidal behaviour. Since this marker of serotonin function is low in relationship to suicidal behaviour in a variety of psychiatric illnesses, it is not merely a marker of these various psychiatric illnesses, but a biological index of the vulnerability to suicidal behaviour associated with these illnesses. We have shown that the more lethal the suicidal behaviour, the lower the level of CSF 5-HIAA and 5-HIAA is proportional to the degree of serotonergic activity in the brain. Some other indices of serotonergic function also include hormone responses to the release of serotonin, such as the prolactin level after the administration of the fenfluramine, a serotonin-releasing agent. Furthermore, platelets have many functions that are mediated by serotonin and provide an easily accessible measure of serotonin function, albeit not in the brain. Both platelet measures and prolactin responses to fenfluramine are indicative of abnormalities in the serotonin system in those who have made suicide attempts compared with psychiatric controls, and the alteration in these serotonin indices is proportional to the seriousness of the suicide attempt in terms of the degree of physical (as opposed to psychological) harm inflicted.

Genetic correlates of neurobiology and suicidal behaviour

Many studies have demonstrated that there are abnormalities in the serotonergic system of individuals who exhibit suicidal behaviour. One approach has been to determine which genes mediate the risk of suicidal behaviour by examining genes that code for proteins involved in the synthesis and metabolism of serotonin—the so-called candidate genes. While many candidate genes, related to neurobiological systems other than serotonin, have been examined in relation to the pathology of suicidal behaviour, we will briefly touch on serotonin candidate genes, as the serotonergic system appears to represent part of the biology of the diathesis or the vulnerability for suicidal behaviour.

Tryptophan hydroxylase (TPH) is the enzyme involved in the rate-limiting step in the synthesis of serotonin. Two isoforms of the enzyme are known: TPH1 and TPH2, found mostly in the periphery and brain, respectively. An abnormality in the production of serotonin may underlie the reduced serotonergic function that is observed in serious suicide attempters. Many studies have demonstrated an association between a polymorphism in the TPH1 gene in intron 7 and suicidal behaviour. While not all studies agree, most report an association between a TPH1 polymorphism and suicidal behaviour in Caucasians.[15] The study of different polymorphisms in the TPH2 gene has yielded no consistent associations with suicidal behaviour. Another serotonergic gene, the serotonin transporter, has a functional promoter polymorphism (5-HTTLPR) and 60% of the studies have described an association between the S allele and violent suicidal behaviour in Caucasians. Studies seeking a relationship between the 5-HT1A or the 5-HT2A receptor genes and suicidal behaviour have yielded mixed results. Other approaches include the dissection of the behaviour into endophenotypes[16] and investigate the association of genetic variants with traits such as aggression and impulsivity, and consider gene–environment interactions and the effect of adversity during early formative years. These studies illustrate the potential of this strategy, whose ultimate goal is to both understand the biological factors that contribute to the risk of suicidal behaviour and develop a blood test that will aid the clinician in identifying patients at higher risk for suicide.

Biological correlates of completed suicide

Completed suicide is the most serious form of suicidal behaviour and one would therefore predict that it would be associated with the most extreme biological abnormalities in terms of the diathesis. This group of patients is also different from suicide attempters in the sense that the brain may be available for study and biochemical analysis. Thus, studies of completed suicide not only look at the most extreme form of this behaviour, but also afford the opportunity to examine brain biochemistry directly instead of using indirect methods, such as CSF, pharmacological challenges, or peripheral measures in blood platelets.

Early biological studies found low levels of serotonin or its breakdown product, 5-HIAA, in the brainstem of suicides.[17] The brainstem contains all of the body's serotonin-synthesizing neurons, which then project to the rest of the brain to innervate millions of other cells. Thus, the observation that there may be modest reductions in serotonin or 5-HIAA in the brainstem suggests that these brainstem neurons are less active in suicide victims. However, a series of studies by our group have reported that, contrary to our initial hypothesis, all the biologic findings in the brainstem indicate it to be hyperserotonergic. There are more serotonin-synthesizing neurons; there is more TPH protein in those neurons, more TPH2 mRNA, and more 5-HT and 5-HIAA.[18]

Most studies have found that suicides have fewer brain serotonin transporter sites. We have reported that this finding is most striking in the ventral or orbital prefrontal cortex, midbrain, and anterior cingulate.[19] Many studies, but not all, have found an increase in prefrontal cortical serotonin-5-HT$_{1A}$ receptor binding in the brain of suicides, particularly in ventral PFC and rostral dorsal raphe nucleus. Moreover, the binding to platelet serotonin-5-HT$_{1A}$ receptors also appears to be increased in suicidal patients. This possible systemic effect raises the possibility of a genetic mechanism. The serotonin transporter decreases and the 5-HT$_{1A}$ binding increases are in overlapping areas of the lateral and orbital prefrontal cortex that has been shown in other studies to be involved in behavioural inhibition, willed action, and decision-making. Binding to these two pre- and postsynaptic sites is inversely correlated. Damage to this area of the brain results in disinhibitory behaviours and potentially an increased risk of suicide and aggressive behaviours.

We have, therefore, postulated that serotonergic input to this orbital area of the brain is involved in behavioural inhibition, and that impairment of this input or damage to this area of the brain results in behavioural disinhibition, thereby increasing the likelihood that an affected person will act on powerful emotions or thoughts or feelings, such as suicidal ideation. The importance of this suggestion is that evaluating this area of the brain using brain-imaging techniques that are currently in development may offer the clinician another way of testing patients to evaluate the possibility of a vulnerability or predisposition to suicidal behaviour.

The role of aggression and impulsivity in suicide risk

It has now been demonstrated by several studies that those who attempt suicide have an increased severity of lifetime aggressive behaviours and suicides have a positive correlation between lifetime history of aggression and 5-HT_{2A} binding in the prefrontal cortex. Impulsivity, on the other hand, is found to decrease with age and the high lethality attempts are carried out by older, less impulsive individuals.[20] These behavioural traits reflect a fundamental predisposition to act on powerful feelings that may be due to an impairment of serotonin input into the ventral prefrontal cortex, as discussed above.[1] It is, therefore, noteworthy that studies of pathologically aggressive patients and of aggression in non-human primates and other species have demonstrated an association with low serotonergic activity. Thus, low serotonergic activity is not only related to the predisposition to suicidal behaviour but also to the predisposition to aggressive and impulsive behaviours in general. Significant aggressive behaviour also has a genetic component, and it may be that there is a genetic element common to both suicidal behaviour and aggressive behaviour. This remains a subject for future research and may centre on regulation of behavioural inhibition.

Conclusion

The study of the biology of suicidal behaviour has provided considerable insights into mechanisms of risk for this behaviour and potential future laboratory tests that may aid the clinician in evaluating suicide risk.

References

1 **Mann JJ**. The neurobiology of suicide. Nat Med. 1998;**4**(1):25–30.

2 **Owens MJ, Nemeroff CB**. Role of serotonin in the pathophysiology of depression: focus on the serotonin transporter. Clin Chem 1994;**40**(2):288–295.

3 **Mann JJ, Malone KM**. Cerebrospinal fluid amines and higher-lethality suicide attempts in depressed inpatients. Biol Psychiatry 1997;**41**(2):162–171.

4 **Malone KM, Corbitt EM, Li S, Mann JJ**. Prolactin response to fenfluramine and suicide attempt lethality in major depression. Br J Psychiatry 1996;**168**(3):324–329.

5 **Delgado PL, Charney DS, Price LH, Aghajanian GK, Landis H, Heninger GR**. Serotonin function and the mechanism of antidepressant action. Reversal of antidepressant-induced remission by rapid depletion of plasma tryptophan. Arch Gen Psychiatry 1990;**47**(5):411–418.

6 **Flory JD, Mann JJ, Manuck SB, Muldoon MF**. Recovery from major depression is not associated with normalization of serotonergic function. Biol Psychiatry 1998;**43**(5):320–326.

7 **Miller JM, Brennan KG, Ogden TR, Oquendo MA, Sullivan GM, Mann JJ, et al**. Elevated serotonin 1A binding in remitted major depressive disorder: evidence for a trait biological abnormality. Neuropsychopharmacology. 2009;**34**(10): 2275–2284.

8 **Brodsky BS, Mann JJ, Stanley B, Tin A, Oquendo M, Green Hill L, et al**. Familial transmission of suicidal behavior: factors mediating the relationship between childhood abuse and offspring suicide attempts. J Clin Psychiatry 2008;**69**(4):584–596.

9 **Mann JJ, Bortinger J, Oquendo MA, Currier D, Li S, Brent DA**. Family history of suicidal behavior and mood disorders in probands with mood disorders. Am J Psychiatry 2005;**162**(9):1672–1679.

10 **Currier D, Mann JJ**. Stress, genes and the biology of suicidal behavior. Psychiatr Clin North Am 2008;**3**(2):247–269.

11 **Roy A, Segal NL, Centerwall BS, Robinette CD**. Suicide in twins. Arch Gen Psychiatry 1991;**48**(1):29–32.

12 **Brent DA, Mann JJ**. Familial pathways to suicidal behavior—understanding and preventing suicide among adolescents. N Engl J Med. 2006;**355**(26):2719–2721.

13 **Lindqvist D, Janelidze S, Erhardt S, Traskman-Bendz L, Engstrom G, Brundin L**. CSF biomarkers in suicide attempters—a principal component analysis. Acta Psychiat Scand 2011;**124**(1):52–61.

14 **Mann JJ, Currier D, Stanley B, Oquendo MA, Amsel LV, Ellis SP**. Can biological tests assist prediction of suicide in mood disorders? Int J Neuropsychopharmacol. 2006;**9**(4):465–474.

15 **Antypa N, Serretti A, Rujescu D**. Serotonergic genes and suicide: a systematic review. Eur Neuropsychopharmacol 2013;**23**(10):1125–1142.

16 **Mann J, Arango V, Avenevoli S, Brent DA, Champagne FA, Clayton P et al**. Candidate endophenotypes for genetic studies of suicidal behaviour. Biol Psychiatry 2009;**65**(7):556–563.

17 **Arango V, Underwood MD, Mann JJ**. Biologic alterations in the brainstem of suicides. Psychiatr Clin North Am 1997;**20**(3):581–593.

18 **Bach H, Huang YY, Underwood MD, Dwork AJ, Mann JJ, Arango V**. Elevated serotonin and 5-HIAA in the brainstem and lower serotonin turnover in the prefrontal cortex of suicides. Synapse. 2014;**68**(3)127–130.

19 **Arango V, Underwood MD, Mann JJ**. Serotonin brain circuits involved in major depression and suicide. Progress in Brain Research, 2002;**136**:443–453.

20 **Oquendo MA, Placidi GP, Malone KM, Campbell C, Keilp J, Brodsky B et al**. Positron emission tomography of regional brain metabolic responses to a serotonergic challenge and lethality of suicide attempts in major depression. Arch Gen Psychiatry 2003;(1):14–22.

Chapter 5

Social dimensions of suicide

Ilkka Henrik Mäkinen

Introduction

Even if suicide is the result of an individual decision, it neither originates nor is it committed in a vacuum. Thus, while social scientists are working on determining the relations between the structure or dynamics of societies and the number of suicides committed in them,[1] it may also be useful for the individual medical practitioner to pay attention to the social environment in which the patient lives and suffers.

These factors are here called social, rather than societal or sociological, because they are clearly recognizable at the individual level. This makes them at least partly dependent on individual decisions. For the sake of convenience, this text may sometimes use expressions that implicate a straightforward causality between various social factors and individual suicides. However, such direct causality should not be inferred. From the doctor's point of view the distinction, even if it is a necessary one for the scientist, is less important. If a patient belongs to a group in which suicide, for one reason or another, is more common than in other groups, then it is a reason for vigilance on the part of the caregiver.

It has been argued that there are three basic determinants of population health in modern societies: material wealth, social structure, and lifestyles. All of these are intertwined. As sheer material wealth in itself does not seem to be of great importance in relation to suicide, the role of the social structure is discussed below. The structure should, however, be understood in the context of the manner in which structural roles (e.g., being married, on disability pension, or having recently migrated) may imply a certain type of lifestyle.

Social categories are inherently dynamic. Although a static mode of description is easier to communicate, one should keep in mind that the human contents of the categories (and sometimes the categories themselves) are constantly changing. Sometimes a person's move into a 'risk category' is the most dangerous moment from the suicidological point of view. Individual-based research shows that many of the stressful or traumatic 'life events' are of social origin.

Many social theories of suicide regard large-scale changes in the social environment as being of major importance for changes in suicide mortality levels in society. An important element in Émile Durkheim's famous theory of suicide[2] was the disruptive effect of rapid modernization. A relatively recent example of such large-scale transformation is the changes in the former Soviet Union, where drastic increases in suicide mortality took place in the 1990s. They have been connected to the 'transitionary' nature of post-communist society, although the causal mechanisms have not been solved in detail.

Social environment in general

The first dimension to be considered is the individual's social network. All previous research points unambiguously to the conclusion that the ties that attach the individual to his or her peers and to the larger society are of utmost importance in relation to his or her propensity to commit suicide. The number, duration, strength, and quality of social relations are all inversely related to suicide risk. People with marital, kinship, occupational, friendship, or other types of social ties are generally at lower risk of committing suicide than those who lack these ties, and people who commit suicide generally possess fewer social ties of any kind than others. This effect has even been shown to exist over time.[3,4]

As with other social factors, the causality question is not clear-cut. A person may commit suicide because s/he lacks social ties, or s/he may experience loneliness because of some third factor (such as mental illness), which ultimately causes isolation and thus influences suicidality in several ways simultaneously. However, there is evidence to suggest that isolation, both physical and psychological, has an effect of its own that is independent of other circumstances.

There are notions of men's suicidality being more influenced by large-scale social circumstances than women's. In times when there are sudden movements in suicide mortality figures, caused by social factors, men's suicide rates seem to both rise and fall more steeply than women's. This could be interpreted as men having a greater propensity to react suicidally to external change. However, there is probably no great difference between the sexes when the crisis touches on the personal sphere.

The presence of other people may mean that social support is available, and even if this is not the case, it may still provide an invisible but nonetheless effective form of social control. Community-oriented life also often implies that one's everyday activities follow a certain routine, which in itself works protectively. Should the worst come to the worst, many suicides are prevented by the purposeful or coincidental intervention of others. Furthermore, the preventive effect of social ties seems to be cumulative: divorced or widowed people have higher suicide rates than married people but among the divorced and widowed those who are not in a position to work or are unemployed, the suicide rates are higher still.

However, the coin has also a reverse side. Social environments in which self-destructive behaviour seems to be valued (e.g., some hard-rock milieus) or in which many such acts are committed and reported may prove to be more detrimental to than protective of the individual. Areas in which there are many suicide attempts are often also those in which various social problems accumulate. Living in a group and following its norms and behaviours is in many ways easier than trying to exist alone, but so too, in this respect, is dying.

Family relationships

Perhaps the most important social environment is the family. While its size may be diminishing and its authority, and even its legitimacy, are sometimes under attack in modern society, it still provides the individual with basic emotional security (or a lack of it) as well as social, and sometimes also financial, support. Furthermore, it still acts as a major institution in people's socialization and the transmission of values and attitudes to the next generation.

There are clear and nearly universal differences in suicidality between people in different marital status groups. Married people generally have the lowest suicide rates, and divorced and widowed people have rates that are two or three times higher. The rate of suicide also seems to vary inversely with the duration of the marriage and the number of children in it. The suicide rates of the unmarried are also generally higher than those of married people.

Marital status (unlike, for example, age) is a voluntary category. Today, it is not automatically assumed that marriage should be lifelong. New categories, such as cohabitation without marriage, have also appeared since the 1960s in many countries.

The difference between marital groups can even be observed at the collective level. Familistic areas, inhabited predominantly by married couples with children, generally have the lowest suicide rates in modern cities. Several factors are involved in the shaping of a familistic lifestyle. First, there is the selection into the married group, which tends to exclude those who are alone and who perhaps are physically and psychologically vulnerable. Second, the fact of being married in modern society usually means that there is a degree of trust between the partners so that they choose to formalize their relationship instead of merely cohabiting. Third, a family-centred life with children often takes place among other couples so that a social environment is created, which especially in the larger cities stands in stark contrast to the more irregular lifestyles in other areas. All these factors are likely to lower suicidality, partly through selection, and partly through protection. Therefore, a status change away from this category (e.g., through divorce) may involve a major risk for the individual.

Being in a family does not automatically mean that a person is protected. As in other social environments, the functionality of the family is essential to its influence on individual suicidality. For example, people with a history of suicide in their families run a considerable surplus risk of committing the act themselves. However, not only the family, but even friends and acquaintances can exercise influence on individual suicidality.

Last but not least, marriage is also a cultural category. While Western marriages are supposedly based on romantic love, this is not an issue, or not at least the main determinant, in many other cultural environments. The opinions of parents and relatives, as well as economic factors, may greatly influence marriage decisions. This implies that the effect of marriage might not be exactly the same across different cultural groups. For example, the high suicide mortality among young females in the rural areas of China has been linked to the arranged marriages that they undergo and to the low status of the bride in her new family. In the past, there have also been societies in which the suicide of the survivors of 'great men' was the social norm. Although these practices are on the wane, the behaviour itself continues even in some contemporary relationships.

Employment

Another main sphere of life is that of one's occupation. There are disparities in suicidality between different categories, among other things, between those who are employed and those who are not. Research suggests that those who are not employed have generally higher risk of both suicide and suicide attempt.[5]

Alike marriage, a work position can provide many things. After the initial selection process, it may offer not only economic resources but also social contacts, social position, support possibilities, and stable routines. Thus, the connection between unemployment and suicide is largely dependent on what exactly unemployment means for the individual. In the crisis years of the 1930s, unemployment peaks in the US and Western Europe would sometimes be visibly followed by peaks in (male) suicide rates, but in modern times, corresponding phenomena are harder to find at an aggregate level in the existing studies. This change can probably be explained by the development of financial support systems, which soften the consequences of unemployment.

However, according to a large comparative analysis, the worldwide crisis in 2008–2010 has been counted to be responsible for having produced 10,000 'economic suicides',[6] cases in which especially unemployment, debt, and foreclosure have had an important role. Greece, a country with one of the lowest suicide mortality rates in Europe, has also been the focus of several debates on the effects on suicide mortality of a long and hard economic crisis. While some researchers have maintained that the crisis has left its mark in the suicide statistics of the country,[7] others[8] argue either that no effects can be shown to exist, or that the causality question is unclear.

Generally, people who are gainfully employed full-time seem to have the lowest suicide rates. The suicide risk of those who are not employed also depends on other factors: it is, for example, difficult to say to what extent the generally higher suicide rates among old people in most European countries can be explained by their retirement from working life alone. However, there are two special high-risk groups for suicide that can be easily recognized, namely those who are outside the labour market for other than home- or career-related reasons (e.g., those on a disability pension); and the unemployed, i.e., persons who would like to have a job but cannot find one. Of these, the first group seems to be at greatest risk.

There are even differences among the employed. Thus, although there may be variation between countries, most European research points at a 'class ladder' in suicide mortality. Among men, those holding higher 'white-collar' positions tend to have the lowest suicide rates; these increase with every successive step down the ladder and are highest on the bottom rung among unskilled workers. The relationship is, of course, confounded by (and also due partly to) other socio-psychological and cultural differences between the holders of the status positions.

For women, the picture is not so clear—there are indications of a U-shaped relationship, where those in the middle positions are at the lowest risk, while women in both the leading and lower positions demonstrate a higher level of suicidality.

Finally, when one person in an interdependent social unit, such as a family, becomes unemployed or otherwise leaves the labour market, it seldom affects her or him alone. Depending on economic or other circumstances, the effect on the whole family may vary from slight annoyance (or even relief) to a major life crisis, which may eventually lead to suicidal acts.[9]

Mobility and migration

It may be generally assumed that all changes in the social environment that cause some important social ties to be disrupted are more or less suicide-promoting. Disregarding the question of causality, it seems that separations, divorces, and negative changes in a person's labour-market status are connected with suicidal crises and ensuing actions. This is also true of geographical movement. A recent or repeated change of residence is often found to be more prevalent among people who kill themselves than among others. Furthermore, areas that are characterized by high levels of mobility often have high suicide rates.

In relation to suicide and geographical movement, most research has focused on emigration–immigration (i.e., the move over international borders). Generally speaking, suicide rates of immigrants tend to be higher in the new country than in the country of origin; a fact that can, in many cases, be accounted for by the 'negative selection' of the migrants (i.e., those with the least to lose move out) as well as by the general stress of immigration along with the psychosocial risks it entails.[10] Recent research has also found that immigrants to Europe from the culturally more distant societies tend to get care different from that of others after a suicide attempt.[11]

With regard to long-term developments, there is no coherent picture—there are reports of converging processes, whereby the suicide mortality of various immigrant groups moves gradually closer to that of the host population over time, but this does not appear to apply to all groups everywhere. For example, immigrant Finns in Sweden still experience a very high level of suicide mortality even after decades in their new country.

This last-mentioned fact illustrates the complexity of the issue. All over the world, people from numerous nations, all with their own migration (and suicide) traditions, emigrate for various reasons to the recipient states, which in turn receive them in different ways. In such circumstances, few general things can be said about the longer-term effects of such multiple processes on suicidality. However, it does appear as if the cultural background of the individual is of great importance. People from nations with low suicide rates (e.g., the Arabic and many Mediterranean and South American nations) tend to maintain the low suicide level in their new environment, while immigrants from Eastern Europe, for example, have a greater risk of suicide in their new countries.

No less important is the path of acculturation that the new immigrant chooses from the options available. A marginalized person, living on the outskirts of the host society, is very dependent on his closest social ties, whereas one striving for quick assimilation risks losing the support of his own group while perhaps not being readily accepted into the group to which he aspires to belong. Immigrants employing a common 'separation' strategy prefer to live among their own ethnic group after moving into the new society, which may very well be beneficial from the point of view of suicidality, as long as the group is large enough to provide support for them.[12]

Culture and religion

Culture, in the sense of salient and more or less collectively held ideas guiding the individual's behaviour, and its perhaps main constituent—religion, are social in the sense that they are most often absorbed in the society of one's origin. Having once been internalized, they often show a surprising ability to subsist in new environments through a process of creative adaptation. It seems that much of the difference in suicidal behaviour between national groups is connected with differences in cultural outlook. Groups differ greatly in the cultural 'visibility' of suicide, the attitude that is taken towards it, and the situations in which it may be considered as an acceptable, or even preferable, course of action.[13-16] While this is not always visible at the individual level, it can be clearly seen at the collective level, where the rates of suicide, the distribution of suicide, and the ways of and motives for committing the act separate different cultural spheres from each other.

An example of this can be found in the remarkable stability of suicide rates in different countries and areas. Even when suicide mortality in general increases or decreases, the *differences* between the units—their rank order, often tend to remain more or less similar.[17] Although there are individual exceptions to this observation, a comparison of the current suicide rates of European nations to those of 100 years ago reveals surprisingly stable patterns, the origin of which must probably be sought in the differences among national and local cultures. The young, however, constitute an exception of this tendency, their suicide rates being more volatile than those of other age groups, perhaps owing to international influences.

Traditionally, religion has been considered to be the 'matrix' of culture. Its relation to suicidality became famous through Durkheim's study, which claimed that Roman Catholics always had lower suicide rates than Protestants. However, in modern societies religion has become individualized to such an extent that its effects can be better discerned between individuals than between societies. Personal religiosity is still the main determinant of *attitudes* towards suicide in Western Europe. In this respect, it seems to be strongly connected with suicidal behaviour, as long as the religious attachment is balanced.[18]

References

1 Mäkinen I. Social theories of suicide. In: Wasserman D, Wasserman C, editors. The Oxford textbook of suicidology and suicide prevention: a global perspective. 1st edn. Oxford: Oxford University Press; 2009: 139–148.

2 Durkheim E. Suicide. London: Routledge; 1992.

3 Maris RW. Social and familial risk factors in suicidal behavior. Psychiatr Clin North America. Review. 1997;**20**:519–550.

4 Rojas Y. Childhood social exclusion and suicidal behavior in adolescence and young adulthood. Stockholm: Department of Sociology, Stockholm University, 2014.

5 Haw C, Hawton K, Gunnell D, Platt S. Economic recession and suicidal behaviour: possible mechanisms and ameliorating factors. Int J Soc Psychiatry. 4 June 2014.

6 Reeves A, McKee M, Stuckler D. Economic suicides and the Great Recession in Europe and North America (2008–2010). BJPsych. 2014;**205**: 246–224.

7 Economou M, Madianos M, Theleritis C, Peppou LE, Stefanis CN. Increased suicidality amid economic crisis in Greece. Lancet. 2011;**378**:1459.

8 Fountoulakis KN, Grammatikopoulos IA, Koupidis SA, Siamouli M, Theodorakis PN. Health and the financial crisis in Greece. Lancet. 2012;**379**:1001–1002.

9 Mäkinen IH, Wasserman D. Labour market, work environment and suicide. In: Wasserman D, Wasserman C, editors. Oxford textbook of suicidology and suicide prevention: a global perspective. Oxford: Oxford University Press; 2009: 221–229.

10 Whitlock FA. Migration and suicide. Med J Aust. 1971;**2**:840–848.

11 Bursztein Lipsicas C, Mäkinen IH, Wasserman D, Apter A, Bobes J . . . Schmidtke A. Immigration and recommended care after a suicide attempt in Europe: equity or bias? Eur J Public Health 2014;**24**:63–65.

12 Zammit S, Gunnell D, Lewis G, Leckie G, Dalman C, Allebeck P. Individual- and area-level influence on suicide risk: a multilevel longitudinal study of Swedish schoolchildren. Psychol Med. Jan 2014;**44**(2):267–277.

13 Farberow NL (ed.). Suicide in different cultures. Baltimore: University Park Press; 1975.

14 Mäkinen IH. Suicide-related crimes in contemporary European criminal laws. Crisis. 1997;**18**:35–47.

15 Wasserman D, Wasserman C, editors. Suicide in religious and cross-cultural perspective (chapters 1–12). In: Oxford textbook of suicidology and suicide prevention: a global perspective. Oxford: Oxford University Press; 2009.

16 **Colucci E, Lester D, editors**. Suicide and culture. Understanding the context. Cambridge & Göttingen: Hogrefe; 2012.

17 **Mäkinen IH, Wasserman D**. Suicide prevention and cultural resistance: stability in European countries' suicide ranking, 1970–1988. Ital J Suicidol. 1997;7:73–85.

18 **Pescosolido B, Georgianna S**. Durkheim, suicide, and religion: toward a network theory of suicide. Am Soc Rev. 1989;54:33–48.

Risk groups for suicide

IIIA Psychiatric disorders
IIIB Personality disorders
IIIC Somatic disorders

IIIA

Psychiatric disorders

Chapter 6

Depression, bipolar disorders, and suicide

Danuta Wasserman

Introduction

In the DSM-5 classification, bipolar and related disorders fall between the spectrum of schizophrenia/other psychotic disorders and depressive disorders. To serve clinical practice, as many bipolar patients experience depressive episodes during their life and were previously studied within the affective disorder spectrum, bipolar disorders are described in this chapter. A systematic review of 50 studies showed that psychiatric disorders were present in 84% of adults and 81% of young people treated in general hospitals due to self-harm.[1] Affective disorders are the psychiatric diagnoses most strongly linked with suicide. It has been demonstrated in a large national psychiatric population sample from Denmark on patients 15–51 years old, that the risk of suicide is highest for bipolar disorders (BDs), affecting 7.8% of males and 4.8% of females, followed by unipolar affective disorder, which affects 6.7% of males and 3.7% of females.[2] Also results from a national survey in China confirmed that patients with BD had a higher suicide risk, than patients with major depressive disorder.[3] The biggest increase in suicide incidents occurs during the first years after the first hospital contact.[2]

Most patients who commit suicide show several symptoms of depression, and up to 60% have fully diagnosable affective disorder. The risk of suicide varies between the different subtypes of depression.[4,5] Suicidal acts occur usually during major depressive episodes or mixed states. Long duration of these states has influence on the overall risk of attempted suicide and completed suicide. Affective temperaments, especially cyclothymic, but also anxious and irritable are associated with both attempted suicide and suicide.[6] These temperaments, as well as rapid mood swings[7,8] contribute to the triggering of suicidal acts. Negative life events (see chapters 14 and 15) such as childhood and adolescent abuse are associated with suicide attempts in persons with depression and other psychiatric disorders.[9] The specific nature of life events is perhaps one of the keys to a deeper understanding of the timing of suicidal behaviour. However, recurrent major depressive episodes are a robust precipitant of suicidal behaviour.[10]

The overwhelming majority of depressed patients do not take their own lives. Depression is, after all, a very common illness. The 12-month prevalence estimate of major depression disorder is 5.5% in high-income countries and 5.9% in low- to middle-income countries, respectively.[11] Global point-prevalence is approximately 4.4 and is higher among females (5.5%) compared with males (3.2%).[12]

It is important to remember that suicide risk is high in untreated patients with severe depression, especially if comorbid disorders, such as alcohol and substance use disorders, anxiety disorders, as well as family history of psychiatric disorders, and previous suicide attempts are present.[1]

Major depressive disorder

In depression, the central experience is despondency, with marked feelings of emptiness, indifference, and hopelessness. Symptoms vary in different age groups and between the sexes.[13] Older depressed people very often show signs of restlessness, have difficulty in sitting still, and have more somatic symptoms. The medication for somatic illnesses can obscure the mental symptoms and make depression more difficult to diagnose. Among middle-aged men, depression may sometimes be manifested by irritability, awkwardness in interpersonal relations, touchiness, sensitivity to criticism, aggression, and even fits of rage.

Adolescents quite frequently take refuge in sleep, shutting out the outside world, and in pathological Internet use.[14] Diagnosing depression in the young is often complicated owing to the interplay with normal developmental stages. The first striking sign of depression could be truancy as well as deterioration in school grades, with concentration difficulties that are perceived as laziness. Feelings of failure and hopelessness are marked. Depressed adolescents' diurnal rhythm may tend to be reversed, and anxiety may sometimes drive them to seek consolation in food. In other cases, they lose weight sharply. Anorexia nervosa or bulimia nervosa often coincides with depression in the young (see Chapter 9). For boys, depression is often associated with behavioural disturbances: they may become rowdy, aggressive and highly irritable, and they may resort to violence. Comorbidity in the form of abuse of cannabis, other drugs, and alcohol is common.

Anhedonia, severe concentration difficulties, anxiety, and alcohol abuse appear to be short-term predictors of suicide and attempted suicide, while mood fluctuations and feelings of hopelessness are long-term predictors.[15]

Melancholia

A melancholic person is entirely indifferent to the outside world: lacking a sense of 'belonging' and involvement even with close family and friends. Typical symptoms of melancholia are being passive, withdrawn, taciturn, and a lack of energy.

Self-belittlement, an exaggerated sense of guilt, and a feeling that life is pointless and that one has failed in everything is very often accompanied by severe recurrent suicidal thoughts and thoughts about death. However, the risk of suicide usually becomes prominent when the patient is in the process of improvement and the psycho-motoric inhibition decreases while, at the same time, perceptions about the capacity to cope with the psychosocial situation are still very negative. For some patients, confrontation with the reality is experienced as being so frightful and filled with anguish that suicide may appear to be the only solution.[13]

Psychotic depression with delusions or hallucinations has been found to be relatively rare among people who commit suicide. However, in suicide prevention and treatment of suicidal patient, attention should be paid to both psychotic and non-psychotic subtypes of depression, as the same risk factors are present in both subtypes.[16]

Depression in males

It is not unusual for men to refrain from seeking professional help even when they are severely depressed. When they finally see a doctor, their depression often remains unrecognized and thus untreated.

It is not deemed compatible with the male role to be weak, to cry, or to be depressed. This may contribute to the fact that men deny their depression and are disinclined to speak of their despondency. It is hardly surprising that depression in men often centres on their occupation and workplace: becoming unemployed means losing not only a job and income, but also colleagues, fellowship, and the structure for life's daily routines. Loss of status is often harder for men to bear than for women, who base their identity to a much larger extent on their families, children, and friends.

Men who become depressed develop different symptoms from women. The depressed man seldom refers to his anxiety, sorrow, or despondency. His depression is manifested in poor performance at work, at home, or in his leisure activities. Quite frequently, he compensates with intense and non-productive activity. Restlessness, irritability, quarrelsomeness, and lack of concentration are typical components. Men probably succumb to depression to a far higher degree than the statistics suggest, but their depression is concealed by alcohol consumption, increased aggressiveness, violence, and suicide.[13]

An untreated depression may become so serious that suicide seems the only way out for a man who has difficulty in confiding in anyone and in seeking medical help. Since depressed men very seldom seek psychiatric help, male depression should be brought to the attention of general practitioners, company doctors, and other somatic physicians (see Chapters 29 and 30). It is recommended that, for men, treatment should be commenced without all the criteria for major depression being fulfilled.

Masked depression

In suicidal patients, it is not unusual for depression to be masked by painful conditions or physical symptoms other than pain, without any underlying physical illness or organ injury. Patients with symptoms of this kind often have difficulty in expressing themselves, in verbalizing their psychological problems, and in describing their life situation. The bodily symptoms are a form of communication, signalling that something is wrong, and these symptoms may be a reaction to a life situation that the patient finds unbearable. Having a physical illness is more accepted, not only in Western culture but also elsewhere. People's inability to get in touch with their own experience can be reinforced by cultures in which mental illness is the object of prejudice.[13]

In suicidal people with masked depression, symptoms may take the form of aches and pains localized to joints, muscles, and other parts of the body, but also tiredness, chronic fatigue, dizziness, numbness in the arms and legs, or a feeling of pressure in the head. It is for these symptoms that these patients consult their doctor. A systematic review of the suicidal patient's life situation often reveals severe conflicts in the family or at work and marked suicidal ideation. General practitioners should be trained to detect masked depression, suicidal thoughts, and various types of suicidal communication so as to be able to prevent suicide attempts and suicide.

Dysthymia

The course of dysthymia is less periodic than that of major depressive disorder. People with dysthymia experience a state of depression that is more or less constant but somewhat mild as compared with major depression. Many dysthymic states start in childhood and are widely regarded as personality disorders with gloom as the keynote; others see them as anxiety disorders. The psychological development of people with dysthymia is often inhibited, since they find it difficult to believe in their own abilities and a bright future for themselves.[13]

Suicide risk in dysthymia may be comparable to that in most severe forms of affective disorders, although the relative importance of the roles played in suicidality by the actual depression, the anxiety component or comorbidity in the form of personality disorder is impossible to ascertain.

Not infrequently, a suicidal patient may have double depression, with major depressive disorder on top of dysthymia.

Bipolar disorders and mania

The majority of patients with a bipolar illness who commit suicide are, at the time of death, in the throes of a major depressive episode or in a mixed depressive state. Suicide during the manic phase is relatively rare. Hypomanic and manic states are often followed by profound depression, with remorse for acts during the manic period.

Male suicides usually take place earlier in the course of the bipolar illness compared with females. However, both suicide and suicide attempts can take place in any phase of a Bipolar Disorder.

The prevalence of suicide attempts appear to be the same among patients with both type 1 and type 2 bipolar disorders.[17] 'Bipolar 1' means a disorder in which mania has occurred on at least one occasion. 'Bipolar 2' refers to a disorder where hypomania has occurred but mania has not. The odds for attempted suicide are higher in patients with many depressed or 'mixed' episodes, compared with manic episodes.[18]

Comorbidity

Concurrent depression and anxiety, which are typical symptoms among suicidal patients, are difficult to separate. Increase of suicide during the seasons of spring and autumn can be associated with an increased occurrence of comorbid depression and anxiety during the same period.[19]

People with major depressive disorder who commit suicide also often show comorbidity of alcohol and other substance misuse, multiple physical diseases, and various personality disorders. Comorbidity varies with sex and age. Older patients have more somatic illnesses than younger ones, while young patients often exhibit various types of personality disorder and men engage in psychoactive substance abuse. Depressive symptoms are also frequently present in schizophrenic patients who commit suicide. Manic–depressive patients who commit suicide are often dependent on alcohol.[20]

Medical consultations before suicide

In more than 60% of cases, people who commit suicide consult psychiatrists in the year before the act and in many cases as late as in the week before the act. Women have more contacts with psychiatric care services, while men more frequently consult general practitioners or other doctors.

Doctors do not always think of suicide risk, since many of the patients they have seen have, before suicide, shown clear calming or masked depression. 'Clear calming' means that suicidal individuals are not anxiety driven because they decided to take their own life and also which method of suicide to use. Male patients seldom spontaneously communicate their suicidal intentions and many of them show signs of masked depression, making it difficult for a correct psychiatric diagnosis.[13]

Antidepressants as means of committing suicide

Concerns are often expressed about the elevated risk of suicide and attempted suicide associated with the treatment of depression with antidepressant drugs. The danger that certain antidepressants are more toxic than others and may, in the event of an overdose, have severe consequences and even be lethal should not, of course, be underestimated.[21]

The older tricyclic antidepressants have relatively high overdose toxicity; the newer antidepressants are less toxic. But, even the newer agents can be used for self-destructive purposes. What counts here, obviously, is not only the properties of the tablets ingested but also the patient's intention as expressed in the quantity of tablets swallowed.

Doctors and relatives alike should bear in mind that there is a risk of suicidal acts at the commencement of treatment with antidepressants before the full effect is achieved (see Chapter 27), since patients' symptoms improve after approximately 2–3 weeks' treatment and their psychomotor inhibitions diminish, while their negative perceptions of the illness and (very often) poor psychosocial situation still persist. Moreover, one should be mindful of the fact that anxiety, which is a powerful impetus towards suicidal acts, is intensified at the beginning of treatment with certain antidepressants. Active follow-up with face-to-face supportive discussions is, therefore, important.

Treatment

Suicide mortality is significantly associated with contact and psychiatric admissions in the preceding year.[22] Mortality due to suicide is highest in persons with bipolar, affective, and personality disorders.[23] In both treatment and prevention, one should also focus on so-called distal risk factors, like low educational achievement, low occupational status and unemployment, along with proximal psychiatric risk factors for suicidality in order to achieve the best effect.[24,25]

Although assessing the suicide preventive effects of various treatments is subject to several methodological difficulties (partly because of the divergent selection factors used in different studies, and partly because of information bias and random fluctuations in suicide rates in small populations), the results of existing studies and clinical experience are clearly promising. Both psychotherapeutical and pharmacological treatments have good effects.[25] (See also Chapters 27 and 28.)

Unfortunately, although some 60% of people seek help shortly before committing suicide, only about 15% receive antidepressant prescriptions and, of these, half show poor compliance to treatment and discontinue their medication 2–3 weeks before the suicide. For others, the dosage is often insufficient. One of the reasons being not only inadequate dosage, but also inherited genetic differences in metabolic pathways. Moreover, psychotherapeutic treatment is not always available. Electroconvulsive therapy is not commonly used and treatment with lithium requires knowledgeable follow-up. According to a Finnish study, only 3% of people who died from suicide had received electroconvulsive therapy and 3% had received lithium treatment.[5]

Prevention

Effective treatment of depression with both pharmacological and psychological methods is the foremost strategy of suicide prevention among young people, the middle-aged, and the elderly alike. Treatment of depression appears, however, to be of more benefit in preventing suicide in women than in men.

Case Study

Keeping problems to oneself
Jussi, age 40

Jussi, a 40-year-old Finnish-born factory worker, had moved to Sweden several years ago in search of a better job. He was engaged to, and lived with, a Finnish woman who was one year his senior and with whom he was expecting a child. The woman's four children from a previous marriage were in their father's care. Jussi was described as taciturn, placid, reliable, helpful, and concerned about his family. Married once previously, he had a child from the marriage, who was looked after by his ex-wife.

In the past six months, his duties at the factory had changed and he no longer enjoyed his job. Although he had not striven to keep his ordinary duties, he felt hurt and disappointed when a colleague was chosen to replace him.

Over the past months, his private life had also changed. He had stopped seeing his siblings, who also lived in Sweden, and he refused to visit his parents in Finland although they had warmly invited him, his fiancée and her children to a big family gathering. From time to time he complained of pain in the same part of his back that he had strained while renovating a boat.

In the past four weeks, Jussi had begun losing interest in everything. Even painting his beloved boat did not appeal to him, although the sailing trips of the spring and summer were approaching. He could be deeply despondent one moment and irritable and restless the next. Previously very even-tempered, he had on one occasion hit his fiancée's 5-year-old son, who was briefly visiting them. This was the impetus for his fiancée's suggestion that Jussi should see a doctor.

Jussi went to see his general practitioner. During the consultation he was reserved and obviously unaccustomed to talking about his situation at work and in his private life. He did not tell the doctor that he felt very lonely and under pressure because of his fiancée's pregnancy, nor did he refer to his worry about how they would cope financially, having to support not only the child from his first marriage but also the baby they were expecting and his fiancée's other children. He shared neither with the doctor nor with anyone else his intensive brooding about what kind of a mother his fiancée would turn out to be, since she had not looked after her own children from her previous relationship.

Jussi also omitted to tell the doctor that everything had felt black and difficult over the past month. The idea of hanging himself kept coming back to him. A colleague had taken his own life one year before and his maternal grandfather, who had been depressed, had hanged himself when Jussi was a child. These ideas were not conveyed to the doctor, who prescribed a painkiller.

The prescription did not help, and the fiancée sensed Jussi's growing dependency and inactivity. Besides backache, he began getting headaches and stomach aches, and his eating habits deteriorated. In three weeks, he lost several kilograms in weight. Jussi became more and more detached from his family. He began resorting to alcohol to get to sleep. No longer interested in anything, he became passive, withdrawn, and sluggish.

One day he refused to see an assistant from the Finnish housing agency whom he and his fiancée had an appointment with to hear about opportunities for getting a better flat. In despair his fiancée turned to the Finnish church, and the parson promised to visit them at home. Jussi always felt uneasy in the presence of the parson, whom he feared and considered stern.

On the day before the parson's visit, Jussi went out early in the morning to the garden and hanged himself. He was found by a passing factory guard and cut down. After resuscitation, he was admitted to a psychiatric unit. After his suicide attempt, Jussi was treated with electroconvulsive therapy, followed by antidepressants, and underwent family therapy with his fiancée.

References

1 Hawton K, Casañas i Comabella C, Haw C, Saunders K. Risk factors for suicide in individuals with depression: a systematic review. J Affect Disord. 2013;**147**(1):17–28.

2 Nordentoft M, Mortensen PB, Pedersen CB. Absolute risk of suicide after first hospital contact in mental disorder. Arch Gen Psychiatry. 2011;**68**:1058–1064.

3 Chen L, Liu YH, Zheng QW, Xiang YT, Duan YP, Yang FD, et al. Suicide risk in major affective disorder: results from a national survey in China. J Affect Disord. 2014;**155**:174–179.

4 Rihmer Z, Barsi J, Arató M, Demeter E. Suicide in subtypes of primary major depression. J Affect Disord. 1990;**18**(3):221–225.

5 Isometsä E. Suicidal behaviour in mood disorders—who, when, and why? Can J Psychiatry. 2014;**59**(3):120–130.

6 Rihmer Z, Gonda X, Torzsa P, Kalabay L, Akiskal HS, Eory A. Affective temperament, history of suicide attempt and family history of suicide in general practice patients. J Affect Disord. 2013;**149**(1–3):350–354.

7 MacKinnon DF, Potash JB, McMahon FJ, Simpson SG, Depaulo JR, Jr., Zandi PP. Rapid mood switching and suicidality in familial bipolar disorder. Bipolar Disord. 2005;**7**(5):441–448.

8 Baldessarini RJ, Undurraga J, Vazquez GH, Tondo L, Salvatore P, Ha K, et al. Predominant recurrence polarity among 928 adult international bipolar I disorder patients. Acta Psychiatr Scand. 2012;**125**(4):293–302.

9 Sokolowski M, Ben-Efraim YJ, Wasserman J, Wasserman D. Glutamatergic GRIN2B and polyaminergic ODC1 genes in suicide attempts: associations and gene-environment interactions with childhood/adolescent physical assault. Mol Psychiatry. 2013 Sep;**18**(9):985–992.

10 Oquendo MA, Perez-Rodriguez MM, Poh E, Sullivan G, Burke AK, Sublette ME, et al. Life events: a complex role in the timing of suicidal behavior among depressed patients. Mol Psychiatry. 2014 Aug;**19**(8):902–909.

11 Bromet E, Andrade L, Hwang I, Sampson N, Alonso J, de Girolamo G, et al. Cross-national epidemiology of DSM-IV major depressive episode. BMC Med. 2011;**9**(1):90.

12 Ferrari AJ, Charlson FJ, Norman RE, Flaxman AD, Patten SB, Vos T, et al. The epidemiological modelling of major depressive disorder: application for the Global Burden of Disease Study 2010. PLoS One. 2013;**8**(7):e69637.

13 Wasserman D. Depression—the facts. Oxford University Press, 2nd edn. 2011: 1–176.

14 Carli V, Hoven CW, Wasserman C, Chiesa F, Guffanti G . . . Wasserman D. A newly identified group of adolescents at 'invisible' risk for psychopathology and suicidal behavior: findings from the SEYLE study. World Psychiatry. 2014 Feb;**13**(1):78–86.

15 Fawcett J, Scheftner W, Fogg L, et al. Time-related predictors of suicide in major affective disorder. Am J Psychiatry. 1990;**147**:1189–1194.

16 Leadholm AK, Rothschild AJ, Nielsen J, Bech P, Ostergaard SD. Risk factors for suicide among 34,671 patients with psychotic and non-psychotic severe depression. J Affect Disord. 2014;**156**:119–125.

17 Novick DM, Swartz HA, Frank E. Suicide attempts in bipolar I and bipolar II disorder: a review and meta-analysis of the evidence. Bipolar Disord. 2010;**12**(1):1–9.

18 Tidemalm D, Haglund A, Karanti A, Landén M, Runeson B. Attempted suicide in bipolar disorder: risk factors in a cohort of 6086 patients. PloS one. 2014;**9**(4):e94097.

19 Partonen T, Haukka J, Nevanlinna H, Lönnqvist J. Analysis of the seasonal pattern in suicide. J Affect Disord. 2004;**81**(2):133–139.

20 Arsenault-Lapierre G, Kim C, Turecki G. Psychiatric diagnoses in 3275 suicides: a meta-analysis. BMC Psychiatry. 2004;**4**:37.

21 Isacsson G, Holmgren P, Wasserman D, Bergman U. Use of antidepressants among people committing suicide in Sweden. BMJ. 1994;**308**:506–509.

22 Hjorthoj CR, Madsen T, Agerbo E, Nordentoft M. Risk of suicide according to level of psychiatric treatment: a nationwide nested case-control study. Soc Psychiatry Psychiatr Epidemiol. 2014; Sep;**49**(9):1357–1365.

23 Nordentoft M, Wahlbeck K, Hallgren J, Westman J, Osby U, Alinaghizadeh H, et al. Excess mortality, causes of death and life expectancy in 270,770 patients with recent onset of mental disorders in Denmark, Finland and Sweden. PLoS One. 2013;**8**(1):e55176.

24 Li Z, Page A, Martin G, Taylor R. Attributable risk of psychiatric and socio-economic factors for suicide from individual-level, population-based studies: a systematic review. Soc Sci Med. 2011;**72**(4):608–616.

25 Wasserman D, Rihmer Z, Rujescu D, Sarchiapone M, Sokolowski M, . . . Carli V. The European Psychiatric Association (EPA) guidance on suicide treatment and prevention. Eur Psychiatry. 2012; **27**(2):129–141.

Chapter 7

Alcohol, other psychoactive substance use disorders, and suicide

Danuta Wasserman

Introduction

The term 'alcohol and other psychoactive substance use disorders (AUDs and SUDs, respectively)' covers problematic use of those substances leading to clinically significant impairment and distress.

Alcohol has been, and is used, on all continents: in both Europe, the Americas, Japan, and Australia and in smaller quantities in the Middle East, Africa, and China.[1] Adults in the West consume alcohol during casual social situations. Some drink to reduce stress or to relieve their inhibitions and anxiety during social occasions because it helps to embolden them. However, excessive alcohol consumption has devastating consequences in the long term.

Since the role of alcohol varies from one setting and culture to another, the level defined as 'high' and deemed to pose risks of developing somatic or psychiatric complications differs from one country to the next and between men and women.

SUDs constitute a considerable global burden of disease and are a prominent risk factor for suicide.[2]

Alcohol use disorders

Figures for alcohol use disorders vary between countries and between social and ethnic groups. According to the National Epidemiologic Survey on Alcohol and Related Conditions in the US, the estimated 12-month and lifetime prevalence of alcohol use disorders (AUDs) was 13.9% and 29.1%, respectively.[3] Prevalence rates differed between regions and were highest among Native Americans.

AUDs are characterized by periods of remission and relapse, with the first episode of alcohol intoxication often occurring in mid-teens and the onset of alcohol use between the ages of 18–25 years. Estimated 12-month and lifetime prevalence of severe AUD among younger people was 26.7% and 37.0%, respectively.[3] AUD has shown to be significantly associated with a broad spectrum of mental health issues, including other substance use disorders, major depressive and bipolar I disorders, antisocial and borderline personality disorders.[4]

Substance use disorders

Based on results from the National Epidemiologic Survey in the US, 12-month and lifetime prevalence of any substance use disorder was 3.8% and 9.9%, respectively.[5] These numbers, however, can be under-estimated. Reliable data on the rates of SUDs from different countries are lacking. SUDs are higher in males and lower in females.[6] Drug users often use a mixture of alcohol and prescription drugs.

Suicide risk

AUDs constitute a considerable global burden of disease. In a meta-analysis assessing mortality rates among individuals with AUD, results showed that people with AUD have a three-fold higher mortality in males and four-fold higher mortality in females compared to the general popu-lation.[7] Moreover, a study performed in the Nordic countries showed that life expectancy was 24–28 years shorter among individuals with AUD compared to the general population.[8] Research shows that AUD is strong-ly associated with suicidal behaviours.[9] A systematic review on AUD and suicidality showed that individuals with AUD had a significantly higher risk of suicidal ideation, suicide attempt, and completed suicide.[10]

Excessive alcohol use promotes adverse life events and induces depres-sion. Acute alcohol and drug use precipitates suicidal behaviours by increasing the impairment of problem-solving skills.[11]

Retrospective studies have shown that AUDs occur in 15–50% of peo-ple who committed suicide depending on the population surveyed and also on sex and age. Alcohol problems are more often observed in young people and middle-aged men who commit suicide than in other groups.

Excessive alcohol use in connection with suicide among women and the elderly is often under-reported, probably owing to shame.[12]

For many people, suicide risk does not necessarily occur as a result of severe dependence. For many, occasions of high consumption or drunkenness can also entail risks of accidents, violence, and suicide when their ability to curb impulses to act, as well as their capacity for constructive thought, is impaired.[13]

The alcohol causes a deterioration in cognitive capacity and, accordingly, in flexibility and the ability to find alternative solutions. Some suicidal excessive alcohol users can possess a fairly good psychosocial coping ability.[14] Their suicides take place when they are in a drunken state and numerous problems have accumulated. Relatively good psychosocial functioning may perhaps explain why alcoholics who eventually take their own lives receive so little psychiatric treatment.

People with a tendency towards anxiety and depression are at high risk of suicide when the effect of alcohol wears off, since these symptoms are exacerbated in conjunction with a hangover. Thus, not only chronic, but also acute alcohol use and heavy episodic drinking should be carefully assessed when evaluating risk of suicidal behaviours.[15,16] Acute alcohol intoxication has been shown to be associated with violent methods of suicide in young and middle-aged adults.[17]

Suicidal process

Suicidal persons with SUDs diagnoses often use direct verbal suicidal communication both immediately before the suicidal act, and long before it. They may, when either intoxicated or sober, accuse members of their immediate family of causing their difficulties and, by implication, their suicidal crises. These accusations are not infrequently expressed during quarrels and in tumultuous circumstances. The purpose of this type of communication may, paradoxically enough, be to satisfy their needs for attention and for support from their nearest family members. The suicidal process is often chronic in substance users, and lasting many years.

Unfortunately, suicidal substance users experience many negative reactions to their suicidal communication from both relatives and health-care staff, who may respond with marked ambivalence and aggressiveness, thereby accelerating the development of the suicidal process towards suicide.

Losing a vitally important relationship in combination with other negative life events are often the immediate factors that precipitate suicide. A suicidal substance user then loses not only love, but also part of his or her already weak self-esteem, since the person who has been lost has often performed the function not only of providing support but also of bolstering suicidal person's self-esteem. The more dependence that suicidal persons experience in their relationships, the greater the risk that separation may push them into chaos, regression, and self-destructive acts.

Hypersensitivity to separation is rooted in the previous life experiences. Suicidal persons have often lacked support in the parental home and had no one to talk to. Early separations due to death, divorce in the family of origin, or a move away from home, as well as social deprivation and parents' excessive alcohol use and, quite frequently, mental illness, contribute to the lack of good identification objects. This impedes development of strong self-esteem and adequate coping strategies. Troubled relationships later in adult life, with the threat of impending separation, are often a repetition of previous patterns and activate earlier feelings of helplessness, hopelessness, and rage. It may then be only a short step to a point at which suicidal behaviour presents itself as the only way out.

Suicidal substance users are also highly sensitive, easily offended, and inclined to interpret everything in negative terms. It is not unusual for them to provoke negative reactions from others, consciously or unconsciously, by their manner and behaviour, and this in turn may result in them feeling rejected, unwanted, and excluded. A vicious circle, with a sense of hopelessness and risk of suicidal behaviour, may easily arise.

When life feels pointless and cheerless, suicidal thoughts and a longing for death may arise even in people who are normally far from suicidality. For most people, however, the step from a suicidal thought to a suicidal act is a long one. In substance users, when their judgement is blunted and impulses are freed from inhibition, the step from thought to act is short. This is why, to a far greater extent than in other people, losses, separations, and various types of offence may be the factors precipitating suicide in substance users.

Comorbidity

Estimating the importance of alcohol or other psychoactive substance use as a single factor in suicide is difficult, since substance users very often have comorbidity of depression, Bipolar Disorders, anxiety disorders, and personality disorders, especially of the borderline type.[18]

Depression is common in alcoholics of both sexes. In women, the onset of major depressive disorder precedes AUD in two-thirds of cases. In men, on the other hand, AUD precedes depression in almost 80% of cases.

Many alcoholics who die from suicide suffer from deep depressions that are quite frequently protracted, with a mean length of one year; unfortunately, they show atypical symptoms, which make detection difficult. Another factor that sometimes impedes diagnosis of depression in suicidal excessive alcohol users is that their personality disorders mask their depression symptoms.

Teenage alcoholics who die from suicide are often characterized by severe and protracted psychiatric morbidity, psychosocial dysfunction, and antisocial behaviour. The same often applies to their families. In some countries such as the Nordic countries, in contrast to others such as the US, the prevalence of AUD and SUD among adolescent female suicides is as high as it is among adolescent males. Young heavy drinkers typically drink during the weekends, and this pattern is reflected in the fact that their suicides are clustered around weekends.[14]

Diagnosis and treatment

Practical guidelines for the assessment and treatment of patients with SUDs have been published by the American Psychiatric Association (APA)[19] and by the National Institute for Health and Care Excellence (NICE),[20] and reported several forms of beneficial therapy including both somatic and psychological treatments.

The duration of treatment may vary, but to bring about changes in moderate alcohol use disorders it should not be less than six months.

Treatment commonly lasts up to two years. It is important to maintain patient contact even if benefits are attained initially. When there is a risk of suicidal behaviour, detoxification should take place on an inpatient basis and for a sufficiently long period.

Suicidal male alcoholics often consult general practitioners or emergency somatic departments for physical ailments. It is sometimes difficult for general practitioners to detect problematic alcohol and substance use if the patient is reticent. Structured forms, such as the CAGE questionnaire,[21] may then be helpful. 'CAGE' stands for cut down, annoyance, guilty feelings, eye opener. The CAGE acronym refers to the four questions: Have you ever felt you should *cut down* on your drinking? Have people *annoyed* you by criticizing your drinking? Have you ever felt bad or *guilty* about your drinking? And have you ever had a drink first thing in the morning to steady your nerves or to get rid of a hangover (*eye opener*)? This questionnaire, which is not intimidating to the respondent, can be used as a possible rapid screening technique. Two or three positive answers are accepted as the criterion.

In dealing with suicidal alcohol users, a timeline follow-back technique, involving a systematic review of the past three months' alcohol and drug consumption in terms of both pattern and quantity, is a helpful tool. Abuse and dependence is often unrecognized in female users (even though many of them are psychiatric patients), owing to women's unwillingness to admit their alcohol habits and doctors' lack of alertness.

Treatment must take into consideration the type and degree of substance use, the somatic status, psychiatric comorbidity, the level of social functioning, and problems in the spheres of life that are affected by those conditions. Measures may range from simple provision of advice or intervention to inpatient care, especially if there is an acute suicide risk.[22]

Medication

Before an alcoholic is diagnosed as suffering from depression, the detoxification process should be completed. In the first few days of 'detox', some 60% of alcoholics show several depressive symptoms. After two weeks, only one patient in five shows signs of depression.

Alcohol users should, therefore, be sober for at least two weeks before their need for antidepressant treatment can be assessed.[23] On the other hand, for persons who have previously been diagnosed as depressed and who are at risk of suicide, antidepressant medication can be commenced earlier.

When alcohol users are treated with antidepressants, not only is their depression relieved but also their craving for alcohol diminishes. There are also studies that show that antidepressants can both remedy depression and prevent a relapse into misuse for drug addicts as well. However, pharmacological treatment must always be combined with psychosocial support and family interventions.

Psychosocial support and psychotherapy

In choosing psychological treatment, personality factors must be taken into account. The treatment objectives should be defined in operational terms, preferably in writing, and followed up regularly. Many suicidal alcohol and drug users have proved to be cognitively more concrete than abstract.

It therefore seems important to link the patient's mental phenomena with highly concrete objectives on a rising scale of difficulty. Relatives should be involved in the treatment process, in view of the frequently present negative emotional climate in families of suicidal substance users. Psychological treatment includes cognitive behavioural therapies, behavioural therapies, motivational enhancement therapies, group and family therapies, community reinforcement, and self-help groups. For adolescents, family therapy is recommended, along with psychotherapy and psycho-educative techniques which have proven to be successful.

When treating patients with different kinds of comorbidities, the underlying psychiatric disorder must always be treated along with the SUD.

In patients with AUD and other comorbidities like psychosis, the risk for suicidality is multiplied and, therefore, both psychosis and AUD should be treated.[24]

Alcohol and drug users often swing between overrating and disparaging themselves and other people—health-care staff included, and they have a tendency to take offence and easily feel hurt and rejected, which can result in a negative attitude to treatment and poor compliance.

Access to alcohol

The easy availability of alcohol and cultural habits that encourage its consumption has a negative bearing on the rate of mortality from suicide. Decreasing accessibility of alcohol, not only on a societal level, but also on an individual level as well as the moulding of social attitudes towards alcohol intake, significantly diminishes the risk of committing suicide (see also Chapter 33).

What should be done?

Pay attention to heavy drinkers in risk situation

When a person suddenly incurs problems in interpersonal relationships, at work or in other contexts, and starts drinking at weekends, others should take notice. The same applies to young people who show a pattern of heavy weekend drinking and come from high-risk families and to alcohol and drug users in workplaces.

Improve diagnostics, treatment, and organization of care

Detection of AUD among female psychiatric patients should be improved, and more attention should also be devoted to psychiatric problems among men who abuse alcohol or drugs and whose psychosocial functioning is fairly good. Only a minority of alcohol and substance users who commit suicide receive adequate psychiatric help in the last month of their lives, despite their obvious psychiatric morbidity.

Although the above facts remain true, both men and women are often in touch with health-care services and communicate their suicidal intent to the staff before committing suicide. The blame may, perhaps, be laid on organizational factors: in many countries, cooperation between AUD and SUD units, general practitioners, and psychiatric departments is very poor; and the same applies to cooperation with social welfare authorities who are responsible for rehabilitation.[25] Setting up special health-care establishments with expertise in treating dual-diagnosis patients may be one solution.

Case Study

Drug initiation
Ann-Marie, age 30

Small and slender, Ann-Marie tended to arouse intense caring feelings in others much of the time but periodically she was provocative, dismissive, and uncommunicative. Her mother had died of cervical cancer when Ann-Marie was 12. Her brother had started abusing drugs, and two years after their mother's death he took his own life by shooting himself. It was Ann-Marie who found his body, and relating the experience still made her quiver with emotion. Her father, 20 years older than her mother and a fisherman by trade, became deeply depressed after his wife's death and his son's suicide, and he isolated himself completely. He was unable to take care of his daughter and took no interest in her schooling, social life, or future.

Ann-Marie had evidently undergone repeated periods of depression with a clearly seasonal pattern since her early teens. During these periods, she had experienced intense suicidal ideation and a pressing feeling that there was nothing to live for. Because of increasing loss of interest in her studies, she had failed to complete her compulsory nine years of schooling. The school psychologist, whom she had met more or less regularly, never diagnosed her depression.

At the age of 16, she had been employed as a nanny, but was dismissed as soon as the family found out that her boyfriend was a well-known drug addict. He introduced Ann-Marie to drugs and alcohol. She was then in contact with the social welfare office, which first arranged hostel accommodation for her and eventually found her temporary employment as an assistant in various shops. She never enjoyed these jobs, and was increasingly drawn into her boyfriend's circle of associates and his drug-taking habits. Every time conflicts arose with the boyfriend or his associates, pitch-black, uncontrollable feelings of hopelessness and suicidal thoughts swept over her.

Between the ages of 18 and 20, Ann-Marie had been admitted several times to various services for drug use treatment, but she had always checked out after a brief stay and returned to the gang. Her life was constantly in chaos, with numerous people—from the psychiatric clinic, the social services, and the police—involved. Ann-Marie was unable to recall the names of various people who bore some kind of responsibility for her and it was obvious that she had not formed any strong ties with any of these carers, or vice versa. They all saw her as a hopeless case.

At the age of 20, she made four suicide attempts in six months. These suicide attempts were triggered by police interrogations that arose because of the involvement of Ann-Marie and her boyfriend Olle in drug trafficking and a burglary that he had roped her into while on parole from prison. A triangular drama that she was unable to resolve (involving herself, Olle, and a temporary boyfriend she lived with during Olle's imprisonment) was another factor that contributed to her suicide attempts.

After the fourth attempt, when she had taken a large number of sleeping pills and was deeply unconscious for several days, she was treated at an intensive care unit. There she came into contact with a female psychiatric nurse, who identified with Ann-Marie's problems and succeeded in motivating her to undergo a long-term cure at a treatment centre for drug users.

After several years of rehabilitation, Ann-Marie continued to have regular sessions with a psychotherapist. Ten years after the treatment, at the age of 30, Ann-Marie was still seeing the therapist a few times a year. She had a job she enjoyed, as an assistant nurse at an old people's home. In her spare time she was committed to her voluntary work, helping to rehabilitate former teenage prostitutes. She was not married but had a steady relationship with a plumber of the same age as herself.

References

1 Degenhardt L, Chiu WT, Sampson N, Kessler RC, Anthony JC, Angermeyer M, et al. Toward a global view of alcohol, tobacco, cannabis, and cocaine use: findings from the WHO World Mental Health Surveys. PLoS Med. 2008;5(7):e141.

2 Ferrari AJ, Norman RE, Freedman G, Baxter AJ, Pirkis JE, Harris MG, et al. The burden attributable to mental and substance use disorders as risk factors for suicide: findings from the Global Burden of Disease Study 2010. PLoS One. 2014;9(4):e91936.

3 Grant BF, Goldstein RB, Saha TD, et al. Epidemiology of DSM-5 Alcohol Use Disorder: results from the National Epidemiologic Survey on Alcohol and Related Conditions III. JAMA Psychiatry. 2015;doi: 10.1001.

4 Ogloff JR, Talevski D, Lemphers A, Wood M, Simmons M. Co-occurring mental illness, substance use disorders, and antisocial personality disorder among clients of forensic mental health services. Psychiatr Rehabil J. 2015;38(1):16.

5 Goldstein RB, Chou SP, Smith SM, et al. Nosologic Comparisons of DSM-IV and DSM-5 Alcohol and Drug Use Disorders: results from the National Epidemiologic Survey on Alcohol and Related Conditions-III. J Stud Alcohol Drugs. May 2015;76(3):378–388.

6 Lev-Ran S, Le Strat Y, Imtiaz S, Rehm J, Le Foll B. Gender differences in prevalence of substance use disorders among individuals with lifetime exposure to substances: results from a large representative sample. Am J Addict. Jan 2013;22(1):7–13.

7 Roerecke M, Rehm J. Alcohol use disorders and mortality: a systematic review and meta-analysis. Addiction. Sep 2013;108(9):1562–1578.

8 Westman J, Wahlbeck K, Laursen T, et al. Mortality and life expectancy of people with alcohol use disorder in Denmark, Finland and Sweden. Acta Psychiatr Scand. 2015;131(4):297–306.

9 Sung Y-k, La Flair LN, Mojtabai R, Lee L-C, Spivak S, Crum RM. The association of alcohol use disorders with suicidal ideation and suicide attempts in a

population-based sample with mood symptoms. Archives of Suicide Research. 2015([Epub ahead of print]).

10 Darvishi N, Farhadi M, Haghtalab T, Poorolajal J. Alcohol-related risk of suicidal ideation, suicide attempt, and completed suicide: a meta-analysis. PLoS One. 2015;**10**(5):e0126870.

11 Brady J. The association between alcohol misuse and suicidal behaviour. Alcohol Alcohol. 2006;**41**(5):473–478.

12 Murphy GE. Why women are less likely than men to commit suicide. Compr. Psychiatry. 1998;**39**:165–175.

13 Taylor C, Cooper J, Appleby L. Is suicide risk taken seriously in heavy drinkers who harm themselves? Acta Psychiatr Scand. 1999;**100**:309–311.

14 Pirkola SP, Isometsä ET, Heikkinen ME, Lönnqvist JK. Suicides of alcohol misusers and non-misusers in a nationwide population. Alcohol Alcohol. 2000 Jan;**35**(1):70–75.

15 Bagge CL, Lee HJ, Schumacher JA, Gratz KL, Krull JL, Holloman G, Jr. Alcohol as an acute risk factor for recent suicide attempts: a case-crossover analysis. J Stud Alcohol Drugs. 2013;**74**(4):552–558.

16 Rossow I, Norstrom T. Heavy episodic drinking and deliberate self-harm in young people: a longitudinal cohort study. Addiction. 2014;**109**(6):930–936.

17 Kaplan MS, McFarland BH, Huguet N, Conner K, Caetano R, Giesbrecht N, et al. Acute alcohol intoxication and suicide: a gender-stratified analysis of the National Violent Death Reporting System. Inj Prev. 2013;**19**(1):38–43.

18 Arsenault-Lapierre G, Kim C, Turecki G. Psychiatric diagnoses in 3275 suicides: a meta-analysis. BMC Psychiatry. 2004;4:37.

19 American Psychiatric Association. Steering Committee on Practice Guidelines. Treatment of patients with substance use disorders, 2nd edn. 2010. American Psychiatric Association. <http://psychiatryonline.org/data/Books/prac/SUD2ePG_04–28–06.pdf>.

20 National Institute for Health and Care Excellence (NICE). Alcohol-use disorders: diagnosis and clinical management of alcohol-related physical complications. June 2010. NICE Clinical Guideline 100. <http://www.guidance.nice.org.uk/cg100>.

21 Mayfield D, McLeod G, Hall P. The CAGE questionnaire: validation of a new alcoholism-screening instrument. Am J Psychiatry. 1974;**131**:1121–1123.

22 Schukit MA. Alcohol-use disorders. The Lancet. 2009 7 Feb;**373**(9662):492–501.

23 Schuckit MA. Drug and alcohol abuse: a clinical guide to diagnosis and treatment, 4th edn. New York, NY: Plenum Publishing; 1995.

24 Batki SL, Meszaros ZS, Strutynski K, Dimmock JA, Leontieva L, Ploutz-Snyder R, et al. Medical comorbidity in patients with schizophrenia and alcohol dependence. Schizophr Res. 2009 Feb;**107**(2–3):139–146.

25 Nordentoft M, Melau M, Iversen T, Petersen L, Jeppesen P, Thorup A, et al. From research to practice: how OPUS treatment was accepted and implemented throughout Denmark. Early Interv Psychiatry. 2013,Apr;**9**(2):156–162.

Chapter 8

Anxiety and suicide

Jan Fawcett

Anxiety symptoms

Anxiety is a complex phenomenon that may include a range of experiences. Patients may experience feelings of fear, anticipation of something terrible happening, impending doom, and worry. These symptoms are called psychic anxiety. Other patients may experience primarily somatic anxiety, symptoms including tightness in the chest, feelings of shortness of breath, nausea, and muscle twitches, to name a few. While it is not uncommon to experience both psychic and somatic anxiety symptoms together, different patients may experience a preponderance of psychic or somatic anxiety symptoms. When inquiring about these symptoms, it is important to use also terms such as fear and worry, in addition to anxiety in order for patients with different backgrounds to recognize the symptoms.

It is common practice to simply accept the patient's statement that they are bothered by anxiety, rather than inquiring about how they experience the symptoms: how *severe* they feel the anxiety is (how much of the day they feel anxious), and when and under what circumstances the anxiety first started. Often the *severity* of anxiety is not assessed, and it is only recorded that the patient complained of anxiety. The patient may experience *severe* anxiety as *intolerable psychic pain*, and because of their depressed state, see the only relief as coming from death.

The DSM classification uses the number of symptoms present, as a proxy for anxiety, and this may lead a clinician to note only the patient's specific symptoms, but ignore severity and changes in severity over time.[1]

A strong reason for assessing the patients' *severity* of anxiety is that complaints of anxiety are common, but the *severity* of the patients' anxiety, not just the presence of anxiety, which is common in mood disorders, is predictive of both poor treatment outcome and suicide risk.

Depression and anxiety

It is an interesting fact that though anxiety is not a criterion symptom for major depression, it is very frequent in its occurrence. Anxiety symptoms lasting three months may meet the criterion for a diagnosis of generalized anxiety disorder (GAD), but since the anxious symptoms frequently occur with the onset of depression, depending on when in the course of depression the patient is clinically assessed, *severe* anxiety may exist that does not meet the criteria for a separate diagnosis.

A study of anxiety associated with 200 patients with major depressive disorder using the SADS-C (Schedule for Affective Disorder and Schizophrenia—measuring Change) rating scale found that 62% of the patients were rated as having anxiety of moderate severity, while 29% were found to have *severe* anxiety symptoms.[2]

Clayton et al.[3] using the sum of six different anxiety sub-scales, like psychic anxiety, somatic anxiety, worry, agitation, etc. studied 327 patients with a primary major depression diagnosis (meaning that no other diagnosis, including GAD, has been made previously). The frequency of anxiety symptoms were plotted against the summed severity of anxiety symptoms from the sub-scales. The outcome showed a very high frequency of anxiety symptoms across the 327 patients, but only 5% of the group had the most *severe* anxiety symptoms, determined in this study by a sum of all six of the SADS-C anxiety scales, including psychic anxiety. This study made the important point that comorbid anxiety is very common in patients with major depressive disorder, but the presence of *severe* comorbid anxiety was relatively rare.

Anxiety is a common comorbid symptom in major depression and one would not expect that it would discriminate between clinical outcomes. Studies have shown, however, that the presence of *severe* anxiety, comorbid with major depression, predicts poor treatment outcomes[4,5] and also a risk for suicide in days, weeks, or the next few months, termed as an acute suicide risk factor.

What is the evidence that severe anxiety is an acute risk factor for suicide?

In 1990, Fawcett et al. published the results from a prospective study of suicide in 954 patients with major affective disorders (major depression, bipolar I and II, as well as schizoaffective disorder, with more than 80% patients hospitalized at the time of assessment) followed for ten years in the NIMH Collaborative Study of Depression.[6] Initial analysis of clinical factors did not separate the 34 suicides from the 920 patients who survived. When the data were analysed statistically, looking at short-term suicides (N = 13), defined as those committing suicide within one year compared with all the 920 patients who survived, and those who died of suicide over years 2–10 of follow-up (N = 21), some interesting findings emerged. One year had to be designated as a short-term follow-up for meaningful analysis because too few suicides, namely 6 has occurred at six months.

As found in other studies, the majority of suicides occurred in the first year after discharge from hospital. Five clinical features listed below were found to be significantly more severe among the short-term suicides compared with the majority sample who survived at one year. *Severity* of psychic anxiety, moderate alcohol abuse, global (*severe*) insomnia (unable to sleep most of the night), diminished concentration, and *severity* of anhedonia, all assessed at baseline, differentiated the suicides within one year from the non-suicides. It was also found that the occurrence of panic attacks and episodes of agitation were significantly more frequent.

In the comparison with suicides occurring over the 'long-term' (2–10 years follow-up), the standard risk factors of severity of hopelessness and severity of suicidal ideation reached significance and a history of recent or past suicide attempt was nearly significant (p = 0.086). This finding led to the first use of acute suicide risk factors vs long-term risk factors. It should also be noted that the acute risk factors are all modifiable with treatment, while only a single long-term risk factor (hopelessness) is treatment-modifiable.

These risk factors were not systematically measured in the prospective study of Pokorny,[7] and the retrospective meta-analysis of Large et al.[8], both of which concluded that no useful short-term risk factors for suicide exist.

Since this study, no further prospective studies of suicide have been published, but several studies with other designs were reported, which support the severity of psychic anxiety and other risk factors as an acute risk factor for suicide.

In 1999, Hall R et al.[9] published a series of 100 suicide attempts seen in an emergency room that were sufficiently severe to require medical or psychiatric hospitalization. These subjects were interviewed with the SADS-C[10] scales. 90% of these patients endorsed *severe* psychic anxiety during the month before their suicide attempt. 70% of patients had 'contracted for safety' with their therapists before their suicide attempts.

In 2003, Busch K et al.[11] published a study of 76 inpatient suicides, with the finding that 79% of these patients had shown charted evidence of *severe* psychic anxiety scored by two of the authors in the week prior to suicide. Interestingly, 78% of these patients had a nursing note recording that denied suicidal ideation or intent as their last communication before their suicides. 28% of these patients had a record of a verbal or written no-suicide contract recorded in their chart.

In 2008, Stordal E et al.[12] published a study from Norway called 'HUNT' (the Health Study of Nord-Trøndelag). This study collected ratings every month (except July) for three consecutive years from 60,995 people. All suicides in 1969–1996, comprising 10,670 males and 3,833 females, were included. One of the rating scales used was the Hospital Anxiety and Depression Scale (HADS), which rated both anxiety and depressive *severity*. This study found that the suicide subjects (males and females combined) rated themselves highest on anxiety in the month of their suicide ($r = 0.72$). It was found that while the anxiety ratings remained high, the depression ratings fluctuated, with highs in June and September.

In 2009, a study by Pfeiffer et al.[13] following 887,859 veterans treated for depression found that the suicides had a significantly increased odds ratio for anxiety disorder NOS, generalized anxiety disorder, and panic disorder. Of particular interest was the finding that patients receiving benzodiazepine or buspirone for anti-anxiety treatment had a significantly elevated odds ratio of suicide (OR = 1.7) and a sub-group treated with high-dosage anxiolytics had a further increased odds ratio of suicide (OR = 2.3), suggesting that *severe* anxiety is related to suicide.

A follow-up study of 96 suicides occurring in 4,441 hospitalized severely ill psychiatric patients found that suicide is likely to occur in a milieu of 'agitation, mixed anxiety and depression, and psychosis'. This description conveys the high likelihood of *severe* anxiety associated with these reported suicides.[14]

An epidemiologic study of suicide attempts by Nock et al.[15] of 109,000 subjects from 21 countries, both developed and developing, demonstrated that suicidal ideation alone did not predict suicide attempts. However, suicidal ideation in disorders characterized by anxiety and impulsivity was predictive of suicide attempts in both developed and developing countries. It has also been shown that anxiety increases impulsivity.

The assessment of anxiety severity

The literature presented above supports the observation that not only the presence of anxiety, but the presence of *severe* anxiety symptoms is an acute risk factor for suicide. Without an assessment of severity, the frequent presence of comorbid anxiety does not reveal anything of clinical importance. The addition of the anxiety specifier, that purports to measure severity of comorbid anxiety were included in DSM-5[1] for the same reason as Goldberg and Fawcett showed previously.[16] The anxiety scale in DSM-5 presents several symptoms of anxiety, which is consistent with the assumption associated with the DSM that number of symptoms is a proxy for severity.

As a clinician who regularly assesses the severity of anxiety symptoms as a routine part of a clinical examination and suicide assessment, I am aware that children and adolescents are often better clinically assessed with the help of scales for this purpose. The Social Anxiety Scale for Children (SAS-C)17,[18] which was used in several of the above studies demonstrating a correlation of anxiety with acute risk of suicidal behaviour, is helpful, for both its simplicity and its demonstrated effectiveness.

The SADS-C[10] psychic anxiety scale is but one of many subscales included in the SADS rating instrument. It lists seven levels of anxiety, two of which are: 0—no information; and 1—not at all. The rest are: 2—slight, conveys the patient occasionally feels somewhat anxious; 3—mild, often feels somewhat anxious; 4—moderate, feels anxious most of the time; 5—severe, feels very anxious most of the time; and 6—extreme, pervasive feelings of extreme anxiety.

The score of 5 (*severe*) and above predicts the most negative outcomes in relation to suicidality.

Clinicians know that different patients communicate different levels of distress and questions must be asked to qualify the most accurate level of severity. For instance, if it is not uncommon for patients to communicate the presence of 'severe anxiety all the time', a clinician might have a dialogue with the patient, as follows:

CLINICIAN: 'What do you enjoy in life?'

PATIENT: 'Nothing.'

CLINICIAN: 'Do you listen to music?'

PATIENT: 'Yes.'

CLINICIAN: 'Enjoy it?'

PATIENT: 'Yes, sometimes.'

CLINICIAN: 'Can it distract you from the anxiety?'

PATIENT: 'Sometimes.'

CLINICIAN: 'How about your puppy or grandson climbing on your lap?'

PATIENT: 'Yes.'

CLINICIAN: 'Are you able to distract yourself to pay your rent or other important actions?'

PATIENT: 'Yes.'

In this situation, the patient's anxiety can be rated as level '4' on severity, not a '5', because the patient can be distracted from the anxiety by a positive event or by the need to do something important immediately. This scaling of anxiety *severity* is quite easy to do in a short amount of time, while correcting for the patient's communication style.

Of course, there are many ways to assess the severity of anxiety, such as the generalized anxiety disorder (GAD-7)[19] scale, etc. The important thing is that the patient's complaint of anxiety is assessed for severity to make a clinical discrimination of importance in the assessment of suicide risk.

Responding to a finding of severe anxiety

It is not uncommon that a patient will be found to suffer from severe anxiety but deny suicidal thoughts or intent. We know that patients frequently deny suicidal intent prior to committing suicide. The patient has severe depression and severe comorbid anxiety, but denies suicidal intent. They will invariably refuse hospitalization—by today's law they are usually not committable if they deny suicidal intent—what then?

It could be, therefore, recorded in the clinician's clinical notes that the patient has a high acute suicide risk, but refuses hospitalization and is not committable. Treatment should be focused on keeping in touch, conveying hope, and trying to reverse the patient's severe anxiety with treatment. Everything should be done to manage a high-risk patient, by making sure they have social support and that they are not left alone. Frequent contact and consultations should be maintained between the patient and clinician during this time. These measures and actions on the part of the clinician can be successful in preventing a suicide or attempt.

The atypical antipsychotic medication quetiapine has been found useful in reducing severe agitation and anxiety as well as depression[20,21,22]. Based on the Pfeiffer study cited above[13], the use of quetiapine, if tolerated, may be a better option than the use of benzodiazepines for agitation and severe anxiety in severely depressed suicidal patients.

Conclusion

Evidence reviewed in this chapter shows that *severe* anxiety that was not assessed in earlier studies, may be a treatment-modifiable acute suicide risk factor, if it is clinically assessed, found to be present and aggressively treated.

The point has been made that the mere presence of comorbid anxiety may not discriminate patients at high acute suicide risk, but the presence of anxiety clinically assessed as *severe* may be both a useful acute or short-term risk factor, as well as a treatment target for reducing suicide and suicidal behaviour.

Case Study

A 47-year-old divorced Caucasian man with bipolar disorder, which, before treatment, had cost him his career as an executive as a result of lapses of insight and judgement, had been stabilized on lithium and fluoxetine when he experienced a recurrence of depression, which occurred when he was under stress in a relationship and at the same time struggling to get a job in a new field. He noted the sudden onset of severe anxiety and feelings of dread and failure; became hopeless and attempted suicide by sitting in a closed garage in a car with the engine running. He was hospitalized and switched to venlafaxine 300 mg per 24 hours and alprazolam 4 mg per 24 hours.

He had described waking up to excruciating anxiety every morning, which worsened when associated with hopelessness and fear of being unable ever to support himself and his children from his previous marriage. He noted the rapid onset of relief of his anxiety directly after the alprazolam doses in the morning, and over a few days his depression remitted. The patient has continued in remission on lithium 1500 mg, divalproex 1500 mg and venlafaxine 300 mg per 24 hours with the alprozolam tapered to an occasional 0.5 mg dose. He has successfully begun a new career.

References

1 **American Psychiatric Association**. Diagnostic and statistical manual of mental disorders. 5th edn. DSM-5. Available at <http://www.dsm5.org>.

2 **Fawcett J, Kravitz HM**. Anxiety syndromes and their relationship to depressive illness. J Clin Psychiatry. 1983;**44**(8 Pt 2):8–11.

3 **Clayton PJ, Grove WM, Coryell W, et al**. Follow-up and family study of anxious depression. Am J Psychiatry. 1991;**148**:1512–1517.

4 **Fava M, Rush AJ, Wisniewski SR, Nierenberg AA, Alpert JE, McGrath PJ, et al**. A comparison of mirtazapine and nortriptyline following two consecutive failed medication treatments for depressed outpatients: a STAR*D report. Am J Psychiatry. 2006;**163**:1161–1172.

5 **Coryell W, Fiedorowicz JG, Solomon D, Leon AC, Rice JP, Keller MB**. Effects of anxiety on the long-term course of depressive disorders. Br J Psychiatry. 2012 Mar;**200**(3):210–215.

6 **Fawcett J, Scheftner WA, Fogg L, Clark DC, Young MA, Hedeker D, et al**. Time-related predictors of suicide in major affective disorder. Am J Psychiatry. 1990; **147**:1189–1194.

7 **Pokorny AD**. Prediction of suicide in psychiatric patients. Report of a prospective study. Arch Gen Psychiatry. 1983 Mar;**40**(3):249–257.

8 **Large M, Ryan C, Nielssen O**. The validity and utility of risk assessment for inpatient suicide. Australasian Psychiatry. 2011;**19**(6):507–512.

9 **Hall RC, Platt DE, Hall RC**. Suicide risk assessment: a review of risk factors for suicide in 100 patients who made severe suicide attempts. Evaluation of suicide risk in a time of managed care. Psychosomatics. 1999 Jan–Feb;**40**(1):18–27.

10 **Spitzer RL, Endicott J**. Schedule of affective disorders and schizophrenia—change version. New York, NY: Biometrics Research; 1978.

11 **Busch K, Fawcett J, Jacobs D**. Clinical correlates of inpatient suicide. J Clin Psychiatry. 2003;**64**:14–19.

12 Stordal E, Morken G, Mykletun A, Neckelmann D, Dahl AA. Monthly variation in prevalence rates of comorbid depression and anxiety in the general population at 63–65° North: the HUNT study. J Affect Disord. 2008;**106**(3):273–278.

13 Pfeiffer PN, Ganoczy D, Ilgen M, Zivin K, Valenstein M. Comorbid anxiety as a suicide risk factor among depressed veterans. Depress Anxiety. 2009;**26**(8):752–757. doi:10.1002/da.20583.

14 Sani G, Tondo L, Koukopoulos A, Reginaldi D, Kotzalidis GD, Koukopoulos AE, et al. Suicide in a large population of former psychiatric inpatients. Psychiatry Clin Neurosci. 2011;**65**:286–295.

15 Nock MK, Hwang I, Sampson N, Kessler RC, Angermeyer M, Beautrais A, et al. Cross-national analysis of the associations among mental disorders and suicidal behavior: findings from the WHO World Mental Health Surveys. PLoS Medicine. 2009; **6**:e1000123.

16 Goldberg D, Fawcett J. The importance of anxiety in both major depression and bipolar disorder. Depress Anxiety. 2012 Jun;**29**(6):471–478.

17 La Greca AM, Dandes SK, Wick P, Shaw K, Stone WL. Development of the social anxiety scale for children: reliability and concurrent validity. J Clin Child Psychol. 1988;**17**:84–91.

18 Chapman E. Confirmatory factor analysis of the social anxiety scale for children. Australian Journal of Educational & Developmental Psychology. 2002;**2**:42–48.

19 Spitzer RL, Kroenke K, Williams JB, Löwe B. A brief measure for assessing generalized anxiety disorder: the GAD-7. Arch Intern Med. 2006;**166**(10):1092–1097.

20 Hershenberg R, Gros DF, Brawman-Mintzer D. Role of atypical antipsychotics in the treatment of generalized anxiety disorder. CNS Drugs. 2014 Jun;**28**(6):519–533.

21 Kreys TJ, Phan, SV. A literature review of quetiapine for generalized anxiety disorder. Pharmacotherapy. 2015 Feb;**35**(2):175–188.

22 Soeiro-DE-Sousa MG, Dias VV, Missio G. et al. Role of quetiapine beyond its clinical efficacy in bipolar disorder: from neuroprotection to the treatment of psychiatric disorders(Review). Exp Ther Med. 2015 Mar;**9**(3):643–652.

Chapter 9

Eating disorders and suicide

Danuta Wasserman

Anorexia nervosa

In a representative sample of US adolescents, 0.3% of teenagers suffered from anorexia nervosa (self-starvation), 0.9% from bulimia nervosa (compulsive overeating with compensatory behaviours to prevent weight gain), and 1.6% from binge-eating disorders.[1] Eating disorders have become more common in the past decades. Anorexia often starts in conjunction with puberty; many children and adolescents go on slimming diets, and it is common for young people nowadays to be dissatisfied with their bodies and concerned with what they may and may not eat.

In a Dutch cohort study, the lifetime prevalence of anorexia nervosa among girls was 1.7%, of bulimia nervosa 0.8%, and of binge-eating disorders 2.3%. Among boys, the lifetime prevalence anorexia nervosa was 0.1%, of bulimia nervosa 0.1%, and of binge-eating disorders 0.3%.[2]

We live in a culture that promotes anorexic behaviour through media and fashion.[3] Information intended to promote health by, for example, encouraging people to reduce their fat intake, cholesterol level, and weight, has a negative impact on some susceptible people who lack the capacity to critically process the media information. They lose control over their own bodies and become inextricably caught up in their compulsive behaviour. Their images and perceptions of their own bodies are markedly disturbed and, in extreme cases, psychotic.

Bulimia nervosa

Certain patients who are diagnosed as anorexic may alternate between anorexia and bulimic phases in which, without discernment and due to an inner compulsion, they consume all kinds of food and then promptly regurgitate it or misuse laxatives and diuretics to prevent weight gain. Bulimics, like anorexics, cannot interpret signals from their body correctly, have difficulty in resisting obsessive impulses to starve themselves or grossly overeat, and lose control over their own body.

Suicidality

Among people with eating disorders, the crude mortality rate range is 6–8%, with suicide as the most common cause of death. It is very common for young anorexics—girls and boys alike—to be depressed at the same time, and the risk of suicide is some ten times higher (in some studies up to 20 times higher) among anorexic girls than among girls in general. Ethnic subcultures do not appear to exert any protective effect against anorexic behaviour.[4] Suicide risk remains high for many years after the initial assessment of eating disorders. Very low weight at the time of the first assessment and frequent hospitalization are clear risk factors for suicide. Boys and girls with eating disorders run a markedly elevated risk of not only suicides but also of suicide attempts.[5–7]

Comorbidity

People with eating disorders often suffer from depression. Substance and alcohol abuse with or without depression are also common. This comorbidity increases the risk of suicide.[8] Girls and boys with eating disorders frequently have personality disorders. Anorexics with an obsessive–compulsive personality are introverted and often depressive. Aggressive retribution is a marked feature of their behaviour. This is the group in which the most severe cases of anorexia nervosa are encountered and in which the self-destructive acts take place. But anorexic patients with borderline and histrionic personalities may also run a risk of suicide despite their apparent openness and verbal skills. This is especially true when the patient is under the influence of alcohol or drugs, when impulse control is weakened.

Prevention and treatment

Beauty ideals that are conveyed in the media and often brought up by vacillating parents must be clarified by information and education at schools. It is natural to have some 'puppy fat' during puberty and for some years after puberty, owing to hormonal development. This natural process should not be counteracted by slimming. The parents should try to stop the slimming process or compulsive overeating in time before the severe compulsive behaviour develops.

In the treatment of suicidal people with eating disorders, the usual methods of behavioural therapy combined with medication are advisable. These techniques should also be combined with some form of insight therapy, depending on the patient's intellectual ability, in order to clarify the psychodynamic aspects on both the individual and relationship level.[9,10]

There are several conceivable psychological explanations for eating disorders. Starving oneself or overeating compulsively means making oneself the focus of attention and receiving care from others, while simultaneously rejecting this strongly. Eating disorders may be seen as a protest against relationships and as a means of controlling them, as well as an expression of a flight from reality and the erection of a barrier between oneself and the rest of the world.

At a symbolic level, not eating or vomiting what one has already swallowed may also mean exerting control of one's intake and thereby meeting and controlling cultural pressure that urges the ideal of abstinence and labels self-indulgence as indicative of inadequacy and laziness. Paradoxically, with this behaviour, which is so much a matter of control, sufferers lose control of their bodies and feelings, and eventually lose their lives.

Another explanation—one that is outside the scope of relationships but that applies to the individual—may be that the growing girl wishes to curb her emerging femininity or the boy his manliness, as a protest against growing up. These young people may perhaps believe that mastering their oral needs to eat may also enable them to curb their sexual urges.

Teaching adolescents to appreciate themselves, to be contented with the way that they look, and to be able to resist the ideals of slimness, which are out of proportion in our culture, may be a protracted process and poor self-image can predict subsequent suicide in individuals with eating disorders. In the prevention of eating disorders it is important to develop awareness about their potentially fatal outcomes.[11]

Case Study: not beautiful enough
Gunilla, age 28

Gunilla had first attempted suicide by slitting her wrists at the age of 17 after her father's suicide. During her childhood, her father had repeatedly attempted suicide. Her mother had alcohol problems. The patient's sister, now a well-adjusted family therapist, had also tried to take her own life after failing on her first attempt to matriculate from upper-secondary school.

Gunilla had lived with her paternal grandmother as a child, between the ages of 7 and 15. Her grandmother, who came from a farming family, had been anxious that Gunilla should eat properly and behave in an exemplary way. Gunilla had felt that her looks were all that mattered and that unless she was well dressed and her hair curled like a doll she was not loved. While living with her grandmother, she had fallen prey to minor eating disturbances. These increased in severity when she moved to live with her parents at 15. She became pregnant at 18 and had an abortion. During that time, she found all food distasteful. She began suffering from anorexia, and successively developed bulimia as well.

Gunilla had always perceived herself as a failure—at school, in sports, as a friend, and as a daughter. She had often changed schools because of her poor study results and she had never completed a course. Gunilla's elder siblings had all been to university. She felt that they had succeeded better in life than she had. Her relationship with her mother was the most fraught with conflict, and her relationships with her sisters were also troubled.

She had made her second suicide attempt at 19, with several tranquillizers and sedatives. In a farewell letter addressed to her sister and mother, she had written that it would be better if she did not exist and wished her family happiness. She was reluctant to undergo any treatment after her suicide attempt.

Ten months later, owing to cardiac arrhythmia after an intense and protracted period of bulimia, she was once more admitted to hospital. Tests showed that she had impaired kidney function and that her arrhythmia was caused by disturbances in electrolyte balance. These somatic problems gave Gunilla a shock, and she now agreed to undergo psychological treatment.

Because she was diagnosed as suffering from severe depression, antidepressants were prescribed and she also embarked on psychotherapy. She realized she had been depressed for as long as she could remember, and she had become faddish about food long before puberty. Gunilla had always suffered from anxiety and been afraid to get too close to people. After two years' treatment, her abnormal eating habits were somewhat normalized. She still alternately went on slimming diets and indulged in overeating from time to time, but not as seriously as before.

At 28, Gunilla married a man from Italy. She resumed her upper-secondary school studies at evening courses but had no specific plans for the future.

References

1 Swanson SA, Crow SJ, Le Grange D, Swendsen J, Merikangas KR. Prevalence and correlates of eating disorders in adolescents: results from the national comorbidity survey replication adolescent supplement. Arch Gen Psychiat. 2011;**68**(7):714–723.

2 Smink FR, Hoeken D, Oldehinkel AJ, Hoek HW. Prevalence and severity of DSM-5 eating disorders in a community cohort of adolescents. Int J Eat Disorder. 2014;**47**(6):610–619.

3 Unikel C, Von Holle A, Bulik CM, Ocampo R. Disordered eating and suicidal intent: the role of thin ideal internalisation, shame and family criticism. Eur Eat Disord Rev. 2012 Jan;**20**(1):39–48.

4 French SA, Story M, Neumark-Sztainer D, et al. Ethnic differences in psychosocial and health behavior correlates dieting, purging, and binge eating in population based sample of adolescent females. Int J Eating Disord. 1997;**22**:315–322.

5 Preti A, Rocchi MB, Sisti D, Camboni MV, Miotto P. A comprehensive meta-analysis of the risk of suicide in eating disorders. Acta Psychiatr Scand. 2011 Jul;**124**(1):6–17.

6 Arcelus J, Mitchell AJ, Wales J, Nielsen S. Mortality rates in patients with anorexia nervosa and other eating disorders. A meta-analysis of 36 studies. Arch Gen Psychiatry. 2011 Jul;**68**(7):724–731.

7 Suokas JT, Suvisaari JM, Gissler M, Löfman F, Linna M, Raevuori A, et al. Mortality in eating disorders: a follow-up study of adult eating disorder patients in tertiary care, 1995–2000. J Psych Res. 2013. **210**:1101–1106.

8 Chesney E, Goodwin GM, Fazel S. Risks of all-cause and suicide mortality in mental disorders: a meta-review. World Psychiatry. 2014 Jun;**13**(2):153–160.

9 Yager J, Devlin MJ, Halmi KA, Herzog DB, Mitchell JE, Powers P, et al. Guideline Watch (August 2012): Practice guideline for the treatment of patients with eating disorders, 3rd edn. American Psychiatric Association (APA); 2012.

10 National Institute for Health and Care Excellence (NICE). Eating disorders: core interventions in the treatment and management of anorexia nervosa, bulimia nervosa and related eating disorders. NICE; 2004. <http://www.nice.org.uk/cg9>.

11 Runfola CD, Thornton LM, Pisetsky EM, Bulik CM, Birgegård A. Self-image and suicide in a Swedish national eating disorders clinical register. J Comp Psych. 2014;**55**:439–449.

Chapter 10

Adjustment disorders and suicide

Danuta Wasserman

Adjustment disorders are associated with an increased risk for suicidal behaviour.[1-5] Apter et al.[2] showed that suicide may occur among young men 'in the absence of apparent psychopathology'. A Finnish study[3] found that young men with the diagnosis of adjustment disorder who committed suicide often communicated their suicidal thoughts to others, but that these thoughts were not taken seriously. These young men had a history of minor depressions of a short-lived nature, and no history of previous psychiatric treatment.

Suicide without recognizable psychopathology also occurs in elderly people who cannot cope with a major change in their life situation. A serious warning sign is an attempted suicide with a violent method in an elderly man or woman. If not appropriately managed, a suicide within a short time after such an attempt often occurs.

An adjustment disorder develops when an individual responds overwhelmingly to a stressor, due to the lack of effective coping strategies, to the point that her/his reaction results in symptoms that are clinically significant and affect the global functioning (see Chapter 2: Stress-vulnerability model of suicidal behaviours).

Common symptoms of adjustment disorder are despondency, a sense of hopelessness, the feeling that one is not functioning as usual, and being close to tears. Anxiety is also common. These symptoms develop within three months in response to the identifiable stressor and normally last no longer than six months. Symptoms usually cease when the person's life situation stabilizes and the stressor is eliminated. However, chronic states may occur, partly because the consequences of a trying life event or the trauma may persist. In a chronic traumatic situation, a new and stressful life event may be the last straw that precipitates the suicidal act.

Studies have shown that up to 25% of adolescents with adjustment disorder display suicidal behaviours,[4] while among adults with adjustment disorder, this figure is 60%.[5] Up to a third of adolescents who commit suicide have adjustment disorder and among suicide deaths in the developing world it appears to be a very common diagnosis.[6] These data show that far from being a mild condition, adjustment disorder is highly likely to lead to a suicidal act.

Both young and elderly persons who commit suicide and have a diagnosis of adjustment disorder are usually fragile, sensitive, easily hurt, and susceptible to stress.[7]

Since boys and men are often poor communicators, it is important to be observant of any signs of suicidal thoughts or depressive symptoms that are conveyed indirectly. The depressed youth refers not to the anxiety, sorrow, or despondency, but to the failure to cope in ordinary situations—in family life, with friends, at school or work, in military service, and in leisure activities. It is advisable to treat depressive symptoms in boys and men without all criteria for the diagnosis of depression necessarily being met.

Longitudinal follow-up studies of patients with adjustment disorder who underwent crisis intervention show that they do not run a higher risk of developing depressive symptoms or dying from suicide than the overall population.[8]

Psychological interventions are likely to be the preferred option for treatment of adjustment disorder. These can vary and depend upon the levels of anxiety, stress, and depression. Due to the risk of suicide, it is important to support the person in managing stress. Families, colleagues, support groups, and psychodynamic therapies alongside relaxation techniques can reduce anxiety. Cognitive therapies are recommended for persons who are prone to deliberate self-harm.[9-12]

Case Study

A rape
Marie, age 24

Marie had undergone a radical change. From being a positive, ambitious extrovert she had been transformed, for the past two months, into a nervous, negative, 'lazy' person with no energy or lust for life.

She had fallen deeply in love with a college student, but had left him because he had turned out to be both manipulative and insincere. Shortly afterwards, she had met a man of her own age through a 'lonely hearts' advertisement. At the end of their first date, he had more or less raped her.

After the rape Marie had felt defiled, disappointed, and filled with anxiety. She had an insistent sense of hopelessness and a marked fear that no man would ever want to live with her. She blamed herself, on the grounds that it had been her fault for letting the man into her flat.

Marie tried to carry on studying, but all the energy that she had once had was gone. Thoughts about the rape kept going round and round in her head. She found it difficult to tell anyone about what had happened, and felt unclean and inferior. She began isolating herself and sought consolation in the Internet. Eventually, the computer took over all her waking hours.

When thoughts about taking her own life became persistent and frightening, she e-mailed a plea for help to an agency that provided professional advice about the body, mind, and health, signing off as 'Young and desperate'. She told the psychologist who contacted her—first by e-mail and, in due course, in person—about her advanced suicide plans and all the details of how she planned to kill herself. All she lacked was the means of doing so.

After three months' supportive psychotherapy, during which she worked through her emotions connected with the rape and her attitude to the opposite sex, she felt better and resumed her studies.

References

1 **Bhatia MS, Aggarwal NK, Aggarwal BB**. Psychosocial profile of suicide ideators, attempters and completers in India. Int J Soc Psychiatry. 2000;**46**(3):155–163.

2 **Apter A, Bleich A, King RA, et al**. Death without warning? A clinical post-mortem study of suicide in 43 Israeli adolescent males. Arch Gen Psychiatry. 1993;**50**:138–142.

3 **Marttunen M, Aro H, Henriksson M, Lönnqvist J**. Adolescent suicides with adjustment disorders or no psychiatric diagnosis. Eur J Child Adolesc Psychiatry. 1994;**3**:101–110.

4 **Pelkonen M, Marttunen M, Henriksson M, Lönnqvist J**. Suicidality in adjustment disorder—clinical characteristics of adolescent outpatients. Eur Child Adolesc Psychiatry. 2005;**14**(3):174–180.

5 **Kryzhanovskaya L, Canterbury R**. Suicidal behavior in patients with adjustment disorders. Crisis. 2001;**22**(3):125–131.

6 **Manoranjitham SD, Rajkumar AP, Thangadurai P, Prasad J, Jayakaran R, Jacob KS**. Risk factors for suicide in rural south India. Br J Psychiatry. 2010;**196**(1):26–30.

7 **Casey P, Bailey S**. Adjustment disorders: the state of the art. World Psychiatry. 2011;**10**:11–18.

8 Bronisch T. Adjustment reactions: a long-term prospective and retrospective follow-up of former patients in a crisis intervention ward. Acta Psychiatr Scand. 1991;**84**:86–93.

9 Gonzales-Jaimes EI, Turnbull-Plaza B. Selection of psychotherapeutic treatment for adjustment disorder with depressive mood due to acute myocardial infarction. Arch Med Res. 2003;**43**:298–304.

10 **Carta MG, Balestrieri M, Murru A, Hardoy MC**. Adjustment disorder: epidemiology, diagnosis and treatment. Clin Pract Epidemiol Ment Health. 2009;**26**:5–15.

11 **Srivastava M, Talukdar U, Lahan V**. Meditation for the management of adjustment disorder anxiety and depression. Complement Ther Clin Pract. 2011;**17**:241–245.

12 **Hsiao FH, Lai YM, Chen YT, Yang TT, Liao SC, Ho RT, et al**. Efficacy of psychotherapy on diurnal cortisol patterns and suicidal ideation in adjustment disorder with depressed mood. Gen Hosp Psychiatry. 2014;**36**(2):214–219.

Chapter 11

Suicide risk in schizophrenia

Alec Roy and Maurizio Pompili

It is estimated that 5–10% of patients with schizophrenia die due to suicide.[1] In a cohort of 176,347 patients who were followed up from their first contact with mental health services until death, immigration, or disappearance, with a median follow-up of 18 years, 6.5% of males with a diagnosis of schizophrenia and 5.9% of males with a diagnosis of schizophrenic-like disorders died by suicide. Corresponding numbers for females were 4.9% and 4.0%.[2] In recent years, research has provided an in-depth analysis of the risk factors for suicide among patients with schizophrenia. Despite the fact that these risk factors often yield too many false positives, it is important to be familiar with them for the proper assessment of suicide risk.

Several studies[3] have determined that the greatest risk for suicide in schizophrenia occurs during the first ten years of illness.

Risk factors

International literature tends to outline a certain profile for schizophrenia patients at risk of suicide: namely being young and male (except in China where studies from certain epidemiological districts show that more women commit suicide than men).[4] Patients who commit suicide are generally Caucasian, unmarried, have good premorbid function, have post-psychotic depression, and have a history of suicide attempts and substance abuse. This latter behaviour complicates the management of patients at risk of suicide.[5]

Clinicians should be aware of what is sometimes called demoralization syndrome in which schizophrenia patients become aware of their illness and its consequences. Patients then may compare their fair premorbid adjustment with their current state and become hopeless and depressed and eventually suicidal.[3]

Hopelessness, lack of social support, and being socially isolated, along with a painful awareness of being ill and being subject to hospitalization, are other important risk factors for suicide in these patients. When health deteriorates in individuals with good premorbid functioning, suicide can result from the awareness that performances previously achieved cannot be maintained. Also, individuals who experience recent loss or rejection, along with limited support from family and community, are at high risk of suicide. These patients usually fear further mental deterioration and experience excessive treatment dependence or loss of faith in treatment.

Studies from international literature[3,6] have described the high-risk patient as a young male, with a history of good adolescent functioning and high aspirations, late age of first hospitalization, high intelligence, with a paranoid or non-deficit form of schizophrenia, who retains the capacity for abstract thinking and the expectations contrast sharply with the declining functional ability, impacting negatively on aspirations and paths of life. Following these findings, Kuo et al.[7] investigated risk factors for suicide among 78 schizophrenia patients in a case-control study and reported that suicide risk was associated with later age of onset in addition to other risk factors.

Pompili and colleagues found that suicide attempts, hopelessness, and self-devaluation were the three variables most strongly associated with completed suicide.[8] Another important risk factor that emerged from this investigation was the presence of sleep disorder, a finding rarely reported hitherto. Furthermore, this study delineated other variables associated with suicide risk, such as agitation, motor restlessness, and mental disintegration. Poor compliance to medication was also predictive of completed suicide in this sample of schizophrenia patients.

Patients with the paranoid subtype of schizophrenia are also more likely to commit suicide. Suicide as a result of command hallucinations, although rare, it has been reported in the literature.[3,4] Kelly et al.[9] reported that a large proportion of schizophrenia patients who committed suicide had poor control of thoughts or thought insertion, loose associations, and flight of ideas as compared with those who died by other means of death.

The risk of suicide peaked not only shortly after discharge from hospital, as reported in the literature, but also shortly after admission. For this reason, Hunt et al.[5] stressed the role of ward safety and close supervision in both inpatient and community settings, especially in the cases of reduced adherence to treatment.

A supportive, supervised living arrangement is ideal. In fact, scientists noted that discharge planning was a proximal factor to suicide in several of their long-stay schizophrenics who had to deal with the painful realization that they were losing the safety of the hospital and the staff and/or that their family was not prepared to have them home. In reviewing the literature, it emerged that[3] the risk for suicide is greatest during the first six months after discharge, but suicide risk is also very high in the five days following discharge as well as in the first 28 days after leaving the hospital.

Staff, and especially nurses, have a crucial role in the process of suicide prevention by delivering information about safety plans. Patients and their families should be instructed on the advisability of a return to the hospital if disturbance occurs again, and they should be encouraged to consider such a return as neither a failure nor a serious setback.[3]

Early recognition of psychotic symptoms is crucial for proper suicide prevention. For instance, in a large cohort of Swedish adolescents followed up longitudinally, Kelleher and colleagues[10] found that psychotic experiences were a strong marker of risk for persistence of suicidal ideation from mid- to late-adolescence/early adulthood, even after controlling for internalizing and externalizing psychopathology and for cannabis use.

Methods of suicide

Schizophrenia patients who die by suicide often use violent means. Kelly et al.[9] found that 73% of the individuals of their sample committed suicide by violent methods, such as jumping from height, drowning, cutting, gunshot wounds, or hanging.

Managing suicide risk with antipsychotic medication

Management of suicide risk through the use of antipsychotics medication is a key factor. Typical neuroleptics do not have much evidence for suicide risk reduction.[11-14] The only atypical antipsychotic approved as an antisuicidal agent is clozapine. However, comparing the characteristics of atypical antipsychotics,[11,12] it is not surprising that also olanzapine, risperidone, and quetiapine have been shown to reduce suicidality among schizophrenia patients.[11] Atypical anti-psychotics have low incidence of extrapyramidal symptoms (EPS) and of akathisia, which is important in the context of reducing suicidality during treatment with these agents.[12-14] The possible role of akathisia in precipitation of suicide risk for patients both treated with antidepressants and antipsychotics has been reported.[14]

According to some reports, the potential decrease in suicide mortality with clozapine treatment is estimated to be as high as 85%. In terms of benefit versus risk, it is estimated that 1.5 of every 10,000 patients with schizophrenia who are treated with clozapine would be expected to die from agranulocytosis (an unfortunate side-effect which needs to be carefully monitored in treatment with clozapine) in comparison with, 1,000 to 1,300 that would have been expected to die by suicide with standard treatment.[3,15]

Apart from clozapine, lithium is the only drug that demonstrates antisuicidal properties in patients with bipolar and major affective disorders.

Managing suicide risk with psychotherapy and psychosocial interventions

Psychosocial interventions are commonly believed to play a role in the management of the suicidal schizophrenia patients. However, due to the heterogeneity and diversity of studies, it is rather difficult to establish whether they play a large role in the prevention of suicide. Schizophrenia patients usually need empathic support; therefore, non-pharmacological strategies do have a role. Clinicians should acknowledge the patient's despair, discuss losses and daily difficulties, and help to establish new and accessible goals. Social isolation and work impairment have been reported as risk factors for suicide in individuals with schizophrenia. Interventions such as social skill training, vocational rehabilitation, and supportive employment are, the prevention of suicide in such patients.

It has become increasingly clear that supportive, reality-orientated therapies are generally of great value in the treatment of patients with schizophrenia; in particular, supportive psychotherapy aiming at offering the patient the opportunity to meet with the therapist and discuss the difficulties encountered in daily activities. Patients are, therefore, encouraged to discuss concerns about medications and side-effects as well as social isolation, economical problems, stigma, etc. Psychosocial programmes should be part of the after-care programmes following a hospitalization. Cognitive therapy has been reported to be helpful.

Case Study

MH was a 26-year-old single, unemployed man. He had his first psychiatric admission at the age of 19 when he began to hear voices and developed paranoid delusions. At that first admission he was also found to be depressed and had marked suicidal ideas. In the subsequent seven years he had six psychiatric admissions—usually through the emergency room because of suicidal ideation or attempts and depression that accompanied exacerbations of the hallucinations and delusions, which occurred when he was non-compliant with his neuroleptic medication. In between admissions he had been unable to find employment.

In his last year of life he was living in a boarding house and had become alienated from his family. His last admission was precipitated when he tried to set fire to himself in his room in the boarding house. At admission he was very depressed, hopeless, and paranoid. During the admission his psychotic symptoms attenuated when neuroleptic medication was reinstated. At discharge he was still somewhat depressed. He failed to attend his first follow-up outpatient appointment. A telephone call to the boarding house revealed that he had hanged himself in his room two days before the scheduled follow-up appointment.

References

1 Palmer BA, Pankratz VS, Bostwick JM. The lifetime risk of suicide in schizophrenia: a re-examination. Arch Gen Psychiatry. 2005;**62**:247–253.

2 Nordentoft M, Mortensen PB, Pedersen CB. Absolute risk of suicide after first hospital contact in mental disorder. Arch Gen Psychiatry. 2011 Oct; **68**: 1058–1064.

3 Pompili M, Amador XF, Girardi P, Harkavy-Friedman J, . . . Tatarelli R. Suicide risk in schizophrenia: learning from the past to change the future. Ann Gen Psychiatry. 2007 Mar;**16**: 10.

4 Phillips MR, Yang G, Li S, Li Y. Suicide and the unique prevalence pattern of schizophrenia in mainland China: a retrospective observational study. Lancet. 2004;**364**:1062–1068.

5 Hunt IM, Kapur N, Windfuhr K, Robinson J, Bickley H, . . . Appelby L. Suicide in schizophrenia: findings from a national clinical survey. J Psychiatr Pract. 2006;**12**:139–147.

6 Fenton WS. Depression, suicide, and suicide prevention in schizophrenia. Suicide Life Threat Behav. 2000;**30**:34–49.

7 Kuo CJ, Tsai SY, Lo CH, Wang YP, Chen CC. Risk factors for completed suicide in schizophrenia. J Clin Psychiatry. 2005;**66**:579–585.

8 Pompili M, Lester D, Grispini A, Innamorati M, Calandro F, Iliceto P, et al. Completed suicide in schizophrenia: evidence from a case-control study. Psychiatry Res. 2009;**167**:251–257.

9 Kelly DL, Shim JC, Feldman SM, Yu Y, Conley RR. Lifetime psychiatric symptoms in persons with schizophrenia who died by suicide compared to other means of death. J Psychiatr Res. 2004;**38**:531–536.

10 Kelleher I, Cederlöf M, Lichtenstein P. Psychotic experiences as a predictor of the natural course of suicidal ideation: a Swedish cohort study. World Psychiatry. 2014 Jun;**13**: 184–188.

11 Keck PE, Jr, Strakowski SM, McElroy SL. The efficacy of atypical antipsychotics in the treatment of depressive symptoms, hostility, and suicidality in patients with schizophrenia. J Clin Psychiatry. 2000;**61**: 4–9.

12 Montout C, Casadebaig F, Lagnaoui R, Verdoux H, Philippe A, Begaud B, et al. Neuroleptics and mortality in schizophrenia: prospective analysis of deaths in a French cohort of schizophrenic patients. Schizophr Res. 2002;**57**:147–156.

13 Meltzer HY. What's atypical about atypical antipsychotic drugs? Curr Opin Pharmacol. 2004;**4**:53–57.

14 Hansen L. A critical review of akathisia, and its possible association with suicidal behaviour. Hum Psychopharmacol. 2001;**16**:495–505.

15 Meltzer HY. Decreasing suicide in schizophrenia. Psychiatr Times. 2001;**18**:1–5.

Personality disorders

Chapter 12

Personality disorders and suicide

Danuta Wasserman

Introduction

The findings of psychological autopsy studies show that 'personality disorder' as the principal diagnosis is reported in approximately 9% of people who take their own lives, and 'abnormal personality' in up to 30%.[1] A review of 50 studies from 24 countries showed that 27.5% of adult self-harm patients who sought hospital care had a diagnosis of personality disorder.[2]

Multiple personality disorders are not unusual, especially among young and middle-aged suicide victims, as well as in suicide attempters, along with psychiatric diagnoses, such as depression, anxiety, alcohol use disorders, conduct disorders, and attention deficit hyperactivity disorder (ADHD).[3] Personality traits like hopelessness, neuroticism, and extroversion correlate to both suicidal ideation, suicide attempts, and completed suicide. Diagnoses of major depressive disorder, substance use disorders, post-traumatic stress disorder, as well as previous self-harm behaviours, sexual assault, affective disability, hostility, and having a caretaker who has completed suicide are clinically important predictors of suicidal behaviours in persons with borderline personality disorder.[4]

The diagnosis of 'personality disorder' poses several methodological problems, and the incidence of personality disorders found among people who commit suicide varies depending on which patients are surveyed and the survey methods used. A restrictive approach is recommended, especially with the borderline diagnosis, more particularly in adolescents, as almost every sign characterized by borderline personality disorder may be manifested in connection with pubertal crises. Pregnant women or people in extreme life situations may also show clear borderline traits that later disappear. Some personality disorders of particular importance in the therapeutic process, in terms of suicide prevention, are described below.

Borderline personality

Borderline personality is characterized by marked identity disturbance, with a chronic subjective sense of emptiness and difficulties in achieving steady, close relationships with others. Self-perceptions are full of contradictions, with repercussions on self-image, sexual orientation, long-term goals, and choice of friends and occupation.

The mechanism known as 'splitting', the purpose of which is to keep bad and good impulses apart, is used as an essential psychological defence by persons with borderline personality. Since borderline personalities have difficulty in distinguishing between their own and others' good and bad impulses and emotions they may use 'projective identifications' i.e., ascribe to others their own rage or the feeling that they wish to get rid of.

Patterns of unstable swings between extremes, with disparagement and overestimation, emotional lability, inadequate control of aggressive impulses, irascibility, and intense efforts to avoid separations—real and imagined—characterize people with borderline personality disorder. Their suicides often take place in a mood of fury mingled with despair triggered by separation from partners or significant others or because of a forced alteration in their accustomed lifestyle.[5]

Antisocial personality

The antisocial person resembles the person with borderline personality disorder in many respects. The specific additional traits of the antisocial personality are defective development of moral and ethical values, with a lack of empathy, an egocentric focus on one's own perceptual world, and contempt for others.

People with an antisocial personality uninhibitedly act out their drives, impulses, and aggressive fantasies. This behaviour is highly resistant to modification. Their dissatisfaction is transformed into aggressive action, sometimes directed against others and sometimes self-directed, rather than into signal anxiety, which has a normative and inhibiting role.

Suicide takes place in the rage that people with antisocial personalities feel when, for example, they are apprehended for offences, embezzlement, or crimes.[1]

Narcissistic personality

The term 'narcissistic' is derived from the Greek myth of Narkissos, who was unable to stop contemplating his reflection in the waters of a spring. He had fallen so much in love with it that he eventually pined away and died.

Characteristic of this personality type is a paradoxical splitting between two entirely opposed self-images—one grandiose, making life a constant quest for confirmation of one's greatness with consequent effort to prove this, the other the antithesis of this, with a self-image full of shame, hate, and terror of self-rejection.

The experiential and conceptual world of narcissistic people is divided into the idyllic and the terrifying, which may alternate. Those in the surrounding world may also be perceived as representatives of one or the other sphere and thus be idealized or disparaged. Ideas or people are rejected when they no longer provide a boost to the narcissistic person's self-image. The narcissistic personality also resembles both the borderline and the antisocial personality, with the major difference being that narcissistic people, when provoked, explode in outbursts of rage or aggressive behaviour only when, according to their judgement, the social situation permits.

Suicide may be the narcissist's reaction to losing the grandiose image e.g., when ageing or illness destroys youthful charm or attractiveness; when a fall in social status or financial loss is incurred, or when a well-regarded job or partner that imparted the reality or illusion of greatness is lost.[6,7]

Histrionic personality

A person with histrionic personality shows a consistent pattern of exaggerated emotionality and an endeavour to gain attention. A poor ability to read other people's intentions and needs contributes to disappointment being felt much more severely than is justified. Adjustment, and contentment may be easily subverted by setbacks. Strains and disappointments bring a depressive, hopeless, and helpless frame of mind.[3,7]

Histrionic people commit suicide as a result of profound disappointment when they perceive strongly that they are no longer needed e.g., because of the death of a loved one, friends, beloved pets or restructuring at the workplace.

Obsessive–compulsive personality

People with obsessive–compulsive personality are highly orderly, conscientious, and responsible but, unfortunately, easily frustrated, vulnerable, depressive, and lonely, owing to their reserved attitude and their endeavours to set themselves apart from their peers. Perfectionist and knowledgeable, they lack tolerance of people who are ignorant and ordinary. There is often a gap between their aspirations and accomplishments, and they suffer from emotional and also intellectual instability, with ups and downs for both 'coping' and intellectual performance.

Many such people feel dissatisfied with their lives and are characterized by a tendency towards counterproductive behaviour, e.g. leaving others in order to avoid others leaving them. This is reflected in both their relationships and at work. Rejecting others before they can be rejected themselves may be these people's guiding principle. Towards themselves, they are denying and non-permissive. Despite their loneliness, they yearn for company and belonging to a group; but this desire may be thwarted by their need to dominate and exert control over others.

Suicidal acts take place when these people are experiencing deep downs and the prospects of bouncing back are perceived to be, or genuinely are, slim.

Other personality traits

The personality disorders described above, together with the emotionally unstable and anxious types of personality, are the most prevalent among people who commit suicide. However personality traits or disorders of avoidant, dependent, paranoid, and schizoid types are also found among suicide victims.[3]

Childhood moulding

Many people with the personality types described above who take their own lives have had a childhood in which they have experienced insufficient parental care, often with a negative emotional climate and neglect of the most profound needs of closeness, contact, warmth, and understanding. Alternatively, they may have been severely restrained, in their need to grow and develop through natural questioning and the ordinary frustrations of life during their upbringing.

Inadequate parental care may be due to the parents' inability to perceive the child's needs, the parents' moodiness or strictness, or the child's lack of a close relationship when the parents die prematurely and there is no one to take their place as a secure substitute and good identification object or role model.

Severely distorted male or female identity, weak self-esteem, and the superego, with elements of strong hostility to the self-image, is the result. Hostility (with risk of suicide) makes itself strongly felt in situations in which the person's low self-esteem is mercilessly exposed.

Genetic make-up

In families in which suicides take place, there are traditions of resolving conflicts or difficult situations by means of suicidal acts. Models like this pave the way for the child to adopt the same self-destructive strategies later in life. But hereditary factors also have a great bearing. Although the extent to which genetic components are implicated in suicide are far from being elucidated (see Chapter 2 on Stress-vulnerability model of suicidal behaviours).

Genetic set-up has consequences in stress-induced situations that call for increased attentiveness. When negative life events pile up, cognition deteriorates and, instead of finding an appropriate strategy, the person reacts, with anxiety, panic, and rigidity. Typically, people on the brink of suicide have tunnel vision, are unable to make subtle distinctions, find solutions, be flexible, and perceive only the dark side of life. Impulsivity is an important factor in suicidality, especially in adolescents and young adults. Personality traits are important predictors of suicidal behaviours and there is evidence of familial transmission of character dimensions from parents to suicidal attempters.[8,9]

Clinical manifestations of genetic predisposition depend on age and on environmental factors, which vary from one phase of the human life cycle to another. This is why negative life events exert influence not only in childhood, but throughout a person's entire life. In the elderly, these events may coincide with other maturation-associated biochemical changes and altered brain functioning.

Suicide risk

People with personality disorders who take their own lives have, to a significantly greater extent than others, experienced a range of highly adverse life events such as troubles at work, unemployment, financial problems, family discord, lack of a permanent home, court convictions, and separations. Problems often come to a head in the last week before the suicide, which precipitates the act (see Chapter 14). Feelings of defeat and entrapment from losing internal and external struggles due to not only external events, but also internal perception are overwhelming.[10]

The suicidal situation in persons with personality disorders[11] is often triggered by a primitive anger or a sense of hopelessness, or a blend of the two, when self-esteem is under severe threat and the usual self-image is unsustainable. When people's images of themselves and their existence collapses and cannot be reinstated in a normal grief process, there is a major risk of suicide. This applies particularly if there have been examples and models of suicidal behaviour in the family. However, suicidal impulses may subside and suicide risk diminish if new circumstances and therapeutic help appear and serve the purpose of providing the support and security that suicidal people are, for the time being, unable to generate for themselves.

Comorbidity

When one or more personality disorders and a psychiatric illness are present at the same time, the suicide risk is high. Some of the males with personality disorders who die from suicide not only suffer from alcohol use disorder and depression, but also from other health problems like somatic illnesses and narcissistic personality disorders.[12]

Depression may sometimes be hard to detect in suicidal people with personality disorders since their feelings of hopelessness are relatively well concealed, even if their depression and despair are profound.

Treatment

Recommendations concerning treatment of borderline personality disorders has been issued by the American Psychiatric Association (APA)[13] and National Institute for Health and Care Excellence (NICE).[14] The APA recommends easier access to hospitalization and pharmacological treatment, while NICE guidelines advocate an integrated clinical approach to patients with borderline personality disorders; i.e., varying combinations of medication and psychotherapy dependent on subtypes of borderline personality disorders and suicide risk.

Pharmacological treatment

In spite of the broad range of possibilities of treating suicidal patients with pharmacological treatment including antidepressants, antipsychotics, and mood stabilizers, data for the effectiveness of pharmacotherapy vary and evidence is not yet robust.[15]

Medication can be helpful in mitigating emotional instability, insecurity, easily aroused emotions, anxiety, and rage.[13] Selective serotonin re-uptake inhibitors (SSRIs) diminish affective instability and impulsiveness. Controlled studies show that low-dose antipsychotic drugs bring an improvement in a broad spectrum of different symptoms in severe borderline personality disorder and schizotypal personality disorder. Those who show aggressive behaviour respond to lithium and there is evidence supporting the antisuicidal properties of lithium. Patients with borderline and histrionic personality disorders who have suicidal tendencies respond to maintenance doses of antipsychotic drugs.

Mood stabilizers like carbamazepine, divalproex, and lamotrigine have proved to be helpful in reducing episodes of lack of control in patients with behavioural disturbances and borderline personality.

Attention should be paid to medications which may cause loss of control and exacerbate suicidality in people with a borderline personality structure[14] (see also Chapter 27).

Psychotherapy

Lasting and severe traumas during childhood affect personality development and have repercussions on experiences and the regulation of emotions. However, it is possible by different psychotherapeutic methods, like dialectical behavioural therapy (DBT), cognitive behavioural therapy (CBT), and psychodynamic and transference focused psychotherapy,[14,16–18] to remedy a constantly recurring feeling of insecurity and unfulfilled emotional needs that are repeatedly brought to the fore in new stressful and traumatic situations that arise later in life.

Other psychological treatments, such as the Systems Training for Emotional Predictability and Problem Solving (STEPPS) programme,[19] psycho-education for persons with borderline personality disorder,[20] and brief dialectical behavioural therapy[21] are examples of psychotherapies used in treatment of patients with personality disorders.

Evidence shows that less time consuming therapies are as effective on suicidal acts and depression as therapies of long duration, which justifies provisions of less time intensive psychological therapies.[22]

During treatment, it is important to work through the old and new traumas and show how the current emotional reactions are a repetition of previous emotional reactions. In this kind of treatment, the cultural factors that influence people's behaviour and emotional expressions must also be taken into account. Efforts to motivate the patient to receive drug treatment, when necessary, should also be included in psychotherapeutic treatment.

Prevention

Research shows that for patients with personality disorders, the prognosis is good with respect to both the psychiatric illness itself and their suicidality if, during the turbulent years of their youth and early adulthood, they succeed in improving their affect and impulse management.

For patients with such characteristics as warmth, charm, attractiveness, talent, and high intelligence, the prognosis is better than for others.

Chronic suicidality, with repeated suicide attempts, does not necessarily mean that the patient will die from suicide. Active and prompt intervention, with both pharmacological and psychotherapeutic treatment, in response to acute problems such as interpersonal or work difficulties, can save the lives of vulnerable and suicidal people. Those who have attempted suicide previously should be taught to seek psychiatric help in time as soon as difficulties or suicidal crisis arises.

References

1 **Isometsä ET, Henriksson MM, Heikkinen ME, et al.** Suicide among subjects with personality disorders. Am J Psychiatry. 1996;**153**:667–673.

2 **Hawton K, Saunders K, Topiwala A, Haw C.** Psychiatric disorders in patients presenting to hospital following self-harm: a systematic review. J Affect Disord. 2013;**151**(3):821–830.

3 **Brezo J, Paris J, Turecki G.** Personality traits as correlates of suicidal ideation, suicide attempts, and suicide completions: a systematic review. Acta Psychiatr Scand. 2006;**113**(3):180–206.

4 **Wedig MM, Silverman MH, Frankenburg FR, Reich DB, Fitzmaurice G, Zanarini MC.** Predictors of suicide attempts in patients with borderline personality disorder over 16 years of prospective follow-up. Psychol Med. 2012;**42**(11):2395–2404.

5 **Kjellander C, Bongar B, King A.** Suicidality in borderline personality disorder. Crisis. 1998;**19**:125–135.

6 **Clark DC.** Narcissistic crises of aging and suicidal despair. Suicide Life Threat Behav. 1993;**23**:21–26.

7 **Ronningstam E, Maltsberger JT.** Pathological narcissism and sudden suicide-related collapse. Suicide Life Threat Behav. 1998;**28**:261–271.

8 **Camarena B, Fresán A, Sarmiento E.** Exploring personality features in patients with affective disorders and history of suicide attempts: a comparative study with their parents and control subjects. Depress Res Treat. 2014:291802.

9 **Wasserman D, Geijer T, Sokolowski M, Rozanov V, Wasserman J.** Genetic variation in the hypothalamic-pituitary-adrenocortical axis regulatory factor, T-box 19, and the angry/hostility personality trait. Genes Brain Behav. 2007;**6**(4):321–328.

10 **Taylor PJ, Gooding P, Wood AM, Tarrier N.** The role of defeat and entrapment in depression, anxiety and suicide. Psychol Bull. 2011;**137**:391–420.

11 **Stanley B, Jones J.** Risk for suicide behaviour in personality disorders. In: Wasserman D, Wasserman C, eds. Oxford textbook of suicidology and suicide prevention: a global perspective. New York, NY: Oxford University Press; 2009: 287–292.

12 Giner L, Blasco-Fontecilla H, Mercedes Perez-Rodriguez M, Garcia-Nieto R, Giner J, Guija JA, et al. Personality disorders and health problems distinguish suicide attempters from completers in a direct comparison. J Affect Disord. 2013;**151**(2):474–483.

13 **American Psychiatric Association**. Practice guideline for the treatment of patients with borderline personality disorder. Am J Psychiatry. 2010.

14 **National Institute for Health and Care Excellence**. Borderline personality disorder (BPD): NICE guidelines. 28 January 2009. Available at <http://guidance.nice.org.uk/CG78≥. Accessed August 2014.

15 Leichsenring F, Leibing E, Kruse J, New AS, Leweke F. Borderline personality disorder. Lancet. 2011;**377**(9759):74–84.

16 Linehan MM, Comtois KA, Murray AM, et al. Two-year randomized controlled trial and follow-up of dialectical behavior therapy vs therapy by experts for suicidal behaviors and borderline personality disorder. Arch Gen Psychiatry. 2006;**63**:757–766.

17 Bateman A, Fonagy P. Effectiveness of partial hospitalization in the treatment of borderline personality disorder: a randomized controlled trial. Am J Psychiatry. 1999;**156**:1563–1569.

18 Kernberg OF, Yeomans FE, Clarkin JF, Levy KN. Transference focused psychotherapy: overview and update. Int J Psychoanal. 2008;**89**:601–620.

19 Blum N, St John D, Pfohl B, et al. Systems Training for Emotional Predictability and Problem Solving (STEPPS) for outpatients with borderline personality disorder: a randomized controlled trial and 1-year follow-up. Am J Psychiatry. 2008;**165**:468–478.

20 Zanarini MC, Frankenburg FR. A preliminary, randomized trial of psychoeducation for women with borderline personality disorder. J Pers Disord. 2008;**22**:284–290.

21 Stanley B, Brodsky B, Nelson JD, Dulit R. Brief dialectical behavior therapy (DBT-B) for suicidal behavior and non-suicidal self-injury. Arch Suicide Res. 2007;**11**:337–341.

22 Davidson KM, Tran CF. Impact of treatment intensity on suicidal behavior and depression in borderline personality disorder: a critical review. J Pers Disord. 2014;**28**(2):181–197.

Somatic disorders

Chapter 13

Physical illnesses and suicide

Jouko Lönnqvist

Health-care staff taken by surprise

The role of physical illness in suicide has received little attention in research and education. Although suicide is a rare event, elevated suicide risk is a known feature of many somatic disorders.[1] Most suicide victims consult health professionals for reasons of physical ill-health in the last 6–12 months of their lives.[2] However, many of them do not express their suicidal ideation, or even their depressive feelings, in clear verbal terms.

Retrospective analysis after a suicide may afford knowledge of the suicidal person's many problems, but in many cases the act of suicide remains enigmatic. Suicide almost always arouses a mixture of feelings among health-care staff—anxiety, a sense of helplessness, anger, rage, sorrow, and guilt among others. Numerous simple explanations may be offered. Suicide reminds health-care professionals of the limits of their care: the best possible help was not available and normal clinical practice was insufficient to prevent suicide. But could the unpredictable have been predicted? Does the suicide carry a message that we can learn for the future?

It is a challenge to improve both understanding of suicide risk and treatment of suicidal patients in clinical practice.

Physical illness and suicide risk

Epidemiological studies have revealed that a number of specific somatic illnesses are associated with elevated suicide risk.[1,3,4] Any physical illness with chronicity, severity, comorbidity, disability, and negative prognosis is correlated with suicide. Only intellectual disabilities are associated with a markedly reduced risk of suicide.[5] Diagnosis of depression is a real challenge for health-care professionals treating patients with physical illnesses and elevated suicide risk.

The physical illnesses most commonly connected with suicide are:

◆ cancer;

◆ human immunodeficiency virus (HIV) infection;

◆ stroke;

◆ coronary heart disease;

◆ delirium;

◆ epilepsy;

◆ Parkinson's disease;

◆ traumatic brain damage;

◆ spinal cord injury;

◆ multiple sclerosis;

◆ Huntington's disease; and

◆ amyotrophic lateral sclerosis.

In addition, some people who eventually commit suicide suffer not only from severe depression but also from an intense fear of severe somatic illness, such as cancer or HIV infection. This kind of somatic symptom disorder usually leads to numerous health-care consultations, with physical examinations yielding negative results and, in turn, bringing disappointment and a growing sense of hopelessness and helplessness. The many faces of depression, especially when many somatic symptoms are present, can mislead even experienced clinicians and cause misunderstandings between patients and their doctors.

Physical illness and the suicidal process

The events that culminate in suicide, which involve suicidal ideation and often attempted suicide as well, are known as the 'suicidal process' (see Chapter 2). Suicide is the fatal outcome of what is, as a rule, a long-term process shaped by various interacting genetic, biological, physiological, cognitive, emotional, behavioural, situational, social, societal, and cultural factors. In this process, physical illness may be seen as either a long-term risk factor or a more immediate, precipitating cause.

In the first five years of cancer, for example, the probability of suicide is elevated. Suicide risk is clearly highest in the first few months after diagnosis, when adaptation to the crisis has not yet occurred. In many other chronic and progressive somatic diseases, the risk may fluctuate depending on the course of the illness. Exacerbation or deterioration of a somatic disease may often also trigger a suicidal crisis. However, most people are capable of living and working through even the most threatening stages of illness if support is available from their significant others and the health-care system. Despite the tremendous acute stress and chronic adaptational demands associated with all major somatic disorders, surprisingly few sufferers from severe physical illness actually commit suicide.

In terms of social background, family status, and previous suicidality, as well as psychiatric diagnoses and personality characteristics, patients with somatic disease who commit suicide are usually clinically very similar to other suicide victims, their main problems being depressive mood and adaptational difficulties. Suicide risk is indirectly associated with physical illness through the anxiety, depression, narcissistic rage, pain, fear (and side-effects of treatment), substance or alcohol misuse, or delirious states experienced by the sick person. Loneliness and isolation that ensue from the illness, access to lethal suicide methods, and imitation of other suicides are other important factors in this context. Elevated suicide risk is not normally directly related to the somatic illness but rather, is due to associated comorbidity. Suicide risk in physically ill people varies by the presence of psychiatric comorbidity.[6] If this comorbidity remains undetected, the patient's distorted behaviour may further accelerate the suicide process.

The best predictive risk factors for suicide among patients suffering from physical illnesses are previous suicide attempts, anorexia nervosa, depression, psychosis, substance misuse, and personality disorder. However, the high suicide risk associated with physical illness is mediated through many mechanisms.

First, since terminal illness makes death an imminent reality, it may prompt patients with incurable diseases to avoid or even flee from the feared end of their lives, with the prospect of pain, anxiety, and annihilation. Some prefer to choose their mode of death actively, by suicide. Proponents of assisted suicide make use in their arguments of these strong emotional reactions that arise in people who know they are dying.

However, the idea of assisted suicide is undoubtedly dangerous, one of the reasons being that adequate somatic and psychiatric treatment has seldom been available to terminally ill suicide victims.

Second, the idea of increasing dependence on others as a result of illness may be the force that drives some patients to commit suicide.

Third, a physical illness often implies the threat of a future in which the health-care system, rather than relatives, will take care of the patient. Separation from loved ones may be a patient's dominant fear. Suicidal ideation that is expressed and openly received by significant others is the most obvious factor prompting early intervention.

Physical illness and comorbidity in completed suicide

The prevalence of physical disorders found in psychological autopsy studies has varied widely between 15 and 80%. A Scottish case-control study identified physical ill-health as one of the major factors that is independently associated with suicide, and treatment of mental disorders comorbid with physical ill-health was seen as an important strategy in suicide prevention.[7] In a nationwide Finnish psychological autopsy study, when the diagnosis of all potentially relevant physical disorders had been included, the incidence of somatic illness was found to be 46%.[8] A Finnish study of elderly suicide victims found that 88% had been suffering from physical illnesses.[9] In a British study physical health problems were present in 82%, and felt to be contributory to death of suicide victims aged 60 and over in 62%.[10] These findings clearly indicate that somatic comorbidity poses a special challenge for preventing suicide to those who treat elderly patients.

4% of all suicide victims in a Finnish study were diagnosed as suffering from cancer, but only a small minority was terminally ill. Only a very small minority of suicide victims suffering from cancer presented no comorbid mental disorder. These findings refute the idea that assisted suicide might serve as an appropriate means of helping severely ill somatic patients. As noted above, such an idea is undoubtedly dangerous, given that adequate somatic and psychiatric treatment is seldom, if ever, available.[11,12]

Suicide prevention through treatment of somatic diseases

Since physical illness is usually a concomitant or precipitating factor in the suicidal process, medical treatment of somatic illness is an important means of suicide prevention. Even a minor positive event may be life-saving when a patient stands on the brink of suicide. Good clinical practice invariably also means effective suicide prevention.

In clinical practice a doctor treats an individual patient, not just a specific illness. A somatically ill patient very often has other comorbid and mental problems, usually anxiety or depression, or both. Accordingly, only a tailor-made treatment strategy—a balanced, optimal treatment plan comprising somatic, psychological, and social elements—can be effective. It is known that suicide victims never suffer from ordinary, simple problems. They tend to have several diagnoses, they are awkward and troublesome patients, and they often have communication difficulties. They have problems in cooperating with health-care professionals and they question the ability of these professionals to help.

Most countries believe in a comprehensive suicide-prevention strategy (i.e., that all available means must be used to achieve an overall impact on suicide rates at the population level). Accordingly, all clinical specialists should be familiar with the high-risk groups in their own fields and the high-risk situations associated with specific somatic illnesses. This means, for example, that neurologists who treat patients with multiple sclerosis must be aware that such patients run a suicide risk that is twice as high as normal: that this risk fluctuates according to the course of the illness and the patients' mood, and that treatment modifies the risk. Likewise, all other specialists and, indeed all health-care workers, have their own specific points to ponder and their own challenges to meet in suicide prevention.

With the growing success of somatic treatments in several somatic illnesses, suicide risk has also declined. The most recent example is HIV infection and AIDS. Suicide risk among people who are HIV-positive has fallen as the outcome has improved.[13] Effective treatment of various physical illnesses will probably further reduce suicide risk. Good medical treatment of underlying somatic disease will undoubtedly improve the scope for successful suicide prevention.

Case Study

'When the bullet hits—suffering in silence'

A middle-aged man who had suffered from urethral stricture for some years was hospitalized for surgery. The stricture was the result of a gonorrhoeal infection that he had contracted before his marriage, more than ten years earlier. The urogenital infection preyed on his mind and he became anxious and depressed.

Shortly after the operation and discharge from the hospital, the patient hanged himself. He had been unable to face the overwhelming threat that he perceived his physical illness to imply. He had received proper surgical treatment for his urethral stricture, but his depression and anxiety had never been recognized or treated—he had been left alone with his fears.

One wonders what the 'reason' for this suicide was: what the precipitating factors were and what kinds of risk factor were present. It emerged afterwards (unfortunately not before or during his stay in hospital) that the patient's brother had committed suicide shortly before the appearance of the urogenital symptoms in the patient. This event had plunged the patient into profound grief. As the urethral stricture had developed, he had begun using painkillers in abundance. It was only discovered after his death that he had been resorting to painkillers occasionally over the past ten years following a severe bullet wound that had caused an open brain injury to the left fronto-temporal sensorimotor region, resulting in post-traumatic epilepsy. The patient had resumed his work but had been obliged to take antiepileptic medication.

Despite his head injury and restricted work capacity, he had succeeded in achieving a happy marriage at the age of over 40 years and supporting his family, including a small child. The psychological autopsy revealed several other traumatic events in the patient's life that had never been worked through in any kind of psychological treatment. His father had died when the patient was 20 years old and his mother had died in childbirth. As a young man, the patient had an illegitimate son, whom he abandoned.

We are still ignorant of the 'reason' for his suicide, since his thoughts and feelings are unknown to us. Was he afraid of losing his happy marriage, fearing that impotence will follow the operation? Did he fear being left alone—as he had been by his mother as a baby, by his father as a young man, and finally, recently, by his brother? These losses and the psychological experience of losing contact with his first child may have aroused in him the fear that his wife might leave him.

No one knows. Nevertheless, the patient's suicide risk could have been recognized if the doctor treating his epilepsy had noted his misuse of painkillers and the signs of depression and anxiety that had developed in connection with the urogenital problems.

References

1 Harris EC, Barraclough BM. Suicide as an outcome for medical disorders. Medicine. 1994;**73**:281–296.

2 Cho J, Lee WJ, Moon KT, et al. Medical care utilization during 1 year prior to death motivated by physical illnesses. J Prev Med Public Health. 2013;**46**:147–154.

3 Stenager, EN, Stenager, E. Physical illness and suicidal behaviour. In: Wasserman, D, Wasserman C (eds). Oxford University Press textbook of suicidology and suicide prevention. OUP, 2009; 293–299.

4 Webb RT, Kontopantelis E, Doran T, et al. Suicide risk in primary care patients with major physical diseases: a case-control study. Arch Gen Psychiatry. 2012;**69**:256–264.

5 Harris EC, Barraclough B. Suicide as an outcome for mental disorders: a meta-analysis. Br J Psychiatry. 1997;**170**:205–228.

6 Qin P, Hawton K, Mortensen PB, Webb R. Combined effects of physical illness and comorbid psychiatric disorder on risk of suicide in a national population study. Br J Psychiatry. 2014 Jun;**204**(6):430–435.

7 Cavanagh JT, Owens DG, Johnstone EC. Suicide and undetermined death in south-east Scotland. A case-control study using the psychological autopsy method. Psychol Med. 1999;**29**:1141–1149.

8 Henriksson MM, Aro HM, Marttunen MJ, et al. Mental disorders and comorbidity in suicide. Am J Psychiatry. 1993;**150**:935–940.

9 Henriksson MM, Marttunen MJ, Isometsä ET, et al. Mental disorders in elderly suicides. Int Psychogeriatr. 1995;**7**:275–286.

10 Michael D, Harwood J, Hawton K, et al. Life problems and physical illness as risk factors for suicide in older people: a descriptive and case-control study. Psychol Med 2006;**36**:1265–1274.

11 Henriksson MM, Isometsä ET, Hietanen PS, et al. Mental disorders in cancer suicides. J Affect Disord.1995;**36**: 11–20.

12 Hietanen P, Lönnqvist J. Cancer and suicide. Ann Oncol. 1991;**2**:19–23.

13 Jia CX, Mehlum L, Qin P. AIDS/HIV infection, comorbid psychiatric illness, and risk for subsequent suicide: a nation-wide register linkage study. J Clin Psychiatry. 2012;**73**:1315–1321.

Section IV

Risk situations
for suicide

Chapter 14

Negative life events and suicide

Danuta Wasserman

Introduction

Feeling loved, a sense of belonging, being needed and respected by others, and an awareness of one's own worth is important to all human beings. Negative life events prevent the satisfaction of these basic needs and may bring some people close to suicide. This applies to those who have no means of regaining what they have lost and who, at the same time, perceive indifference, rejection, or aggression among the people around them.

In a suicidal person, life and death wishes vie for supremacy. The person's ambivalence in other respects may be just as marked. Current negative life events are often superimposed on the experience of similar events in childhood or on occurrences that relate to the same emotional and intellectual sphere that may have been experienced over many years, causing chronic stress. What matters is not only the occurrence of a negative life event as such, but how a person perceives it, the absence of protective factors, the presence of diathesis for suicidal acts, as well as gene and environment interactions (see Chapters 2 and 3).

Traumas

Violence, physical and mental abuse

Bullying, victimization and harassment at school or the workplace are risk situations for suicide. Risk situations also arise when there are acts or threats of violence against significant others in the at-risk person's surroundings. Traumatic events, such as sexual molestation and assault, rape, and physical and mental abuse, are connected with suicide. The same applies to incest, torture, and any occurrence that brings to the fore memories of incest, torture, or other traumas.

Childhood traumas, are often unresolved if the child lived in a dysfunctional family that was incapable of looking after him or her. Suicidal people often come from broken homes or homes in which one or both parents were emotionally disturbed or mentally ill. Depression and/or alcoholism are typical features.[1-4]

Negative life events

An unexpected change in a person's life situation (an actual or threatened loss, or failure at home or at work) may bring to the fore memories of similar situations and perceptions of injury. This is a clear risk situation for suicide. Several studies have shown that negative life events act both as catalysts in the suicidal process and as factors that precipitate suicide.[5-9] Both childhood adversity and recent negative life events increase the risk for suicide attempts and suicide. In a major Finnish study of 1,067 suicide victims,[10] recent negative life events were found to have occurred in 80% of cases. The most frequent life events were problems at work, family discord, somatic illness, financial problems, unemployment, separation, death of a family member, and illness in the family. The women had often experienced more negative life events than the men. However, not only life events, but also major depressive episodes are key precipitants for suicidal behaviours.[8]

Young people undergo separations more often than their elders and also have more severe problems in relationships with the family. An increasing problem of setbacks in terms of finances, work, and unemployment affecting individuals' mental health and suicidal behaviours is observed among young and middle aged persons.[11] Among elderly people who commit suicide, on the other hand, somatic morbidity and problems connected with retirement are more prevalent. Life events that act as both acute and chronic stressors in suicide appear to have a cumulative effect.

Suicide rates are elevated among workers in certain occupations—chemists, farmers, police officers, artists, doctors, and mental health-care staff.[12] The relatively high propensity of these groups to commit suicide may be the result of complex interaction between stress factors at work, the access to the means of suicide and other risk factors, such as psychiatric and personality disorders.

Actual and threatened losses

Apart from separation from a partner or friend, a separation or loss may involve the loss of possessions, functions, or relationships that have afforded security. For some people, when everyday life changes no longer provide a purposeful existence, suicide risk is high. This applies particularly to those who have difficulty in finding a new purpose in everyday life and settling into new routines.

Loss of a significant other

The loss of a key person (e.g., a partner, relative, friend, neighbour, or a home help (for an elderly or disabled person)) who provided practical help and a boost to the suicidal person's self-image may be a major loss. The frustration is particularly acute for people with marked dependency needs. Goethe, in 'Westöstlicher Divan' has described so aptly this kind of reaction: 'When he keeps my hands full, my self seems important and dear . . . he goes, and instantly I am lost.' ('*Wei sie sich an mich verschwendet,/Bin ich mir ein wertes Ich;/Hätte sie sich weggewendet,/Augenblicks verlör ich mich.*') The loss of love, activities, meaningful experiences, financial benefits, and status that were associated with the lost person may expose an inner sense of emptiness. With simultaneous frustration of security needs, a high-risk situation may arise. A separation that reminds of similar events in the childhood also implies an elevated suicide risk.

After the death of a parent or spouse, suicide risk rises more among men than women and remains elevated for 4–5 years. After suicide of a close family member, the risk of suicide is elevated for other family members during a grief process that is usually long and difficult.

Loss of a national or cultural affiliation

Suicide rates are elevated among refugees and immigrants who have not yet adjusted to their new country (see Chapter 17). Separation from the old culture and the shock of sudden confrontation with the new culture tell part of the story. However, separation from the rest of society that is not the entirely voluntary choice of a group or an individual seems also to boost the suicide risk. This applies to many indigenous ethnic groups, such as the American Indians, the Aborigines, and the Inuit.[13]

Loss of health

Falling ill or suffering a relapse, whether the illness is somatic or mental or consists in substance misuse, is experienced as a disappointing and negative life event. A new acute phase of a chronic illness forces the sufferer to learn, once more, to live with the illness. Not all people can cope with such a burden (see Chapter 13).

Hospitalization

For psychiatric patients and elderly people who are chronically ill, admission to hospital may be perceived as a threat to personal autonomy. The risk of a suicidal act before treatment starts can be high.

Temporary leave from hospital

Temporary leave from hospital after a suicide attempt or in the course of treatment for mental illness, when the patient's suicidal ideation is still pronounced, constitutes a risk situation. Such problems may be particularly severe if the ward staffs have fragmented perceptions of the patient. Marked processes that involve group dynamics may begin when the patient is perceived in disparate ways by different members of staff. In such situations, suicide risk assessment must be carried out along with the analysis of staffs' attitudes.

Discharge from hospital

Discharge from hospital may also be a risk factor. Both repeated suicide attempts and completed suicides often take place shortly after patients are discharged from hospital care. Not only suicide mortality but also the rate of death from other causes is particularly high in the first weeks and months after attempted suicide, and they remain elevated for as much as one year afterwards. This is probably due to the lack of properly thought-out rehabilitation and follow-up measures. These measures should be planned well in advance of the patient's discharge in cooperation between the hospital, the family, and community service providers.

Loss of health or life by significant others

Illness, whether sudden or chronic, and death of a family member or significant other is a risk situation. For young women, abortion (whether they have chosen it of their own free will or have been compelled by circumstances to undergo it) may arouse a strong sense of guilt and loss.

Loss of employment, study opportunities, home and financial position, and fear of change

The loss of one's home, failure in studies, unemployment, financial difficulties, and bankruptcy are common negative life events among people who commit suicide.

For some people, a change of workplace and even a return to work, which most people regard as something positive, may be risk factors. These events may remind them of previous unsolved problems at the workplace or of their own inability to cope with the duties concerned.

For sensitive young people, choosing an occupation, education, home, and partner may constitute a risk situation. Students embarking on higher education, especially during the first and second year, and conscripts in the armed forces at the start and end of their military service can also experience severe stress. This stress, when combined with psychiatric and psychological risk factors, contributes to the elevated suicide rates in these groups.

Sudden wealth or economical loss, due to bankruptcy, gambling, etc. may also involve risk if the person has very low self-esteem and is afraid of not meeting the demands of the new situation (see Chapter 5).

Relationship problems

Suicide is often immediately preceded by various types of problems in relationships with close family members, especially spouses and partners, friends, and colleagues. Loneliness, despondency and depression caused by these problems are exacerbating factors. Spouses who are not supportive and who act as a reminder of parents' negative behaviour are a risk for a suicidal person, who is often engaged in a lifelong quest for love, consolation, and a supportive existence.

Change in activities due to public holidays

Fluctuations in suicide rates in connection with all major public holidays have been described in several studies.[14,15] The phenomenon involves a fall in the incidence of suicidal acts before the holiday and a rise after it. In the West, this pattern is particularly marked at Christmas, New Year, Easter, and Whitsun and in the US also in connection with Independence Day, Thanksgiving, and Labour Day. It is strikingly similar for suicide and attempted suicide. The pattern is similar in other cultures; i.e., risks are around major holidays.

The factors involved may include not only the change in the content of everyday activities but also disappointment, thwarted expectations, cumulative relationship problems, and abstinence due to overconsumption of alcoholic beverages during leisure days.

Suicide may take place in connection with a 'red-letter day'. The date may be of particular significance to the person concerned, such as when a family member committed suicide, the person's own birthday, or some other emotionally loaded anniversary.

Seasonal patterns, with more suicides during the spring and summer than during the winter, are also characteristic.

Changing phases of life

Entering or leaving a phase of development, such as puberty, middle age, the menopause, or old age, may be perceived as problematic and constitute a risk situation, possibly owing to the loss of the previous content of life before a new one is found or due to a loss of good relationships. People whose happiness has been based on their youth and success in their career may experience ageing as a loss of the youthful, successful self-image and, as such, experience ageing as a process damaging to their self-esteem.

Change caused by contravention of law or norms

A legal problem, being caught breaking the law, having one's driving or gun licence confiscated, being exposed as an embezzler, or any other disclosure that arouses shame will elevate the suicide risk.

Change caused by imprisonment

Immediately after going into prison or in periods when new legal problems arise (e.g., new charges being brought, a sentence being modified, or an appeal to a higher court being rejected), people are in a suicide risk situation that is often overlooked. When a prisoner receives news of illness in the family or the loss of a loved one, or experiences some type of narcissistic injury or rejection, this too is a risk situation for suicide. Otherwise, risk factors for prison inmates do not deviate from those for suicide victims in general. The usual psychiatric, psychosocial, somatic, and personality factors, as described previously in this book, apply (see Chapter 18).

War and natural disasters

The role of war and suicides in the armed forces is described in Chapter 19. Natural disasters, such as floods, hurricanes, and earthquakes may also precipitate suicidal ideation and culminate in suicide among victims.[16]

Narcissistic injury

All the life events described above may contribute to a perception of injury and attack on one's self-worth. Of paramount importance is the way in which a suicidal person perceives the negative life event—the loss, change, or trauma—and, in particular, whether it induces feelings of helplessness and hopelessness. A person's coping strategies and the availability of help (whether others offer it, fail to do so, or even show a negative or hostile attitude) are other crucial variables, together with the inborn and acquired vulnerability. Therapeutically bolstering confidence is an important preventive stratregy.[17]

Sexual and gender minorities and suicidal behaviours

Identity issues as sexuality and sexual orientation are common during adolescence. The term sexual minorities is used for individuals who have lesbian, gay, or bisexual identification (LGB), and the term gender minorities for persons who identify as transgender (T). The term queer is an umbrella term connoting individual identities that fall outside the realm of heterosexuality (LGBTQ). Research has shown that LGBTQ populations are at a greater risk for suicidality compared to their heterosexual counterparts.[18,21]

In an Irish cohort of more than 1,000 students with a mean age of 14 years, five percent reported to have concerns regarding their sexual orientation. When compared to their peers, these students had higher levels of depressive symptoms, anxiety, and markedly increased prevalence of attempted suicide (29% vs. 2%), physical assault (40% vs. 8%), sexual assault (16% vs. 1%), and substance misuse.[19] LGBTQ adolescents are to greater extent victimized, bullied, and harassed verbally, electronically, and physically than their peers. They are more likely to report suicide ideation, regardless of their gender or ethnicity.[20]

Similar findings are reported for adults.[18,21] LGBTQ adults experience often chronic stressors like victimization, bullying, and different kinds of harassment, which have negative effects on their mental health and have serious effects on suicidal ideation and behaviours. Experiencing discrimination is related to suicidality for LGBTQ persons. Persons with LGBTQ identity have several barriers to seeking support, and therefore they are in need of sensitive health services and early preventive interventions specifically addressing their needs. It is also important to provide in different settings, a non-judgemental approach to discuss sexual orientation and mental health issues.

References

1 **Krysinska K, Lester D**. Post-traumatic stress disorder and suicide risk: a systematic review. Archives Suicide Research. 2010;**14**(1):1–23.4.

2 **Zetterqvist M, Lundh LG, Svedin CG**. A comparison of adolescents engaging in self-injurious behaviors with and without suicidal intent: self-reported

experiences of adverse life events and trauma symptoms. J Youth Adolesc. 2013 Aug;**42**(8):1257–1272.

3 Sokolowski M, Ben-Efraim YJ, Wasserman J, Wasserman D. Glutamatergic GRIN2B and polyaminergic ODC1 genes in suicide attempts: associations and gene-environment interactions with childhood/adolescent physical assault. Mol Psychiatry. 2013 Sep;**18**(9):985–992.

4 You Z, Chen M, Yang S, Zhou Z, Qin P. Childhood adversity, recent life stressors and suicidal behavior in Chinese college students. PLoS One. 2014;**9**(3): e 86672.

5 Foster T. Adverse life events proximal to adult suicide: a synthesis of findings from psychological autopsy studies. Arch Suicide Res.2011;**15**(1):1–15.

6 BurónP, Jimenez-Trevino L, Saiz PA, García-Portilla MP, Corcoran P, Carli V, et al. Reasons for attempted suicide in Europe: prevalence, associated factors, and risk of repetition. Arch Suicide Res. 2013;31.

7 Liu RT, Miller I. Life events and suicidal ideation and behavior: a systematic review. Clin Psychol Rev. 2014 Apr;**34**(3):181–192.

8 Oquendo MA, Perez-Rodriguez MM, Poh E, Sullivan G, Burke AK, Sublette ME, et al. Life events: a complex role in the timing of suicidal behavior among depressed patients. Mol Psychiatry. 2014 Aug;**19**(8):902–909.

9 McFeeters D, Boyda D, O'Neill S. Patterns of stressful life events: distinguishing suicide ideators from suicide attempters. J Affect Disord. 2015 Apr;**175**:192–198.

10 Heikkinen ME, Isometsa ET, Aro HM, et al. Age-related variation in recent life events preceding suicide. J Nerv Ment Dis. 1995;**183**:325–331.

11 Nordt C, Warnke I, Seifritz E, Kawohl W. Modelling suicide and unemployment: a longitudinal analysis covering 63 countries, 2000–11. The Lancet Psychiatry. 2015;**2**(3):239–245.

12 Milner A, Spittal MJ, Pirkis J, LaMontagne AD. Suicide by occupation: systematic review and meta-analysis. Br J Psychiatry. 2013 Dec;**203**(6):409–416.

13 Lester D. Native American suicide rates, acculturation stress and traditional integration. Psychol Rep.1999;**84**:398.

14 WooJ-M, Okusaga O, Postolache TT. Seasonality of suicidalbehavior. IJERPH. 2012;**9**(2):531–547.

15 Beauchamp GA, Ho ML, Yin S. Variation in suicide occurrence by day and during major American holidays. J Emerg Med. 2014 Jun;**46**(6):776–781.

16 Kõlves K, Kõlves KE, De Leo D. Natural disasters and suicidal behaviours: a systematic literature review. J Affect Disord. 2013;**146**(1):1–14.

17 Rowe CA, Walker KL, Britton PC, Hirsch JK. The relationship between negative life events and suicidal behavior: moderating role of basic psychological needs. Crisis. 2013 Jan;**34**(4):233–241.

18 Mereish EH, O'Cleirigh C, Bradford JB. Interrelationships between LGBT-based victimization, suicide, and substance use problems in a diverse sample of sexual and gender minorities. Psychol Health Med. 2014;**19**(1):1–13.

19 **Cotter P, Corcoran P, McCarthy J, et al**. Victimisation and psychosocial difficulties associated with sexual orientation concerns: a school-based study of adolescents. Ir Med J. 2014 Nov–Dec;**107**(10):310–313.

20 **Mueller AS, James W, Abrutyn S, Levin ML**. Suicide ideation and bullying among US adolescents: examining the intersections of sexual orientation, gender, and race/ethnicity. Am J Public Health. 2015 May;**105**(5):980–985.

21 **Grant JE, Odlaug BL, Derbyshire K, Schreiber LR, Lust K, Christenson G**. Mental health and clinical correlates in lesbian, gay, bisexual, and queer young adults. J Am Coll Health. 2014;**62**(1):7578.

Chapter 15

Suicidal people's experiences of trauma and negative life events

Danuta Wasserman

Early years leave their mark

Suicidal people's reactions and attitudes to current negative life events must be seen in the light of the frustration of their fundamental needs. Their needs—to be seen, loved, and acknowledged—are not only being frustrated in the current situation but have been since early childhood.[1]

Suicidal people's relationships, past and present, have often been characterized by frustration, narcissistic injury, and rejection. Similarly, their current emotional and cognitive perceptions and reactions are usually loaded with memories and feelings associated with early object losses and a negative emotional climate in the family home. Their parents may have been strict, quick to punish, lacking in empathy, and sometimes indifferent, unemotional, or overprotective, thus overstepping the normal limits of the parental role and failing to respond to the child's needs. With a lack of good examples of communication skills and behaviour during childhood and with suicidal behaviour experienced as a model in the family home, suicidal people tend towards self-destructive acts as a 'way out' when negative life events bring their lack of self-confirmation to the fore.[2–5]

Lack of self-love

Much has been written about narcissism among suicidal people, and there are numerous interpretations of the Narkissos myth. For people who are close to suicide, however, the problem is their lack of self-love rather than any exaggerated 'love of self'. What they experience is a thirst for confirmation from others, and they are devastated by its absence.

Suicidal people long for love, intimacy, and appreciation. Their hunger to satisfy these needs is often masked by their efforts to concealing it. This behaviour may be misinterpreted by others as showing that they are provocative, self-sufficient, cold, and rejecting. Close up, however, the fragility of the deeply distressed and dissatisfied suicidal person's psychological defence mechanisms become apparent.

Shame

Morbid shame about not being loved and appreciated and not being able to live up to the high ideals and standards that suicidal people have usually imposed on themselves is common. They feel inferior, of little worth, weak, and uncertain, while at the same time dreaming of being loved, cherished, and valued. However, their dream of strength and security is thwarted by negative life events. Shame permeates their personality, and arises when their 'shortcomings' are laid bare by a situation of loss and/or offence.

However, suicidal people may be tormented by shame even when they are in fact loved, successful, and good at what they do. They are constantly plagued by an innermost feeling, which stems from their early years, that no one can love them since what is below the surface is so terrible. They cannot enjoy their successes. Their feelings that any acknowledgement they receive is given for something that they have not deserved, and that they have in fact deceived others, reinforces their shame.

The shame pushes them to become different, to 'reinvent' themselves, and if this proves impossible, suicidal impulses become stronger. A desperate urge to wipe out a part of oneself that is perceived as bad can lead to suicidal acts.

Narcissistic injury

Grave injury to self-respect often precipitates suicidal behaviour. Suicidal persons have a disastrous propensity and talent for provoking constant repetitions of various types of injury or offence. Not infrequently, these appear to confirm that they are not loved, needed, or wanted. Many suicidal people are, moreover, sensitive to take offence in situations that would never be perceived as hurtful by other people. This tendency may sometimes be so marked that a long series of trivial or even imaginary offences can be interpreted as a coherent pattern, and suicidal people, therefore, adopt a paranoid attitude towards others. The narcissistic injury does not result in grief and working through, but in bitterness, longing after revenge and furious outbursts, with self-destructive acts as a result.

This does not exclude the possibility that suicidal people may, in fact, be ill-treated by others, including health-care staff. This can be blamed on the individuals' tendency to take offence, which in turn makes them even more implacable and filled with resignation and hate.

Anger and rage

The step from narcissistic injury and shame to anger and rage can be a short one. Suicidal situations are precipitated when people feel that they have been 'revealed' and their innermost beings have been laid bare. This exposure may take place with the disappearance of, for example: a much-loved partner who has contributed greatly to the suicidal person's self-confidence; the caring parent who has looked after the schizophrenic child all his life; wealth or one's beloved country, together with the security that people, circumstances, and things provided. Anger and rage is close when real-life circumstances that have held at bay the undesired self-image no longer exist, since the undesired self-image cannot be fended off solely by means of fantasies. If a person's affect-neutralizing ability is poor, losses and offences are perceived as being so severe, injurious, and insurmountable that the longing to die can seem the only way out.

Guilt

Guilt is another feeling that dominates suicidal people's consciousness.[6] High self-ideals and strict, almost archaic and rigid moral norms contribute to self-reproach, which readily arises when negative life events occur. The next step easily leads to anxiety and guilt about not succeeding, in contrast to others. The sense of guilt may grow strong and prompt efforts to make amends that may sometimes be directly contrary to the suicidal person's own interests and instinct of self-preservation.

A vicious circle may arise when others call this behaviour in question and are surprised or show a non-committal attitude, instead of being grateful—as the suicidal person expects.

Guilt can also be experienced as a result of unconscious or conscious hostile or revenge feelings towards an 'ambivalent' (loved and at the same time hated) lost object.[7]

Guilt caused by hatred of parents, spouse, or other key persons may make a person feel so wicked that suicide may present itself as a deserved punishment. Feelings of guilt and shame also reinforce negative self-perception, with the result that suicide is chosen as a means of escape from this painful awareness.

Despair and hopelessness

Despair and hopelessness concerning the future are often felt by suicidal persons when they experience losses, traumas, and other major life changes. Fantasies of rebirth or reunion with a lost object through suicide can be strong, along with ideas of worthlessness.[8]

Paradoxical behaviour

Suicidal people's behaviour may sometimes be paradoxical, and it is not unusual for this behaviour to bring about negative life events. A suicidal person may have a fear that his or her dependence on confirmation from others, his or her innermost sense of worthlessness, and his or her shame about being abandoned will be discovered. The suicidal person may, therefore, compensate by deluding family members and hospital staff into a false sense of security and may succeed in convincing surrounding people that he or she can manage without their help while at the same time feeling unable to do so. Through rejection of people whom he or she loves or needs, a suicidal person may create an illusion of control over an interpersonal relationship.[9-11]

To avoid disclosure and the need to feel shame for the 'unworthiness' that suicidal people perceive inside themselves, they mask their vulnerability with such defences as fantasies of greatness that emphasize their independence and invulnerability, despite their great dependency and vulnerability.[3]

Denial of real-life circumstances, which results in brutal confrontations that boost the risk of suicide, is another means of self-defence against the own vulnerability. By failing to re-examine their own emotional and cognitive perceptions, suicidal people bring ruin on themselves and put their own lives at stake.

Suicidal people's ambivalence can be used to save their lives, not to hasten death

But what guilt, shame, or hurt can be so great as to make people choose death? There is no universal answer to this question, since individual experience cannot be easily translated from one person to another, or from one person to a group. No generalizations can be made. However, a suicidal person is almost always ambivalent about the choice between life and death to the very last. Ambivalent feelings are mixed feelings. Paralysing doubt alternates with thoughts cast hither and thither, resignation, misgivings, and cancellations. Tunnel vision, which restricts and distorts perceptions, is typical for suicidal individuals.

There is a difference between the healthy ambivalence that is a basic human emotion, the healthy doubt that leads us forward, and the pathological ambivalence that paralyses a person. This pathological ambivalence is a matter of inadequate integration of different affects and their cognitive and intellectual contents. Good and evil identification objects, the wish to live and the wish to die, a need to be extremely dependent and a need to be extremely independent, and love and hate often strongly coexist and compete with each other in suicidal people. Contradictory feelings do not readily become integrated and serve as guidance in how to live a more harmonious life. Even minor negative life events and instances of inadequate support from family and friends may therefore be fatal for suicidal people.

It is essential to listen and respond to the shame, hurt, and guilt expressed by people who have severe suicidal ideation, refer to suicide plans, or tried to attempt suicide. By listening, one may help to detect the ambivalence that is always present in those who are contemplating taking their own lives. This ambivalence can be used to arrest the negative development of the suicidal process and prevent a premature and unnecessary death.

If we are 'deaf' to the suicidal communication and vulnerability of those who are close to suicide, their self-destruction may ensue.[12]

References

1 **Shneidman ES.** The suicidal mind. New York, NY: Oxford University Press; 1996.

2 **Apter A, Plutchik R, Sevy S, et al.** Defense mechanisms in risk of suicide and risk of violence. Am J Psychiatry. 1989;**146**:1027–1031.

3 **Hendin H.** Recognising a suicide crisis in psychiatric patients. In: Wasserman D, Wasserman C (eds). The Oxford textbook of suicidology and suicide prevention: a global perspective. Oxford University Press; 2009: 327–331.

4 **Ronningstam E, Weinberg I, Maltsberger JT.** Psychoanalytic theories of suicide: historical overview and empirical evidence. In: Wasserman D, Wasserman C (eds). The Oxford textbook of suicidology and suicide prevention: a global perspective. Oxford University Press; 2009: 149–158.

5 **Hendin H.** The psychodynamics of suicide. J Nerv Ment Dis.1963;**136**:236–244.

6 **Hendin H, Haas A.** Suicide and guilt as manifestations of PTSD in Vietnam combat veterans. Am J Psychiatry. 1991;**148**:586–591.

7 **Freud S.** Mourning and melancholia. In: Strachey J (ed.). The standard edition of the complete psychological works of Sigmund Freud, volume **XIV**. London: Hogarth Press; 1957: 243–258.

8 **Maltsberger JT, Bui DH.** The devices of suicide: revenge, riddance, and rebirth. Int Rev Psychoanal. 1980;**7**:61–72.

9 **Maltsberger JT, Bui DH.** The psychological vulnerability to suicide. In: Jacobs D, Brown H (eds). Suicide: understanding and responding. Madison CT, US: International Universities Press; 1989:59–72.

10 **Lifton R.** Suicide. In: Jacobs D, Brown H (eds). Suicide: understanding and responding. Madison CT, US: International Universities Press; 1989:459–469.

11 **Duilt RA, Michaels R.** Psychodynamics and suicide. In: Jacobs D (ed.). Suicide and clinical practice. Washington, DC: American Psychiatric Press; 1990: 44–53.

12 **Wolk-Wasserman D.** Attempted suicide: the patient's family, social network and therapy (doctoral dissertation). Stockholm: Karolinska Institute; 1986.

Chapter 16

Attempted suicide as a risk factor for suicide

Lars Mehlum

Introduction

Attempted suicide is a major public health problem in most countries. Prevalence figures vary depending on age, gender, and context (clinical or general population). Population studies generally report much higher rates; young people report higher rates and suicide attempts are generally more prevalent in females than in males. For example, the Irish National Registry of Deliberate Self Harm, established in 2002, reported[1] in 2012 an overall rate of such self-harm at 211 per 100,000 with more presentations among women (228 per 100,000) than men (195 per 100,000), higher rates among younger people with a peak rate for women in the 15–19-year age group and higher rates in cities than in rural districts. Drug overdose was the most common method of self-harm (69%), followed by cutting (23%). Attempts peaked in the hours around midnight and alcohol was involved in 38% of cases.

In addition to suicide attempts the increasing prevalence of non-suicidal self-injury (NSSI) (self-harm without any suicide intent) particularly in the young is a huge public health challenge, with far higher prevalence estimates than the ones mentioned above. There are some significant differences in the way attempted suicide and NSSI should be understood and managed by clinicians, but the boundary between the two is not easy to draw in every case.

Risk factors for completed suicide

Attempted suicide is the strongest and probably most universal of all known predictors of suicide. According to follow-up studies, approximately 10% of those who have been admitted for psychiatric treatment after a suicide attempt will eventually commit suicide. An additional 10–50%, depending on population characteristics, will repeat their suicide attempts. Within the group of suicide attempters the following characteristics seem to indicate a higher risk of later suicide:[2–5]

+ male sex;
+ age above 45 years;
+ separated, divorced, or widowed status;
+ unemployment or old-age retirement;
+ chronic somatic illness;
+ major psychiatric disorder;
+ personality disorder;
+ alcohol or other substance use disorder;
+ use of violent methods for suicide; and
+ leaving of a suicide note.

Mood disorders, such as major depression or bipolar disorder and schizophrenia, certain personality disorders, and substance use disorders are all well-documented risk factors for suicide. Severe anxiety disorders such as panic disorder may also lead to an increased risk of suicide. The danger of completed suicide is generally greatest in the first year (and particularly in the first three months) after the suicide attempt,[2–5] as many people will be more vulnerable to stress during this period. Psychiatric disorders often lead to a suicide attempt despite the fact that treatment may have reduced the symptom level. Most suicide attempters will need protection and support and this should be sustained throughout the first year after the suicidal crisis.

Despite the evident danger of suicide, it is important to remember that on average 90% of suicide attempters will survive according to follow-up studies.[6] For many suicide attempters the suicidal crisis was the turning point for them to be offered or to be able to receive help and psychiatric treatment. However, many suicide attempters do not seek further treatment after they have been discharged from emergency medical care and they have a high tendency of dropping out of the treatment even if they accept trying it. Clinicians should, therefore, make every effort to actively engage these patients in follow-up treatments and try as much as possible to reduce obstacles to receiving such treatment. The crisis should be regarded as a window of opportunity for patients, with support from health-care personnel, to solve problems that would otherwise not be identified or available for change.

Clinical challenges

When working with suicide attempters, clinicians are faced with several challenges:

- keeping the patient safe, by protecting the patient against suicide or irreversible injury;
- reducing the patient's profound feeling of hopelessness;
- re-establishing a sense of connectedness to other people;
- engaging the patient in treatment and motivating change; and
- helping the patient increase their subjective experience of the quality of life.

Although it will depend on the nature of the injury, patients who have attempted suicide will often initially require treatment in an emergency room and then need to be observed for the next 1–3 days in an acute medical ward. A psychiatric examination, in which an adequate history is taken and the suicide intent and the risk of suicide is evaluated, should be conducted as early as possible during this early treatment phase and in any event before the patient is discharged from hospital.

The psychiatric consultation should provide information that is necessary for treatment planning, and it should also serve as a clinical intervention focusing on the patient's most critical problems and psychological needs. Establishing a therapeutic alliance, even in the case of short-term emergency treatment, is of utmost importance for the prospect of successful treatment of patients in suicidal crises. While patients must get the opportunity to recover from their medical condition (e.g., the intoxication) in an atmosphere of kindness and reassurance, most patients also need to give verbal expression to their problems and emotions, with the therapist's help. Sometimes, these expressions of emotions or expectations or demands from the patient may make therapists feel uncomfortable, helpless, or angry and negative 'transactions' between the patient and therapist may develop. Therapists should not neglect to actively validate how hard it must feel for the patient to go through all of the problems having led to the crisis and to comply with the requirements in the treatment. It is important to remember that whereas the therapist needs to validate the patient, they should not validate the suicidal behaviour.

After the initial medical treatment is completed, some patients can be discharged and followed up on an outpatient basis. Before discharge, the clinician should re-evaluate the suicide risk and a 'safety plan' should be made in collaboration with the patient.[7] A safety plan is a step-by-step list of measures to be taken when the risk of suicidal behaviour increases and it spans from what the patient can do alone to what the patient can do with the help from family or friends and with help from health-care personnel. It should also include a list of warning signs that this particular patient typically experiences when the risk is on the rise. The safety plan will often help the patient more effectively tolerate distress and suicidal feelings without acting on them. Before patients are discharged from emergency treatment it is important to involve the family, if possible, in order to organize protective measures, motivation for treatment, increase the patient's compliance, and to give emotional support. The family must be given proper information (provided that the patient does not object to this).

Hospital treatment

The presence of one or more of the following characteristics indicates that the patient should be transferred without delay for psychiatric inpatient treatment:

◆ suicide attempt made with a high degree of suicidal intent;

◆ continued desire or plan for suicide;

◆ symptoms of severe mental disorder, such as major depression or psychosis, and alcohol or other substance use disorders;

◆ poor impulse control or weak barriers against suicide;

- poor social support; and
- recent severe social stressors, loss, or emotional trauma.

Sometimes, the patient refuses to be hospitalized. If in such cases there is imminent danger to the patient's life, involuntary inpatient treatment is often necessary. When the patient is transferred to a psychiatric inpatient unit there is a need to promote the establishment of a new therapeutic alliance through measures mentioned above. A clinical re-evaluation should be conducted immediately and, depending on the results, all necessary safety measures should be undertaken to place the patient in a secure room with safety windows and to remove the patient's belt, razors, and other dangerous objects. Some patients must be observed continuously; in any case, frequent observations are needed. Control measures have the potential of threatening the patient's personal integrity and should, therefore, be implemented with care and respect.

Before free exit or home leave is permitted, careful evaluation must be performed and the patient's family should be informed. The patient's safety plan should be revised or if no such plan has been made, there is a need to do it now and help the patient make use of it. To a certain extent the patient's impulse control can be strengthened, symptoms alleviated, and the tendency of substance abuse reduced through effective use of antidepressant or antipsychotic agents (or both). If a patient who has signs of major depression does not respond to antidepressants or if it is too risky to wait for several weeks for the antidepressants to become effective, a trial of electroconvulsive therapy may be appropriate.

Suicide attempts in the elderly

The suicide rate in single men over 80 years of age is particularly high. The mortality from suicide increases with social isolation and particularly after loss of a spouse. Previous suicide attempts, particularly suicide attempts using highly lethal methods, in elderly men and women generally imply a much higher risk of subsequent completion of suicide than they do in young people.

Elderly patients who attempt suicide, often suffer from major depression, which is frequently related to social isolation or a sense of worthlessness linked to a reduced physical or mental capability.[8] Somatic illness or polypharmacy may also give rise to depression or pharmacological side-effects. It is extremely important that, in addition to the psychopharmacological treatment of depression, these challenges are dealt with psychotherapeutically or through social work or family interventions by personnel who are sensitive to the existential aspects of these complex problems. Somatic problems must also be diagnosed and treated. In the short term it is seldom possible to invoke radical changes for the better in the patient's life. However, even minor changes may have the potential of reducing the patient's feeling of hopelessness; this is an important objective in all clinical interventions with suicidal patients.

Young suicide attempters

In young suicide attempters, depression is often prominent. In some cases the depressive symptoms are part of a pervasive pattern of emotion dysregulation linked to personality dysfunction.[9] This pattern will often lead to additional problems with interpersonal functioning, academic performance, substance abuse, and physical health. Some of these young people have developed a pattern of chronic suicidal behaviour, and in these cases there is a need for specialized psychiatric treatment, such as dialectic behavioural therapy[10] or mentalization-based treatment[11] after the acute crisis has subsided.

Young females who have developed suicidal feelings seem generally to possess better help-seeking skills and to be more easily available for assessment and treatment than young males that are often more avoidant and reluctant to seek treatment. Active strategies to engage these young people in treatment and to counteract treatment interfering behaviours such as not showing up for therapy sessions, not taking prescribed medication, or not completing inter-session homework assignments, are necessary. Parents and/or other family members should be involved in the process of treatment of minors unless there is a special reason to avoid this (e.g., the patient having been sexually abused by one of the parents) and to adopt a family format is often recommendable.

Outpatient treatment

After discharge from emergency medical care or from psychiatric inpatient treatment, there is normally a need for follow-up care, the duration of which must be adapted to each patient's need. Depending on the clinical picture there may be a need for follow-up of medication, referral for alcohol or drug rehabilitation, and individual or family therapy. Some patients can rely on their family doctor to coordinate the various treatment components. In many cases, however, patients have difficulties seeking help or complying with the treatment that is offered to them. This calls for an active and rehabilitative approach from the therapist's side. In some agencies organized teams follow-up suicide attempters through home visits and practical and problem-solving-oriented assistance during the first few weeks after discharge from hospital.[12] It is very important to create a continuous chain of care, beginning with the emergency phase of the treatment, continuing with hospital treatment and leading eventually to some form of after-care programme.

Systematic reviews[13] examining the effectiveness of psychosocial interventions in reducing repetition rates of suicide attempts have indicated that brief structured psychotherapies, more specifically cognitive behaviour therapy,[14] problem-solving therapy,[15] and interpersonal psychotherapy[16] have shown reduced repetition rates of suicide attempts and increased patient adherence to the active treatment compared to standard care. Furthermore, as mentioned above, several treatments specifically developed for patients with borderline personality disorder with a pattern of repetitive suicide attempts, such as dialectical behaviour therapy[10] and mentalization-based treatment[11] have proven successful in reducing subsequent rates of suicide attempts.

Case Study

Jill is a 45-year-old woman who discovers that her husband has had an affair with a younger woman during the last six months. She tells him to leave and files for divorce. Gradually, however, she feels increasingly depressed, hopeless, and suicidal. After having ingested all of her sleeping pills, she is brought to the general hospital emergency room in a drowsy state by her sister. After the acute medical procedures have been completed,

Jill is very sleepy and she is kept under close observation at the acute medical ward. Next morning she is seen by the consultant psychiatrist who listens carefully to her story at the same time as he makes diagnostic evaluations and assesses the risk for further suicidal behaviour.

Although Jill is clearly depressed, she is glad that she survived the suicide attempt. It seems that there is a clear need to treat the depression with a suitable antidepressant and that Jill will need psychotherapeutic support to cope with the loss and the conflict and the profound changes going on in her life. Before she is discharged from hospital, a safety plan is worked out together with Jill, an appointment at an outpatient psychiatric clinic is made, and Jill's sister comes for a brief meeting with Jill and the psychiatrist. A year later when Jill has her last appointment at the outpatient clinic, she has fully recovered from her depression and there have been no further suicide attempts.

References

1 Griffin E, Arensman E, Wall A, Corcoran P, Perry IJ. National Registry of Deliberate Self Harm Ireland. Annual Report 2012. Cork, National Suicide Research Foundation; 2013.

2 Goldacre M, Seagroatt V, Hawton K. Suicide after discharge from psychiatric inpatient care. Lancet. 1993;342:283–286.

3 Haw C, Bergen H, Casey D, Hawton K. Repetition of deliberate self-harm: a study of the characteristics and subsequent deaths in patients presenting to a general hospital according to extent of repetition. Sui Life Threat Behav. 2007;37:379–396.

4 Angst F, Stassen HH, Clayton PJ, Angst J. Mortality of patients with mood disorders: follow-up over 34–38 years. J Affect Disord. 2002;68:167–181.

5 Suominen K, Isometsa E, Suokas J, et al. Completed suicide after a suicide attempt: a 37-year follow-up study. Am J Psych. 2004;161:562–563.

6 Retterstøl N. Long-term prognosis after attempted suicide. Thomas: Springfield; 1970.

7 Stanley BH, Brown GK. Safety planning intervention: a brief intervention to mitigate suicide risk. Cogn Behav Pract 2012;19(2):256–264.

8 Fässberg MM, van Orden KA, Duberstein P, et al. A systematic review of social factors and suicidal behavior in older adulthood. Int J Environ Res Public Health. 2012;9(3):722–745.

9 Mehlum L, Friis S, Vaglum P, Karterud S. The longitudinal pattern of suicidal behaviour in borderline personality disorder: a prospective follow-up study. Acta Psych Scand. 1994;90: 124–130.

10 Linehan MM, Heard HL, Armstrong HE. Naturalistic follow-up of a behavioral treatment for chronically parasuicidal borderline patients. Arch Gen Psych. 1993;50:971–974.

11 Bateman A, Fonagy P. Effectiveness of partial hospitalization in the treatment of borderline personality disorder: a randomized controlled trial. Am J Psych. 1999;156:1563–1569.

12 **Mehlum L, Mork E, Reinholdt NP, Fadum EA, Rossow I.** Quality of psychosocial care of suicide attempters at general hospitals in Norway—a longitudinal nation-wide study. Arch Sui Res. 2010;**14**(2):146–157.

13 **Crawford MJ, Kumar, P.** Intervention following deliberate self-harm: enough evidence to act? Evid-Based Ment Health. 2007;**10**:37–39.

14 **Brown GK, Ten HT, Henriques GR, et al.** Cognitive therapy for the prevention of suicide attempts: a randomized controlled trial. JAMA 2005;**294**:563–570.

15 **Salkovskis PM, Atha C, Storer D.** Cognitive-behavioural problem solving in the treatment of patients who repeatedly attempt suicide. A controlled trial. Br J Psych. 1990;**157**:871–876.

16 **Guthrie E, Kapur N, Kway-Jones K, Chew-Graham C, et al.** Randomised controlled trial of brief psychological intervention after deliberate self-poisoning. BMJ. 2001;**323**:135–138.

Chapter 17

Immigrant populations and suicide

Ahmed Hankir and Dinesh Bhugra

Setting the scene: a narrative offering a qualitative insight into suicidal behaviour in refugees

> Imagine that you are an Afghani refugee. You are a single mother with two children who has fled an abusive marriage, and survived two rapes, including one in a refugee detention centre that resulted in pregnancy. You have endured separation from your supportive parents, who die in Afghanistan while you are still awaiting asylum. While attempting to cope with all this, together with unemployment, isolation and ostracism from your ethnic community, you hear that your refugee claim has been denied. In despair, you threaten to kill yourself and your children.
>
> (Reproduced from *Lost in Translation: Mental Health of Newcomers*, written for New Canadian Media by Aparna Sanyal (2014))

Introduction

Culture plays a crucial role in the crafting of a community's collective character. Moreover, the cultural community that a person is embedded in ineluctably has an influence on that individual's cognitive schema, behaviour, occupational and social functioning, and modus operandi. Culture can also have an effect on how vulnerable or resilient people are responding to psychiatric disease, stress, and other factors that can precipitate suicidal behaviour. Culture, conversely, can also confer protection against suicidal behaviour.

Culture has been defined as the 'Learned, shared and transmitted values, beliefs, norms and life ways of a particular group [of people] that guides their thinking, decision-making, and actions in patterned [stereotypical] ways'.[1] We know that culture is integrated; people acquire and assimilate culture. Although culture can change (gradually or abruptly), culture also ensures generational continuity.

It is society and culture—through the proxy of policymakers—that determines the provision of physical and mental health-care services (and the parity or *dis*parity of esteem between the two) and those who may receive and use them. A given culture can also determine what is considered to be mental illness (i.e., Muslims have been known to attribute mental and psychological phenomena to Jinn possession and/or the 'evil eye'; the explanatory models that a cultural group formulates can influence why they may, for instance, consult a faith healer as opposed to a general practitioner and, hence, not receive the benefits of early intervention).

Birthplace is an index of migration and as such can form part of the definition of a migrant ethnic population. Immigrants, particularly refugees, have long been treated as a marginalized, stigmatized, and socially excluded people from their destination culture. This and other issues that immigrants can encounter (i.e., acculturation stress, poverty, unemployment, and the inability to speak the dominant language, to name but a few) can have profound effects on their mental well-being, so much so that they may resort to tragically ending their lives with their own hands.

The lack of culturally competent health-care practitioners and culturally sensitive and personalized mental health services can present as major barriers for immigrants to accessing and engaging with the relevant services. This, consequently, and in no small measure, can cause immigrants to resort to suicidal behaviour.

The focus of this chapter is suicidal behaviour in migrant groups and refugees. We will discuss and analyse the social and cultural factors that influence suicidal behaviour in this population, the obstacles to treatment and early intervention, and prevention and management strategies targeted at this specific group.

Suicidal behaviour in immigrant groups in Europe

There are various terms describing self-harm, such as attempted suicide, parasuicide, deliberate self-harm (DSH), and non-suicidal self-injury (NSSI).[2] It is not only a simple matter of theoretical concepts, but perceptions of those behaviours vary dramatically across cultures. In some settings it is likely that the self will be more socio-centric and, therefore, will include others who may be 'harmed' in some way whereas in other cultural settings the self-harm may be directed at one self in an ego-centric way. Despite controversy surrounding the term deliberate self-harm, we use it interchangeably with attempted suicide in this chapter since we are explaining and describing suicidal behaviour as a whole.

Bursztein[3] et al. compared the frequencies of attempted suicide among immigrants and their European hosts, between different immigrant groups in Europe, and between immigrants in Europe and their countries of origin.

Data on 27,048 persons, including 4,160 immigrants, were collected from the WHO/EURO Multicentre Study on Suicidal Behaviour (the largest database available in Europe) from 11 European centres between 1989 and 2003. Person-based suicide-attempt rates (SARs) were calculated for each of the 56 immigrant groups. Completed suicide rates of their countries of origin were compared with the SARs of the immigrant groups.[3]

This landmark study revealed some important findings: 27/56 (48.2%) of the immigrant groups studied showed significantly higher—and only 4/56 (7.1%) significantly lower—SARs than their hosts. Interestingly, immigrant groups tended to have similar rates across different centres. Moreover, there was a positive correlation between the immigrant SAR and the country-of-origin suicide rate. However, Chileans, Iranians, Moroccans, and Turks displayed high SARs as immigrants despite low suicide rates in their home countries.[4] A similar trend was found in another European study involving ten countries (Turkey, Switzerland, Belgium, Finland, Israel, the Netherlands, Italy, Sweden, Estonia, and Germany). This study also revealed that the highest rates of suicide attempts among immigrants generally corresponded to higher rates of suicide in the country of origin.[4]

Bursztein and colleagues concluded that the generally higher suicide attempt rates among immigrants compared to host populations and the similarity of the rates of foreign-born and those immigrants who retained the citizenship of their country of origin point to difficulties in the acculturation and integration process. Most importantly, perhaps, is the positive correlation found between attempted and completed suicide rates which suggests that the two are related, a fact with strong implications for suicide prevention.[3]

Specific factors in suicidal behaviour

Self-harm and suicidal behaviour have existed for millennia across the different cultures, albeit each specific culture may attach its own unique meaning to these acts. Thakur[5] discusses two types of suicide: religious suicide and general suicide. Religious suicide has been observed in both the Hindu and Jain religions.[6] General suicide encompasses social, economic, and political dimensions. Politically motivated suicides tend to be dramatic and carried out in public.[7]

Some cultures glorify suicide (i.e., historically the notorious Japanese Kamikaze pilots and more contemporarily the radicalized suicide bombers with their own interpretations of religious scripture and ideologies); others prohibit it (i.e., certain religious groups such as Islam and Catholicism). Both the person's cultural background and the destination culture that the individual is migrating to can influence their 'cultural identity' and his or her proclivity towards suicidal behaviours.

The term self-harm evidently incorporates the word 'self' and the concept of 'self' has great variation across cultural groups. A culture that has a socio-centric concept of self would mean that a member of that culture who engages in self-harm behaviour can unintentionally 'harm' those who may encompass him or her since the socio-centric concept of self transcends the plane of the egocentric self. This can be a protective factor since the person contemplating suicidal behaviour may not want to harm those who have his or her best interests in their hearts and hence this would preclude them from carrying out the act.

Conversely, the concept of the self as being socio-centric can also be a risk factor since acts of self-harm can be aimed towards certain individuals in order to antagonize them and/or to communicate a message to them. For example, in an arranged marriage, a young Asian female who has migrated to a British culture and left her family behind her in India may feel isolated, trapped, and 'voiceless'. She may feel that the only way of getting her voice heard is by killing herself as has tragically been noted in case studies. Indeed, the results of a prospective study revealed that females of Asian origin who migrated to England who attempted suicide reported arranged marriages to be a contributory factor for their suicidal behaviour.[8]

There are studies that have implicated both age and gender as risk factors for completed suicide. Kliewer examined the factors influencing the suicide rates of numerous immigrant groups in a number of developed cosmopolitan countries, such as Australia, Canada, England and Wales, and the US. Age-specific suicide rates indicated that relative to the native-born, foreign-born older males, 65 years and older had substantially elevated risk of suicide. Overall, however, there were higher rates of suicide in native-born males than that for the foreign-born. By contrast, with the exception of ages 25–39 years, the foreign-born females had higher rates than the native-born females.[9]

There are a number of factors which may contribute to the deleterious effect of migration on females. For example, in many instances, the decision to migrate is made by the man. In a patriarchal culture, women may have little if any influence on the decision to migrate. Moreover, they are frequently less cognizant and less prepared for the difficulties they may encounter in the destination culture.[9]

'Culture conflict' and 'culture shock'

The term 'culture conflict' describes tensions between individuals or even the struggle that an individual has with oneself when they attempt to resolve and integrate perceived or real irreconcilable values.[10]

An individual may have with oneself a conflict concerning one's own 'soul'. Take, for example, a single Muslim Saudi Arabian man who has migrated to a Western destination culture where prostitution and alcohol are legal. That very man must, if he cares to abide by the tenets of Islam, attempt to resist these temptations which are seemingly ubiquitous. Despite the fact that he may be a pious and devout individual he is, after all, a human being and as such it is only natural for him to have a desire to succumb to the temptation. He may not be able to resist this powerful impulse and by capitulating to it be engulfed by remorse and pathos for (in his perception) betraying his faith. A possible consequence of this is the development of suicidal ideation and behaviour in the context of a severe depressive illness as has been evidenced in clinical case studies.[11]

Regarding tensions between individuals we can use the example of when a younger member of a migrant family is attracted to the destination culture he or she is thrust into. This young immigrant may individuate and deviate from the culture of origin and imitate the prevailing culture. The family may then attempt to reel the perceived maverick youth back into the fold and inculcate him or her with traditional cultural values. Here, we have a clash between the ostensibly dichotomous orthodox values of the origin culture and the less traditional values of the destination culture. This can result in the renegade individual feeling melancholic, isolated, ostracized, and, in extreme cases, suicidal. This would be consistent with the findings of research into intergenerational conflict in young people of Asian origin in the US which showed that intergenerational conflict increased the risk of suicide by thirtyfold, especially in less-educated young people.[12]

Culture conflict should be distinguished from 'culture shock' which is what individuals may experience after migration as their adjustment to the destination culture may occur over a prolonged and protracted period. There is, however, a degree of overlap between the two. Culture shock has been defined as the 'Sudden unpleasant feelings that violate an individual's expectations of the new culture [they have migrated to] and cause them to value their own culture negatively'.[13] Oberg identified six aspects of culture shock: strain; a sense of loss or feelings of deprivation; rejection by members of the new culture; role expectation and role confusion; surprise, anxiety, and indignation; and feelings of impotence.[14]

Refugee mental health

It is important to differentiate between groups who have migrated voluntarily and those who have migrated through compulsion; for example, the exodus of Syrians into Turkey due to the conflict in their country of origin. Refugees are perhaps the most vulnerable group of all immigrants. According to the Geneva Convention (1951), a refugee is a person who has a 'well-founded fear of being persecuted for reasons of race, religion, nationality, membership of a particular social group or a particular political opinion, is outside the country of their nationality and cannot, or will not, because of fear, benefit from the protection of that country'.

Conflict in the refugee's country of origin may result in the development of severe psychopathology such as post-traumatic stress disorder and major depressive disorder. Severe psychiatric illnesses in refugees may be a prelude to suicidal ideation. This and the way in which they are received by the destination country, dilapidated living conditions, and lack of social support and isolation all contribute and conspire to rendering this immigrant group particularly vulnerable to suicidal behaviour.[15]

Some migrant populations (including refugees) are wealthy, whereas others are in abject poverty. We should, therefore, realize that the phenomenon of migration is complex and we should not come to any simple conclusions about the way in which migration influences social experience and health.

Prevention and management strategies for suicidal behaviour in immigrants

Sometimes the clinician has a stereotyped approach, has not had interpreters available, or is unaware of crucial cultural factors when they encounter an immigrant who may have suicidal ideation pervading and permeating their mind. In order to tackle these issues, many models are available. These include culture brokers and cultural mediators as well as cultural liaison workers. The underlying principle, by and large, is that they will function as interlocutors and communicate between the services and the community the services are catering for. In Canada, for example, cultural consultation is always done with an interpreter and, if needed, a culture broker (Jaswant Guzder, Associate Professor, Department of Psychiatry, McGill University—2014 personal communication) and that the primary aim is to establish cultural safety, and to explore all aspects of the presenting complaint.

The lack of translation services is a factor that severely impacts immigrant patients and prevents the completion of a thorough assessment and the offering of therapy. The provision of translation services may enable mental health service providers to detect the early warning signs of suicidal behaviour in immigrant patients and consequently facilitate timely intervention to prevent completed suicides from occurring.

There have been further developments addressing the language barrier issue with many organizations developing leaflets in different languages. Indeed, there is evidence that supports the efficacy of leaflets in educating immigrant, cultural, and religious groups about mental illness and distress.[16]

Assessment of suicide risk in immigrants

Mental health practitioners are expected to perform a thorough and comprehensive assessment of suicide risk on an immigrant who presents to services in a crisis as they would do with any other service user. There are, however, other factors that are unique to this population and that must also be taken into consideration:

- It reflects good practice to obtain knowledge about the minority group that the service user belongs to—particularly their cultural stance on suicide—prior to initiating the interview process. Confer with a colleague who may be familiar with (or indeed from the same) cultural background as the service user. Consult the hospital religious services which should be able to provide vital information and advice on suicidal behaviours, from the perspective of different religious groups.

- Be aware that individuals from minority groups may be less likely to disclose information on suicidal behaviour (i.e., out of shame and stigma from being ostracized from society and the negative effects their suicidal behaviour can have on their family's social standing in their cultural community).

♦ Respect and be extremely sensitive to cultural differences when assessing risk of suicide in an immigrant. Above all else you are duty bound to behave professionally regardless of what your own personal views on suicidal behaviour may be.

A personalized approach to suicidal behaviour in immigrants

To the world you may be just one person but to one person you may be the world.

(Bill Wilson)

Dignity is in the heart of everything that we do in the provision of mental health-care services. It can be all too easy to be prescriptive when assessing and treating a service user and the person can be lost in the protocol. By all means we condone and commend adherence to treatment algorithms and guidelines formulated by a robust evidence-base in the management of suicidal behaviour in immigrants; however, there can never be a replacement for personalized treatments (and perhaps in no other specialty is this more possible than in psychiatry). Although there may be a wealth of data that supports the efficacy of pharmacotherapy in the management of severe mental illness that can precipitate suicidal behaviour, some service users may not opt to 'popping pills' because their culture perceives this to be a sign of. There are case studies that support the use of cognitive behavioural therapy in immigrants who present with severe psychiatric illnesses.[17] We encourage mental health-care service providers to take a holistic and personalized approach in the assessment and treatment of immigrants who present with suicidal behaviour, to deploy the 'soft skills' of listening and empathy to allow the narratives to unfold and flow, and, consequently, a rapport and therapeutic alliance to become established. Sometimes, just being made to feel that someone is genuinely listening to you with all earnestness and compassion and that someone actually cares can be the antidote that a lonely and forlorn human being needs, to nourish their soul with. In this scenario, non-verbal (and non-judgemental) communication and tranquil silence can be more efficacious than any drug and offer a safe sanctuary where deep and seemingly indelible wounds can heal.

Conclusion

Culture is dynamic and affects all aspects of illness and behaviour (including suicidal behaviour). The 'idioms of distress' that immigrants use may not necessarily match diagnostic criteria and although culture is being homogenized by globalization, there are no universal models of psychotherapy or pharmacotherapy for the treatment of mental illness that may be heralded by suicidal behaviour. To summarize succinctly: one size does *not* fit all.

Assessing the mental health needs of immigrants includes openness to exploring cultural formulations to elicit the meaning of symptoms. A presenting complaint has to be explored to understand the suffering behind the symptom. Indeed, Oliver Sacks in the preface of his best-selling book *The Man who Mistook his Wife for a Hat* argues that '. . . in order to restore the human subject at the centre, the suffering, afflicted, fighting human subject, we have to deepen a case history into a narrative or tale'.

As in other areas of medicine, education is key and training in cultural competency should be part of the curriculum for all mental health pro-fessionals, including teachers, nurses, and medical students in attempts to fathom the idioms of distress of immigrant groups, to detect psy-chopathology that may be a prelude to suicidal behaviour, and to offer timely intervention to prevent attempted or completed suicide from tak-ing place.

References

1 **Leininger M, McFarland M**. Transcultural nursing: concepts, theories, research, and practice. 3rd edn. New York, NY: McGraw-Hill; 2002.
2 **Brunner R, Kaess M, Parzer P, Fischer G, Carli V, . . . Wasserman D**. Life-time prevalence and psychosocial correlates of adolescent direct self-injurious behavior:

a comparative study of findings in 11 European countries. J Child Psychol Psychiatry. 2014;**55**(4):337–348.

3 **Bursztein-Lipsicas C, Mäkinen IH, Apter A, De Leo D, Kerkhof A, . . . Wasserman D**. Attempted suicide among immigrants in European countries: an international perspective. Soc Psychiatry Psychiatr Epidemiol. 2012 Feb;**47**(2):241–251. doi: 10.1007/s00127–010–03363–6. Epub 1 Jan 2011.

4 **Voracek M, Loibl LM**. Consistency of immigrant and country-of-birth suicide rates: a meta-analysis. Acta Psych Scan. 2008;**118**(4):259–271.

5 **Thakur U**. The history of suicides in India. Delhi: Mushiram Manohar Lal publications; 1963.

6 **Embree L**. Phenomenology of the cultural disciplines. Springer; 1994.

7 **Bhugra D**. Politically motivated suicides. Br J Psychiatry 1991;**159**:594–595.

8 **Bhugra D, Desai M**. Attempted suicide in South Asian women. Adv Psychiatr Treat. 2002;**8**:418–423.

9 **Kliewer EV, Ward RH**. Convergence of immigrant suicide rates to those in the destination country. Am J Epidemiology. August 1987;**127**(3):640–653.

10 **Bhugra D, Becker M**. Migration, cultural bereavement and cultural identity. World Psychiatry. February 2005;**4**(1):18–24.

11 **Hankir A, Zaman R**. Jung's archetype, 'The Wounded Healer', mental illness in the medical profession and the role of the health humanities in psychiatry. BMJ Case Rep 2013;2013:pii: bcr2013009990

12 **Bursztein LC, Makinen IH**. Immigration and suicidality in the young. Can J Psychiatry 2010;**55**(5):274–281.

13 **Bhugra D, Ayonrinde O**. Depression in migrants and ethnic minorities. Adv Psychiatr Treat. 2004;**10**:13–17; doi:10.1192/apt.10.1.13.

14 **Oberg K**. Culture shock: adjustment to new culture environments. Practical Anthropology. 1960;**7**:177–182.

15 **Bhugra D, Gupta S, Bhui K, et al**. WPA guidance on mental health and mental health care in migrants. World Psychiatry. 2011;**10**(1):2–10.

16 **Bhugra D**. Migration and mental health. Acta Psychiatrica Scandinavica. 2004;**109**(4):243–258.

17 **Walsh K, Hope DA**. LGB-affirmative cognitive-behavioral treatment for social anxiety: a case study applying evidence-based practice principles. Cogn Behav Pract 2010;**17**:56–65.

Chapter 18

Suicide in the criminal justice system

Marco Sarchiapone

Introduction

People who have contact with the criminal justice system (with or without jail or prison sentence) represent a high-risk group for suicidal behaviour, with a significantly higher rate of suicide than in the general population. Detention and restraint of freedom may be considered to be proximal risk factors for suicidal behaviours, since they may act as a trigger in people vulnerable to suicide, such as those with psychiatric and personality disorders, with impulsive/aggressive traits or with a history of childhood trauma.[1] The rate of suicide attempts and completed suicide seems to be higher among offenders who have experienced childhood trauma, especially emotional or physical abuse, or emotional neglect.[1]

Socio-demographic characteristics

Several socio-demographic factors are associated with a risk for suicide in people in contact with the criminal justice system.[2]

Gender: Fazel et al.,[3] collecting data on suicides and undetermined deaths in prisons in 12 countries, found that of 861 suicides in prison, 810 were men, with a rate of suicides among males around three to seven times higher than in the general population. It was shown that men show a higher risk of suicide than women after discharge from prison.[4]

Age: The rate of suicidal behaviour increases with the age of the inmate.[5] Mumola found that inmates aged 18–24 had the lowest probability to commit suicide; this rate steadily increased for the age ranges 25–34 and 35–44. The highest rate of suicide was found for the inmates aged 55 plus. However, the average age of suicide among prisoners is lower than in general population.[6]

Ethnicity: Several researchers reported a higher rate of suicidal behaviours among white prisoners. White prison inmates, compared with black inmates, showed an 86% higher death rate and their death rate was twice as high as the rate of Hispanic inmates.[7] Pratt et al.[8] confirmed a lower risk of suicide for offenders with non-white ethnicity.

Marital status: Research shows a positive association between suicidal behaviour and single status of prisoners.[9]

Psychiatric diseases

The prevalence of psychiatric disorders among prisoners is higher than in the general population.[10] Suicidal behaviours in prisoners are significantly associated with higher rates of psychosis, depression, history of alcohol misuse, and/or drugs misuse. Schizophrenia and personality disorders, especially antisocial personality disorder, increase the risk of suicide among offenders.[11]

Rivlin et al.[1] showed that compared with controls, prisoners had higher levels of impulsivity, aggression, and hostility, and significantly lower self-esteem. Also, in a sample of 1,265 Italian male prisoners, higher levels of impulsivity and aggression were reported in offenders with suicidal behaviours, in comparison with those who did not display such behaviour.[12]

Suicide risk assessment and treatment of prisoners

The critical period for suicidal behaviour among prisoners is within seven days of admission into prison. For this reason a risk assessment for suicide should be performed as soon as possible. The screening should preferably be conducted by trained professionals, with specific expertise in psychology and psychiatry. It should be taken into account that the presence of one or more of the following factors may be indicative of an increased risk of suicide and highlight a need for intervention: current thoughts about suicide and/or previous suicide attempts; history of substance abuse; high levels of shame, guilt, and worry; hopelessness, crying, lack of emotions, lack of verbal expression, fear about the future; signs of psychiatric disorders, such as depression, psychosis, anxiety, and/or aggression; history of trauma; previous treatment for a mental health problem; current use of psychotropic medication, and poor support from the family.[13] Self-harm in prison is also a clear a risk factor for suicide—especially among women who self-harm several times per year.[14] Even if suicide among prisoners has specific characteristics, the indications for their prevention can follow the recommendations for general suicidal behaviour treatment.[15] Establishing a therapeutic alliance is fundamental in order to increase the possibility of successful treatment of the prisoner. If possible, social interaction should be facilitated and segregation or isolation cells should be avoided. In some cases, hospitalization should be considered, especially in case of high suicidal intent, suicide plans, symptoms of severe mental disorders, poor impulse control, and poor social support. Moreover, it is fundamental to involve the patient's family and facilitate contact with them.

Effective programmes for suicide prevention in prison

Suicidal behaviour in prison is a serious problem with a great impact on the prison society. For this reason, different suicide preventative programmes have been developed to curb the phenomenon. Barker et al.[16] conducted a systematic review on the effectiveness of suicide-prevention actions in prisons. The authors indicate that multifactored suicide-prevention programmes are the most effective, especially those who include mental health screening, with particular attention to risky periods and providing psychological support for inmates by avoiding the isolation of suicidal inmates. Other effective measures are those which suggest removing potentially dangerous items from the inmates, providing access to psychiatric hospitalization in case of psychosis offering follow-up treatment, and ensuring appropriate levels of observation. Also, adequate staff training on suicide prevention and refresher courses each year are recommended. Hawton et al. suggest that counteracting clustering in time and location of prisoners who self-harm is important in self-harm management and prevention of suicide. The response to self-harm should be extended to other inmates in the same wing or prison as well, as they could also be at risk.[14]

Two programmes seem to be particularly effective. Real Understanding of Self-Help (RUSH), was adapted from dialectical behaviour therapy (DBT), with the aim of reducing suicidal and self-harming behaviours through the teaching of adaptive coping skills. During the programme a reduction of borderline personality disorder symptoms was seen, especially among vulnerable violent offenders and first time offenders under the age of 25.

The second programme, Skills-Based Training on Risk Management (STORM), was adapted for the prison staff with the aim to increase knowledge about suicide prevention and demonstrated an improvement in attitudes, knowledge, and confidence.

Conclusions

Suicide is a heterogeneous phenomenon, with specific risk factors. Offenders represent a high-risk group for suicide and suicidal behaviour, as in this population, as compared with the general population the presence of risk factors such as psychiatric disorders, namely anxiety, depression, substance use, personality disorders, as well as impulsive personality traits is very high. Nevertheless, many prisoners with mental illnesses, who consequently are at great risk of suicide, remain undetected and untreated. Furthermore, suicide-prevention interventions for prisoners should be extended beyond the discharge of the inmates, since several studies reported high risk of suicide also in this period.[8]

References

1 Rivlin A, Hawton K, Marzano L, Fazel S. Psychosocial characteristics and social networks of suicidal prisoners: towards a model of suicidal behaviour in detention. 2013. PLoS One;**8**(7). doi:10.1371/journal.pone.0068944.

2 Fazel S, Cartwright J, Norman-Nott A, Hawton K. Suicide in prisoners: a systematic review of risk factors. J Clin Psychiatry 2008;**69**(11):1721–1731.

3 Fazel S, Grann M, Kling B, Hawton K. Prison suicide in 12 countries: an ecological study of 861 suicides during 2003–2007. Soc Psychiatry Psychiatr Epidemiol. 2011;**46**(3):191–195. doi:10.1007/s00127–010–01841–4.

4 Kariminia A, Law MG, Butler TG, Levy MH, Corben SP, Kaldor JM, et al. Suicide risk among recently released prisoners in New South Wales, Australia. Med J Aust 2007;**187**(7):387–390.

5 Mumola CJ. Suicide and homicide in state prisons and local jails. Bureau of Justice Statistics; 2005.

6 Liebling A. Suicides in prison. Routledge; 2002.

7 Haycock J. Race and suicide in jails and prisons. J Natl Med Assoc. 1989;**81**(4):405–411.

8 Pratt D, Appleby L, Piper M, Webb R, Shaw J. Suicide in recently released prisoners: a case-control study. Psychol Med. 2010;**40**(5):827–835. doi:10.1017/S0033291709991048.

9 Hayes LM. National study of jail suicides: seven years later. Psychiatr Q. 1989;**60**(1):7–29. doi:10.1007/BF01064362.

10 Sarchiapone M, Carli V, Giannantonio MD, Roy A. Risk factors for attempting suicide in prisoners. Suicide Life Threat Behav 2009;**39**(3):343–350. doi:10.1521/suli.2009.39.3.343.

11 Richard-Devantoy S, Olie J-P, Gourevitch R. Risk of homicide and major mental disorders: a critical review. L'Encéphale. 2009;**35**(6):521–530. doi:10.1016/j.encep.2008.10.009.

12 Carli V, Jovanović N, Podlesek A, Roy A, Rihmer Z, Maggi S, et al. The role of impulsivity in self-mutilators, suicide ideators and suicide attempters—a study of 1265 male incarcerated individuals. J Affect Disord 2010;**123**(1–3):116–122. doi:10.1016/j.jad.2010.02.119.

13 World Health Organization (WHO). Department of Mental Health and Substance Abuse. Preventing suicide in jails and prisons; 2007.

14 Hawton K, Linsell L, Adeniji T, Sariaslan A, Fazel S. Self-harm in prisons in England and Wales: an epidemiological study of prevalence, risk factors, clustering, and subsequent suicide. Lancet. 2014 Mar 29;**383**(9923):1147–1154.

15 Wasserman D, Rihmer Z, Rujescu D, Sarchiapone M, Sokolowski M, Titelman D, et al. European Psychiatric Association. The European Psychiatric Association (EPA) guidance on suicide treatment and prevention. Eur Psychiatry. 2012 Feb;**27**(2):129–141.

16 Barker E, Kõlves K, De Leo D. Management of suicidal and self-harming behaviours in prisons: systematic literature review of evidence-based activities. Arch Suicide Res. 2014;**18**(3):227–240. doi:10.1080/13811118.2013.824830.

Chapter 19

Suicide in the armed forces

Vsevolod A Rozanov

Introduction

Suicide in the military has been known since ancient times. Warriors committed suicide to avoid defeat or when under threat of humiliation. To a certain extent, for a long period of time, suicide in such situations was even a part of the officers' code. On the other hand, it should not be confused with the self-sacrifice of military personnel as a heroic act, which is usually aimed to save the lives of fellow combatants, or the culturally conditioned act of '*seppuku*' in Japan.

Suicide in the armed forces can be seen as a self-destructive phenomenon within a specific social and occupational group. Of course, armies are not the same as century ago. Today, more and more military people are operating through and analysing information. However, soldiers who carry weapons account for the greater part of all armies, and land operations are still common. Regular military forces include about 20 million people worldwide and this number is growing: including reservists and other militarized organizations, the number of people affiliated with armed forces is approximately five times higher. This gives a good impression of how important the topic may be, especially taking into consideration that the overwhelming majority of military staff are males, who commit suicide much more often than their female counterparts.

It is also important to remember that armies in both different countries and historical periods have deep distinctions. For instance, there are armies based on conscription, or fully professional, or mixed. There is also a difference between high commanders, officers, and soldiers, between active duty military and veterans, between those who were not involved in action and combat and those who have gone through real war, and between different types of forces, etc. There are many factors that influence suicide in the armed forces that must be taken into consideration, which makes the possibility of generalizing conclusions rather complicated. On the other hand, there is always a common factor; i.e., belonging to a special social group with specific internal regulations, cultures, and traditions.

Durkheim's explanations of military suicide and comparative rates

Emil Durkheim, in his classical work, dedicated a substantial part of his sociological monograph to suicides in the armies of different European countries.[1] Within his classical sociological concept, suicide is a phenomenon that depends on two broad factors: social integration and social regulation. In accordance with this concept, suicide in the army may be understood as a result of very high social integration (a military person regards himself to be a small but integral part of a large group and this may lead to altruistic suicide) and very high social regulation (a military person is deprived of many personal freedoms and this may lead to fatalistic suicide) (Fig. 19.1).

In Durkheim's time, suicide in the military was reported in Europe to be substantially higher than in the general population,[1] which is not the case today. In Table 19.1, suicide rates in the military environment are compared with suicide rates in males in the general population

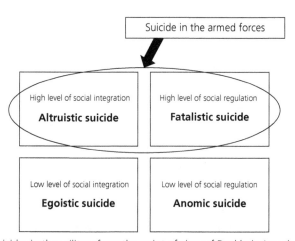

Fig. 19.1 Suicides in the military from the point of view of Durkheim's sociological concept

in the same country. Results show that suicide rates within military forces are substantially lower, than in men in the general population, with the exception of the US. It coincides with our usual perception of a military person as having a more disciplined, trained, self-reserved, and generally healthy personality with special psychological traits and higher resilience towards stress. Service in the army usually helps one to acquire a healthier lifestyle and develop constructive coping strategies. The army protects itself from unstable personalities and/or people with mental health problems, which are screened for at pre-admittance stage. Due to this selection process, in many cultures military people are often perceived as the best representatives of the nation. This perception coincides with the so-called 'healthy soldier effect'. On the other hand, it must be taken into consideration that this effect, which is borrowed from the occupational health concept of the 'healthy worker effect', can be well observed if such indicators as cardiovascular mortality are considered, but it is often not the case when mortality from external causes is taken into consideration.[2] Moreover, the level of stress in the armed forces may exacerbate mental health problems.

Table 19.1 also reveals, to some degree, a correlation of suicides in the armed forces with the level of suicide among the general population. It is well known that, despite some fluctuations, suicide rates are

Table 19.1 Male suicide rates per 100,000 persons in the military forces compared with the suicide rates of the same age and sex in the general population*

##	Country	Military (different forces)	General population (males < 65)	Source
1	Italy	1.10–2.03	6.9–9.8	Mancinelli et al., 2001
2	UK	3.0–15.0	18.0	Mickelwright, 2005
3	France	14.0–18.0	22.0	Desjeux et al., 2001
4	Norway	13.6	28.1	Hytten, 1985
5	Ireland	15.3	22.0	Mahon et al., 2005
6	US	20.2	19.5	Kuehn, 2009
7	Russian Federation	14.0–32.0	50.0–70.0	Litvintsev et al., 2003

*Rather wide range of suicides within one national military community depicts varying situation in different types of forces, from elite highly educated (like air forces) to land brigades

comparatively stable in different countries, which is sometimes referred to as 'cultural resistance.'[3] It is, therefore, no surprise that suicide rates in the armed forces more or less correlate with general suicide rates. Moreover, in spite of easy access to firearms in all armies, the predominant methods of suicide in the armed forces correspond with the most common methods used in society. For instance, in the US it is the use of a firearm, while in Slavonic countries, it is hanging.

On the other hand, suicides in the military may have some peculiarities and may differ from national rates changes[4] which may be explained by internal processes in the military, social or economic problems, changes in the moral state, prestige of the military service, etc. The army is a part of society, but it also has its own internal life, problems, and peculiarities which can influence actual change in suicide rates within military forces.

For instance, recent reports from the US have shown that the situation regarding suicides within the military forces can change at an alarming rate within a short historical period. There is disconcerting information about high suicide rates in both the US Army and among veterans. For the first time in the history of the US military forces, suicide rates among military personnel in 2008 appeared to be higher than in the general population and increased further. Specialists, who have been monitoring the situation in the US for many years, consider that the most recent increase in suicide rates among war veterans also warrants attention and requires urgent action.[6]

From the data presented in Table 19.1, one may draw the conclusion that the military is generally a 'low-risk' occupation. Such a conclusion may be misleading or based on wrong assumptions. It is, therefore, necessary to take into consideration a full set of complex factors when assessing comparative risk in different professions. These differences are often understood on the basis of the concept of occupational stress. On the other hand, it is possible, for example, that in alleged 'high-risk' occupations a person may have a high suicide risk not because of occupational stress but because of the demographic composition of the people in the profession.[5] This is very relevant for military personnel.

To better understand the reasons for differences in suicides among the military and civilians, specific risk and protective factors that may exist within military units should be carefully scrutinized.

General and specific risk factors

The risk factors and situations known for attempted and completed suicides, of course, have the same impact in the army as in a civilian population. For instance, demographic factors (sex, age, ethnicity, marital status, region of the country) are very important. It has already been mentioned that military suicides are mostly males (though females are increasingly represented in the military forces too), young soldiers who complete suicides are mostly bachelors, while officers are more likely to be married, the majority of suicide victims in the military are comparatively young people, etc. So-called distal (long-standing) risk factors, like past suicide attempts, depression, and alcohol abuse problems are also important in case they are not identified among military personnel. Of course, proximal (immediate) risk factors are very important and quite common; for instance, stressful personal events may act as a risk factor. In the case of servicemen, most often it is bad news from home (break-up with the spouse or girlfriend, illness or death of a relative, financial loss, etc.).

On the other hand, there are some specific risk factors that exist in the military environment. The following factors may be associated with an increased risk of suicide in the military context: (i) the loss of or lack of personal freedom experienced by people entering such a closed and authoritarian system as the armed forces; (ii) the aggressive masculine culture in many military communities which may leave little room for self-disclosure and peer support; (iii) the risk of personal traumatic stress exposure due to taking part in a combat situation and subsequent traumatic stress reactions or disorders; (iv) the easy access to firearms; (v) the military lifestyle with frequent relocations and the break-up of supportive social structures; (vi) changes in social structures due to reorganizing processes often taking place in armed forces; and (vii) the danger of suicide contagion and clustering of suicides in military units.[7]

In spite of the existence of these risk factors (that must be added to usual risk factors in the general population), suicide rates in military populations remain, in most cases, lower than in the civilian population of men of the same age. This could possibly be attributed to the existence of protective factors that balance the situation. These factors will be discussed in due course.

Combat stress and suicide in combatants

It was noted by Durkheim that during wars when social integration in the society is more pronounced, suicide in the general population usually drops. There is no consensus regarding suicides in the acting military at war. During war conflicts in the last century which involved huge contingents of soldiers, suicides in the military forces were not well registered in relation to massive combat mortality. Some authors have hypothesized that suicidal soldiers during the war were 'seeking death' and were killed in combat, while their suicides were not understood as such.[8] Recent war conflicts are very different; human life has much higher value and suicides in the armed contingents which are deployed to active duties are better registered. The situation in the US Army, which has recently been involved in several conflicts far outside its native country, imparts a great deal of important information.

In the US Armed Forces, suicide rates among military personnel have doubled since the initiation of military operations in Afghanistan and Iraq. It became especially clear after the 2nd Iraq War, which started in 2003. Since 2004, the number of suicides by military personnel has steadily increased, surpassing in 2008 the suicide rate of the general US population for the first time in history.[9] This negative tendency is usually explained by combat stress and mental health consequences of severe traumatic experiences and war exposure in general. The extent of the problem is apparent from the following figures: a survey of 1,700 soldiers and marines serving in Iraq since 2003 revealed that 94.5% saw dead bodies or human remains, 92% reported being attacked or ambushed, 86.2% knew someone killed or seriously wounded, and 55.7% caused the death of an enemy combatant.[7]

The main consequences of this stress may be seen in the high incidence of post-traumatic stress disorder (PTSD), depression, anxiety disorders, and substance abuse among US military personnel. All these conditions may contribute to elevated suicide risk, as well as brain trauma, which is also rather common.[10] There are many studies providing clear evidence that suicide risk is especially elevated in those military personnel who developed PTSD (in US personnel returning from their missions this disorder is diagnosed in 12–15% of persons).[11] Notwithstanding, depression is considered the leading underlying disorder for suicide. Recent studies suggest that PTSD has a pronounced effect on risk mostly if comorbid with depression. Individuals with comorbid PTSD and depression are characterized by a greater severity of symptoms, increased suicidality, and a higher level of impairment in social and occupational functioning.[12]

The model of suicidal behaviour in those who have been involved in direct combat and have developed such comorbidity has been proposed, which consists of the following components: (i) genetic factors; (ii) prenatal development; (iii) biological and psychosocial influences from birth to mobilization/deployment; (iv) mobilization/pre-deployment stress; (v) combat stress, traumatic brain injury, and physical injury; (vi) post-deployment stress; (vii) biological and psychosocial influences after the deployment; (viii) trigger (precipitant) of a suicidal act; and (ix) suicidal act. The first four components, according to the proposed model, determine the vulnerability to combat stress; whereas, the first seven components ascertain a predisposition to suicidal behaviour, so they overlap. Concerning the three key components of the suicidal process (i.e., biological, personality/psychological, and social/environmental), this model is congruent with the more general stress-vulnerability model[13] and takes into account specific social interactions and stressors of the military.

This model may also explain risk that exists in the modern US military forces due to specific features of deployments of the troops which are placed in the combat zone for several months and then return home to be later sent overseas again. It can be applied to military forces of several other countries which are involved in campaigns far from the homeland.

So, it is not universal but useful for understanding the role of combat stress in exacerbating suicidal tendencies.

Suicide in war veterans

One of the most serious problems that exists is suicides in those who have finished their service and returned to civilian life, especially if they were directly involved in actions. In former military personnel that are discharged after being at war, called here 'war veterans', psychological and emotional consequences of war as well as mental health consequences of war exposures are present.[14] This topic started to attract attention in the US after the Vietnam War when suicides in war veterans became a social problem that was widely discussed in the mass media. Though some initial studies did not confirm that suicide rates in veterans were higher than in non-veterans of the same sex and age, very soon psychosocial problems of those who have experienced war conflicts became a hot topic for the general public. The same problems were identified not only in the US but also in other countries; for instance, in the Russian Federation, among Afghanistan veterans, and in Croatia among veterans of local conflicts. Finally, in the US after both the Afghanistan and Iraq conflicts, studies indicated that veterans returning from war zones had significantly higher standardized mortality ratio (SMR) compared with the general population.[15] In another important study, about 104,000 veterans comprising of different ages from the Vietnam and post-Vietnam conflicts were compared with more than 200,000 non-veterans. Results confirmed that the risk of suicide among war veterans was higher than in non-veterans.[16]

High risk of suicide among veterans may be explained by combat stress and mental health consequences of being at war—PTSD, depression, substance abuse, etc. On the other hand, veterans experience various psychosocial problems even in spite of fairly good social and medical support in civil life. They may have feelings of guilt, remorse, and anguish; they may have chronic pain due to physical injuries and invalidity. All this may lead to mental health problems of ex-military which are diverse, polymorphic and are combined with psychosocial consequences. As a result domestic and occupational breakdown, social exclusion, criminality, homelessness, substance-misuse, and mental illnesses are rather prevalent in war veterans.[17] Psychosocial, physical, and mental health problems are clustering together, constituting high risk factors for completed suicide.

A valuable insight into a psychological mechanism that is especially relevant for veterans is provided by the Interpersonal-Psychological Theory of Suicide.[18] This concept puts forward three important factors, which may lead to suicide: (i) feelings that one does not belong to the group (thwarted belongingness); (ii) feelings that one is a burden on others or society (perceived burdensomeness); and (iii) an acquired capability to overcome the fear and pain associated with suicide (acquired capability of lethal self-injury). A person discharged from the armed forces loses relations with comrades, can have problems during the transition period, and feels excluded from civilian life which has changed while he was absent. Stressful experiences from the war zone, seeing and experiencing painful and fearful events are also important underpinnings of suicide risk. During military missions, soldiers are trained to develop certain aggressive and impulsive behavioural automatisms in order to deal with the stressful environments. It is quite possible that combat training and military exposures may cause habituation to fear of painful experiences, including suicide. Veterans who commit suicide are a heterogeneous group, wherein they are differentially exposed to social, psychological, or psychopathological risks. Combat stress and experiences of war may be the unifying factor. This, again, emphasizes that stress is the main mechanism that exposes existing vulnerabilities which, in combination with some personal features and in situations of low social support, may lead to suicide.

Young soldiers' suicidal behaviour

Young soldiers constitute the majority of personnel in conscription armies. There is a global tendency regarding growing numbers of suicide particularly in younger males which is linked to existential and emotional problems, substance misuse, impulsivity, risky behaviours, and other factors. No surprise that when the time comes for the military service they may 'import' their risks to the army. This raises several important questions: (i) how military forces can protect themselves from drafting personalities with hidden suicidal tendencies; (ii) how to prevent exacerbation of these tendencies in the stressful military environment; and (iii) what actions must be taken if suicide attempts have occurred.

Every conscription is accompanied by the screening process of conscripts, recruitment to the professional army is followed by even more exacting examination. The instruments of screening may vary, yet they are generally based on psychological testing (cognitive, psychological performance) and clinical interviews. Direct questions regarding risk of suicidal behaviour are usually not used, while main attention is paid to depressive symptoms (including suicidal ideation and hopelessness), alcohol and drug misuse, and signs of reduced coping. In the search for possible signs of impaired resilience the Sense of Coherence (SOC), a concept developed by Antonovsky is suggested. Low SOC score was found to be a strong predictor of suicidal behaviour, higher suicidal ideation, and other mental health problems, such as alcohol and drug abuse.[7]

There are also some other indirect signs that may help to suspect suicidal risk. For instance, poor self-rated health, low intelligence tests results at the age of 18, and short stature in correlation with poor, low scores in logic tests were found to be associated with the risk of attempted suicide in conscripts.[19] These signs may reflect problems associated with early periods of life, stressful experiences in early childhood and adolescence, and impaired development of a young person's abilities. This, in turn, may be the reason for the feeling of basic inferiority of such person in the military environment, which can, together with low educational level, possible family problems, and poor integration into a military unit, be strong determinants of soldier suicide. These factors help to outline the so-called 'psychological portrait' of the suicidal soldier.

On the other hand, suicidal behaviour may be linked to very contrasting traits of personality. For instance, an Israeli study compared psychological characteristics (from army records) of combatant and non-combatant soldiers who committed suicide, with others who did not commit suicide. It was found that combatant soldiers who committed suicide showed proof of greater behavioural adjustment, motivation to serve, and a greater sense of duty. Those who were involved in combat had fewer referrals for psychological evaluation and fewer unit changes. This may reflect the tendency for perfectionism in these soldiers. The authors came to the conclusion that excessive motivation and the tendency to be autonomous and independent may account for suicide in combatant soldiers, while in non-combatant soldiers the main predisposition for suicidal behaviour may be driven by other personality characteristics.[20]

One of the most recent studies from the US has revealed tendencies that support the role of factors besides combat stress and the importance of better screening of recruits. It was revealed that while suicide rates for soldiers who served in Iraq and Afghanistan more than doubled from 2004 to 2009 to more than 30 suicides per 100,000, the trend among those who were never deployed nearly tripled to between 25 and 30 suicides per 100,000. Rates for a civilian population of similar age and sex remained steady at 19 suicides per 100,000 during this time. These results, as the authors say, 'argues indirectly against the view that exposure to combat-related trauma is the exclusive cause of the increase in Army suicides', pointing to problems among modern youth. There were concerns that the rise in suicides was the result of two recent US Army trends designed to recruit or retain personnel. One trend was the liberalization of screening rules and enrolment of recruits with poor education or conduct records. The other was the practice of forcing soldiers to remain in service beyond their enlistment. The study did not directly confirm the role of these practices, but suggested a higher prevalence of mental health problems among the modern younger generation. About one in four soldiers in the army appear to suffer from at least one psychiatric disorder and one in ten has multiple disorders. Most importantly—about a third of soldiers who attempted suicide are associated with mental disorders developed before they joined the army: an indication that more professional efforts are needed while screening for mental health problems among recruits.[21] The question remains, however: what is the reason for growing mental health problems among the younger generation? This is a global problem.

Protective factors and suicide prevention in the armed forces

The following factors can protect against suicide in military units: (i) the military is a highly organized structure which can make prevention programmes part of routine activities, and implement them in a prompt and effective way; (ii) preliminary and ongoing medical and psychiatric controls of those who are dealing with weapons facilitates early recognition of mental health problems; (iii) special prevention units may be organized and special means of reporting may be implemented which may provide quick identification of suicidal persons along with their referral to specialists; (iv) the military can discharge those with suicidal ideations or actions and this may reduce suicide risk in the contingent; and (v) every case of completed or attempted suicide can be thoroughly investigated, thereby obtaining important information for further prevention models.[7] In general, military organizations have many possibilities to control the situation with suicides and suicidal behaviour, and to implement prevention programmes.

As in civilian life, such programmes in the armed forces have primary, secondary, and tertiary components. Primary prevention is aimed at the whole military community and explores factors such as general psychological climate in the military, morale, psychological well-being, and management of work stress. This may also include wide organizational measures aimed to prevent legal and disciplinary problems, such as bullying and harassment. It may also include increased awareness about mental health promotion, suicide prevention, and a stress resilience training as part of the general training of soldiers. Secondary prevention measures target those groups at higher risk, which may be young conscripts shortly after inclusion, active-duty military personnel involved in actions, and veterans. Tertiary prevention is aimed at those who have revealed themselves; for instance, suicide attempters. They constitute a target for special psychosocial interventions and psychiatric examination.

Prevention measures exist in every army. They usually include such components as information/education, leadership interventions, medical interventions, and (in some armies) crisis telephone services. Information and education are the key elements of many programmes. They aim to both enhance knowledge about suicide among all military personnel and, in a more targeted way, teach commanders and responsible staff such as medical specialists, psychologists, or special training officers. There is a general consensus that suicide-prevention programmes in military organizations should use proactive and complex approaches with an emphasis on taking advantage of the special opportunities that exist within military organizations.[22]

Much attention is paid to leaders' competence. Positive leadership, empathy, and deep concern for soldiers are crucial for suicide prevention in the military. It is important for leaders to know their soldiers and their concerns, and to be prepared to refer a soldier in need of professional help. The key to preventing suicide in the unit is to respond to any verbal, behavioural, or situational cues. This means that commanders should possess both awareness and good knowledge of suicide. Prevention efforts are usually the personal responsibility of commanders and leaders. On the other hand, private soldiers also need to be taught to take any suicidal statement by a fellow soldier seriously, and to inform the chain of command immediately. In this case, they are playing a special role as 'gatekeepers'.

An example of this is a suicide preventive intervention targeting Ukrainian Air Force units with about 10,000 personnel, which was based on the model of gatekeepers' education. It included education/information of the responsible personnel, military psychologists, and medical staff, with further dissemination of information via special training for soldiers. By introducing suicide-prevention education, the rate of suicides quickly dropped, giving rise to enthusiasm and satisfaction among commanders. Nevertheless, it became rapidly apparent that only constant education and consultations of specialists ensures success.[23]

Another example is an ambitious programme developed within the US Air Force that consisted of measures aimed to encourage personnel to seek help for mental health, psychological, or relationship problems, and of enhancing a general understanding of mental health issues as well as changing policies and social norms. One of the important aspects of the intervention was training (education) in suicide prevention. It was found that implementation of the programme was associated with a sustained decline in the rate of suicides and other adverse outcomes (homicide, family violence). A 33% relative risk reduction was observed for suicide after the intervention; reduction for other outcomes ranged from 18 to 54%.[24] These results are encouraging. On the other hand, suicide-prevention measures based on help-seeking behaviour may be useful for young conscripts, but not for officers, as many referrals to mental health facilities can be seen as the end of a career.

In the modern armed forces throughout the world, the importance of mental health issues is growing, with suicide prevention being one of the most important topics. Knowledge enhancement and awareness regarding risk and protective factors of suicide involving all military staff is one of the most effective components of suicide prevention in the armed forces. Further accumulation of the scientific knowledge regarding suicide will provide a wider and deeper understanding of how to educate military communities in mental health promotion and suicide prevention.

References

1 Durkheim E. Suicide. A study in sociology. Routledge, London; 1992/1987.

2 Waller M, McGuire AC. Changes over time in the 'healthy soldier effect'. Popul Health Metr. 2011;9:7.

3 Makinen IH, Wasserman D. Suicide prevention and cultural resistance: stability in European countries' suicide ranking, 1970–1988. Ital J Suicidology. 1997;7(2):73–85.

4 Litvintsev SV, Shamrey VK, Fadeev AC, Reznik AM, Arbuzov AL. On the state of psychiatric aid in the Russian Federation Armed Forces. Voen-Med Journ. 2003;324:13–20.

5 Stack S. Occupation and suicide. Soc Sci Q. 2001;82(2):384–396.

6 Kang HK, Bullman TA. Is there an epidemic of suicides among current and former US military personnel? Ann Epidemiol. 2009;19(10):757–760.

7 Rozanov VA, Mehlum L, Stiliha R. Suicide in military settings. Combatants and veterans. In: Wasserman D, Wasserman C, eds. Oxford textbook of suicidology and suicide prevention. New York, NY: Oxford University Press; 2009: 258–265.

8 **Lester D**. Suicide during war and genocide. In: Wasserman D, Wasserman C, eds. Oxford textbook of suicidology and suicide prevention. New York, NY: Oxford University Press; 2009: **31**, 215–218.

9 **Department of Defense**. Task Force on the Prevention of Suicide by Members of the Armed Forces. The challenge and the promise: strengthening the force, preventing suicide, and saving lives department of defense. Washington, DC; 2010.

10 **Brenner LA, Betthauser LM, Homaifar BY, Villarreal E, Harwood JE, . . . Huggins JA**. Post-traumatic stress disorder, traumatic brain injury, and suicide attempt history among veterans receiving mental health services. Suicide Life Threat Behav. 2011;**41**(4):416–423.

11 **Kang HK, Natelson, BH, Mahan CM, Lee KY, Murphy FM**. Post-traumatic stress disorder and chronic fatigue syndrome-like illness among Gulf War veterans: a population-based survey of 30,000 veterans. Am J Epidemiol. 2003;**157**(2):141–148.

12 **Sher L**. A model of suicidal behaviour in war veterans with post-traumatic mood disorder. Med Hypotheses. 2009;**73**:215–219.

13 **Wasserman D**. A stress-vulnerability model and the development of the suicidal process. In: Wasserman D, ed. Suicide. An unnecessary death. London: Martin Dunitz; 2001: 13–27.

14 **Rozanov VA, Carli V**. Suicide among war veterans. Int J Environ Res Publ Health. 2012;**9**(7):2504–2519.

15 **Kang HK, Bullman TA**. Risk of suicide among US veterans after returning from the Iraq and Afghanistan war zones. JAMA. 2008;**300**:652–653.

16 **Kaplan M, Huguet N, McFarland BH, Newsom JT**. Suicide among male veterans: a prospective population-based study. J Epidemiol Comm Health. 2007;**61**:619–624.

17 **Deahl MP, Klein S, Alexander DA**. The costs of conflict: meeting the mental health needs of serving personnel and service veterans. Int Rev Psychiatry. 2011;**23**:201–209.

18 **Selby EA, Anestis MD, Bender TW, Ribeiro JD, Nock MK, . . . Joiner Jr. TE** Overcoming the fear of lethal injury: evaluating suicidal behaviour in the military through the lens of the Interpersonal–Psychological Theory of Suicide. Clin Psychol Rev. 2010;**30**:298–307.

19 **Jiang G-X, Rasmussen F, Wasserman D**. Short stature and poor psychological performance: risk factors for attempted suicide among Swedish male conscripts. Acta Psychiatr Scand. 1999;**100**:433–440.

20 **Bodner E, Ben-Artzi E, Kaplan Z**. Soldiers who kill themselves: the contribution of dispositional and situational factors. Arch Suicide Res. 2006;**10**:29–43.

21 **Schoenbaum M, Kessler RC, Gilman SE, Colpe LJ, Heeringa SG, . . . Cox KL**. Predictors of suicide and accident death in the army study to assess risk and resilience in service members (Army STARRS). JAMA Psychiatry. 2014;**71**(5):514–522.

22 **Zamorski MA**. Suicide prevention in military organizations. Int Rev Psychiatry. 2011;**23**:172–180.

23 **Rozanov VA, Mokhovikov AN, Stiliha R.** Successful model of suicide prevention in the Ukraine military environment. Crisis. 2002;**23**:171–177.

24 **Knox KL, Litts DA, Talcott GW, Feig JC, Caine ED.** Risk of suicide and related adverse outcomes after exposure to a suicide prevention programme in the US Air Force: cohort study. BMJ. 2003;**327**:1376–1380.

Section V

Age-related suicide

Chapter 20

Adolescent suicide and attempted suicide

Alan Apter and Yari Gvion

Epidemiology

Violence is by far the most common cause of death in young people. This may take the form of suicide, homicide, or motor vehicle accidents. Different countries have different rates of each of these phenomena; in most countries suicide rates are higher than homicide rates, and in many industrialized nations the number of young people dying from suicide is higher than the number of fatalities from road accidents. Although there has been a decrease in fatal suicide among young people in the West, perhaps due to increasingly effective prevention measures, youth suicide continues to pose a major public health problem, as among young people aged 15–29 years, suicide is the second leading cause of death globally.[1]

In addition to deaths among young people from suicide, many young people make non-fatal deliberate attempts to kill themselves. This phenomenon (also known as 'attempted suicide', 'parasuicide', 'non-suicidal self-injury', or 'deliberate self-harm') is at least 10–100 times more common than suicide, although the exact prevalence of such acts is unknown. The relationship between attempted suicide (parasuicide) and suicide is controversial but non-fatal suicidal behaviour remains an acute clinical problem.[2]

An increase in the numbers of young people in the West who take intentional overdoses or deliberately injure themselves has been observed over the last half-century. As a result, deliberate self-poisoning has become the most common reason for acute hospital admission among adolescent women. Attempted suicide (parasuicide) is more common in females than in males, the sex ratio being highest during adolescence. The highest rates for females are in the age range of 15–19 years. Rates of attempted suicide are inversely related to social class. In some developing countries such as India, young women are highly vulnerable for completed suicide and thus the 'gender paradox' does not apply to these geographical areas.[1]

Most statistics on attempted suicide (parasuicide) are derived from hospital samples, which represent only about one-third of actual attempted suicides. In a series of studies conducted on a general population (Saving and Empowering Young Lives in Europe—SEYLE study) the prevalence of risk factors for suicidal behaviour was explored among a sample of 12,395 adolescents recruited in randomly selected school across 11 European counties. Three groups of adolescents were identified: a low-risk group (57.8%)—this group reported low to very low frequency of risk behaviours; a high-risk group (13.2%) who reported high on all risk behaviours; and there was a third group—'invisible' risk (29%)—who reported similar prevalence of suicidal thoughts, anxiety, subthreshold depression, and depression compared with the high-risk group. This group reported high use of Internet/TV videogames, sedentary behaviour, and reduced sleep. The prevalence of suicide attempts in the 'invisible' risk group was 5.9% and 10.1% in the high-risk group.[3]

Risk factors for youth suicide

One of the major risk factors for youth suicide is the presence of a diagnosable psychiatric disorder, especially affective disorder and borderline personality disorder. As in adults, attempted suicide is an important risk factor for suicide.[4–6]

Borderline personality disorder is traditionally associated with nonfatal suicide attempts but there is increasing evidence that suicide is common in these patients as well. Intentional self-damaging acts and suicide attempts are the 'behavioural speciality' of these patients. About 9% of patients with borderline personality disorder eventually kill themselves. Females with anorexia nervosa are also at very high risk for suicide, which is now the major cause of death in this condition.

Former adolescent psychiatric patients are at special risk of eventual suicide (10% for males and 1% for females). A family history of psychiatric disorder is also common (25–50%) in adolescent suicide victims, as is the presence of substance or alcohol abuse (33–70%). The comorbidity of affective disorder, personality disorder, and substance abuse is especially lethal. The presence of firearms in the home and issues of gender identity such as homosexuality are also well-recognized risk factors for adolescent suicide.

Low socio-economic status (SES) has shown to be a significant risk factor for suicidal behaviours among youth. Among adolescents, there is evidence suggesting that the implication of socio-economic factors and mental disorders on suicidality are equivalent in nature.

Four comorbid constellations can be identified as having special significance for suicide in adolescent populations:

◆ the combination of schizophrenia, depression, and substance abuse;

◆ the combination of substance abuse, conduct disorder, and depression;

◆ the combination of affective disorder, eating disorder, and anxiety disorders; and

◆ the combination of affective disorder, personality disorder (cluster A, paranoid and schizoid personality disorder), and dissociative disorders (disruption in integrated functions of consciousness, memory, identity, or perception of the environment).

These constellations require vigorous psychiatric intervention.

Depression

Among teenagers, both attempted and completed suicides are, in the great majority of cases, preceded by depressive symptoms. There are considerable differences between depressed children and young people who have made suicide attempts and those who have not. Depressed young people who attempt suicide often come from broken families and have had one or more relatives who have committed or attempted suicide. They have also, relatively often, run away from home and thus been brought up without favourable role models. Physical and mental abuse, as well as sexual assault, is also more common in this group. Young people who have attempted suicide often have lasting problems at school and also difficulties in achieving workable relationships with their peers compared with young people who are depressed and have not attempted suicide. Abuse of alcohol and drugs, impulsive behaviour, reduced hours of sleep, and asocial behaviour are additional risk factors for attempted and completed suicide among depressed young people.[3,7,8]

Owing to the high incidence of depression among young people who have attempted suicide, it is important to make a diagnosis and provide adequate treatment at an early stage. Studies show that depressive disturbances are more common among children and young people than was previously believed. In the SEYLE study comprising 12,395 adolescents from 11 European countries, it was found that 29.2% of the adolescents were sub-threshold depressed, and 10.5% depressed with high comorbidity with anxiety. Both sub-threshold and threshold depression and anxiety were related to suicidality and functional impairment.[7]

Unfortunately, many young people with depression are not identified, partly because their depressive symptoms are often atypical and partly because adults do not readily recognize depressive symptoms in the young, owing to their wish to see their children as happy and healthy. Since the number of young people with depression appears to have increased since the Second World War, and the age of onset of depressive disturbances has decreased, it is important to increase the effort to detect depressions in order to be able to prevent suicidal behaviour.[9,10]

Major depression is most easily diagnosed when it appears acutely in a previously healthy child; in such cases the symptoms closely resemble those seen in adults (see Chapter 4). Often, however, the onset is insidious and the child may show many other difficulties such as attention deficit disorder or separation anxiety disorder before becoming depressed.

Mood disorders tend to be chronic when they start at an early age and the child comes from a family in which there is a high incidence of mood disorders and alcohol abuse.

In some cases the depressed adolescent may also be psychotic and have hallucinations and delusions, which are usually mood congruent. When the psychotic themes are related to suicide, as occurs in command hallucinations or delusions of guilt, the risk of suicide is very high.

Bipolar disorder

Bipolar disorder was once thought to occur only rarely in youth. However, approximately 20% of all bipolar patients have their first episode during adolescence, with a peak age of onset between 15 and 19 years. Developmental variations in presentation, symptomatic overlap with other disorders, and lack of clinician awareness have all led to under-diagnosis or mis-diagnosis in children and adolescents. Therefore, clinicians need to be aware of some of the unique clinical characteristics associated with the early onset form. Similarly, it is important to recognize the various phases and patterns of episodes associated with bipolar disorder. The first presentation may be with either manic or depressive episodes. Between 20 and 30% of young people with major depressions go on to have manic episodes.

Adolescents with bipolar disorder are at increased risk of completed suicide.[11] 20% of adolescents with bipolar disorder made at least one medically significant suicide attempt. In the literature relating to adults, a large review of studies that examined depressive and manic–depressive disorders found that the mean rate of completed suicides was 19%. Patients who are male or who are in the depressed phase of their illness are at the highest risk.

Schizophrenia

Schizophrenia is a common psychiatric disorder of adolescence (hence the term 'dementia praecox'). Because schizophrenia is a serious disorder with ominous prognosis and social stigma, some clinicians are hesitant to make this diagnosis even when there is sufficient evidence to do so. This potentially denies the child and family access to appropriate treatment, knowledge about the disorder, and specialized support services. However, despite diagnostic criteria being met, the initial diagnosis may be inaccurate given the overlap in symptoms between schizophrenia, affective disorders with psychotic features and, possibly, personality and dissociative disorders.

The differentiation between schizophrenia, psychotic depression or mania, and schizoaffective disorder is not always easy in adolescence. The patient must be followed longitudinally, with periodic diagnostic reassessments, to ensure accuracy. Patients and families should be educated about these diagnostic issues.

Depression in schizophrenia may be related to the fact that the young person feels that he or she is 'falling apart' and becoming mentally ill, and there is indeed evidence that suicidality and depression in these patients is related to good premorbid function, better insight, higher intelligence, and preservation of cognitive function. Post-psychotic depression and depressive states caused by neuroleptic medications may also have a role to play in this dangerous condition.

Many schizophrenic patients are depressed and suicidal, especially if they are young and have not been ill for a long time. At least two-thirds of the suicides are related to depression and only a small minority to the psychotic symptoms such as hallucinations.[5],[12] The suicide often occurs shortly after discharge and thus may be related to lack of social support.

Finally, many adolescents with schizophrenia also abuse drugs and alcohol, thus increasing their risk of suicide. Sometimes, the abuse is an attempt at self-medication. Anticholinergic medications given for the relief of extrapyramidal symptoms give some adolescent patients a 'high' to which they become addicted, and some patients may simulate extra-pyramidal symptoms in order to obtain these drugs. Child-onset and adolescent schizophrenia are often preceded by difficulties of attention and learning, for which stimulant medications are given. In the context of a developing schizophrenic condition there is, again, a potential for abuse and drug-induced depression.

Alcohol and drug abuse

Adolescents with psychoactive substance abuse disorder (PSUD), especially males, are more likely to commit suicide with guns than other adolescents. Adolescent suicide also seems to be related to more chronic

PSUD in subjects who have not sought treatment. In one study, PSUD was typically present for at least nine years before the suicide.

Intoxication for the purpose of self-medication of anxiety and despondency, which often follows a crisis, may trigger suicide in an adolescent who feels shame, humiliation, or frustration. It has been suggested that adolescents may use psychoactive substances to bolster their courage to carry out the suicide attempt or suicide. Intoxication may also lead to impaired judgement and decreased inhibition and may thus facilitate suicidal behaviour.[13]

Eating disorders

There has been recognition of the very definite increased risk of suicidal behaviours in girls with eating disorders such as anorexia and bulimia.[14]

Psychological characteristics of adolescent suicide attempters

Impulsivity

An important finding shows that a combination of depressive symptoms and antisocial behaviour is the most common antecedent of teenage suicide. 'Assaultiveness' and instability of affect as reflected in borderline personality disorder may also be important correlates of adolescent suicidal behaviour, especially in combination with depression. Impulsivity has frequently been described as a risk factor for suicide and a personality characteristic of adolescent suicide attempters. Lack of impulse control has been found to distinguish adolescent suicide attempters from adolescents with an acute illness. However, impulsivity does not seem to characterize all suicide attempters, since group comparisons have found no difference between suicidal patients and controls on measures of cognitive impulsivity. Instead, impulsivity may be important in identifying high-risk subgroups.[15]

Pathological Internet use (PIU) is considered to be an impulse control disorder, thus conditions associated with impulsivity were found among PIUs. Furthermore, suicide attempts proved to be significantly and independently linked with PIU.[16]

Anger

Several authors have indicated that anger is an emotional state that is often associated with adolescent suicide attempts. Suicide attempters in the emergency room report intense anger before the attempt, and adolescent suicide attempters often exhibit a wide range of aggressive behaviours.[17]

Anxiety

Anxiety has been identified as an important risk factor for suicidal behaviour in adolescents.[7] Compared with psychiatric outpatients, suicide attempters exhibit higher levels of anxiety. In a large community sample of adolescents,[18] a significant association between anxiety disorders and suicide attempts was found in males but not in females.

Psychodynamic aspects of adolescent suicide

We live in a world in which we are faced everywhere with evidence of conflict. Humans live in a dangerous world surrounded by sickness and accidents, beasts and bacteria, the malignant forces of nature, and the vengeful hands of their fellows. One would expect that in the face of these overwhelming blows from all sides, people would unite in a universal brotherhood of beleaguered humanity. However, this is not so. Instead, we are faced with an enemy behind the lines, for one of the forces that threatens our existence is self-destruction, that extraordinary propensity of human beings to join hands with external forces in the attack upon their own existence. People say that they want life, liberty, and happiness, and yet they sacrifice themselves to injure others and expend time, trouble, and energy to shorten the lives of others. Moreover, there are some who, as if lacking something else to destroy, turn their weapons upon themselves. Such observations led to Freud's formulation of the death instinct: a strong impulse to self-destruction that exists from birth in all people. This impulse may lead to suicide in exceptional cases only, as it is opposed by a parallel constructive life force within the personality.[19]

Psychoanalytic theory hypothesizes that, in the unconscious, it is possible to regard one's body as not being part of one and it is also possible to treat the body as if it included the body of someone else. This latter phenomenon is called 'introjection' because a person with whom the individual identifies very much appears to be 'introjected' into the self. Therefore, any desired treatment of the other person can now be carried out on oneself. This turning back of hostile feelings on the self thus serves the psychological usefulness of displacing unacceptable wishes onto the self (i.e., 'kicking the cat' with one's own body). Menninger proposed that a dynamic triad underlies all aggressive behaviour, whether directed inwards or outwards: the wish to die, the wish to kill, and the wish to be killed. Thus, many suicides in adolescents represent a revenge on parents since the adolescent was too afraid or felt too guilty to kill someone else.[20]

One of the important dynamics in adolescent suicide is narcissistic injury, in which even a 'cry for help' is felt to be unacceptable to the ego ideal. Psychological autopsies of 18–21-year-old male soldiers showed that many of the inexplicable suicides occurred among the most highly functional and successful youngsters, who had committed suicide after the most minimal failures. In addition, many of these youngsters were described as being very 'private' people for whom the 'stiff upper lip' code did not allow complaints or requests for help. 'Crying for help' may be more acceptable for girls, and this may partly explain why attempted suicide is more common in girls and completed suicide is more common in boys.[21]

Clinical assessment of suicidal risk

Suicidal adolescents should undergo a comprehensive psychiatric and psychological evaluation. It may be advisable to hospitalize most attempters to reinforce the seriousness of the problem to the child and the family and to ensure evaluation, since lack of compliance with treatment is characteristic of suicidal adolescents who are brought to emergency rooms.

Often what appears at first to be an impulsive over-reaction to a transient interpersonal problem turns out, on more thorough evaluation, to be symptomatic of more chronic difficulties. An attempt of low lethality may be more indicative of miscalculation than of low intent, so it is important to assess what result the child expected. A child with low intent or attention-seeking motives may be at higher risk as a result of impulsivity or a miscalculation in the direction of higher lethality.

In young people, in whom assessment takes time, emergency room personnel tend to take a rapid history of present circumstances and briefly assess for depression, and the mistaken diagnosis of adjustment disorder is often made. A careful history of impulsive behaviour and conduct problems should be taken. This is especially important in adolescents who are identified as being school drop-outs, truants, or unemployed. A history of drug and alcohol use as well as questions of identity and sexual orientation must be sought in all patients.

Suicidal intent is often secretive in nature; therefore, it is critically important to establish rapport during the initial interview. Children and adolescents are more likely to respond to an active and responsive clinician. Although confidentiality may be a concern, it is wise to avoid promises of blanket confidentiality. Discussing with the child ahead of time what will be discussed with parents and, if possible, having the child present during the discussion with the parents helps maintain rapport and increases the chance of future compliance. Delineating specifically what further evaluation or treatment modality will address the problem can increase compliance. Because about half of suicide attempters fail to keep their first appointment, having the child and family meet the future therapist and having an appointment made for them may improve the attrition rate.

In addition to asking about suicidal intent, attitude towards death, recent stressors, availability of suicidal means, level of protection at home, the presence or absence of previous attempts, and exposure to suicide, psychiatric diagnoses require systematic evaluation. The symptoms associated with major depressive disorder, bipolar disorder, oppositional-defiant disorder (especially with impulsivity and aggression), substance or alcohol abuse, and psychosis should be assessed. The presence or absence of these symptoms, as well as the youngster's psychological and psychodynamic personality structure, is important in formulating a treatment plan.[22]

Treatment

Treatment must encompass the acute management of suicidal behaviour as well as treatment of associated mental disorders and psychological problems.[22–29]

Acute management

A major problem in the management of adolescent suicide attempters is the failure of adolescent attempters to attend and complete treatment. It has been suggested that about half of the adolescent suicide attempters do not receive adequate psychotherapy after their attempt. Parental denial and psychopathology may interfere with treatment planning. Some clinicians have attempted to deal with this problem by mandating the admission of all adolescent suicide attempters to a general hospital for brief therapy and evaluation. This policy has been widely adopted and has been made compulsory by law in Israel.

Since family relationship difficulties are extremely common in adolescent attempters, one might expect that family therapy would be the most productive way of helping suicidal youngsters. This approach appears, however, to be severely limited in effectiveness in many cases because of the high rejection rate by parents, as reflected by high levels of non-attendance at treatment sessions.

Several experts have tried to develop systematic 'manualized' therapies for adolescent suicide attempters based on evidence that shows deficiencies of problem-solving abilities in adolescents shortly after the attempt. Some of these therapies have been shown to be of value in randomized controlled trials.

Hospitalization

Clinicians should be prepared to hospitalize suicide attempters who express a persistent wish to die or who are psychiatrically ill until their mental state or level of suicidal behaviour has stabilized. A relationship with the suicidal adolescent and his family should be established in the emergency room and the importance of treatment should be stressed. An appointment and a follow-up plan should be scheduled before discharge. A 'no-suicide contract', in which the child or adolescent agrees not to engage in self-harming behaviour and to tell an adult if he or she is having suicidal urges, may be useful but should not be relied on. The contract should never decrease a clinician's vigilance or curtail monitoring of the child or adolescent. Clinicians should also be aware of suicide contagion in the case of exposure to suicidal behaviour on a ward.

Discharge home

Suicidal adolescents should only be discharged home if the clinician is satisfied that adequate supervision and support will be available over the next few days and if a responsible adult has agreed to dispose of potentially lethal medications and firearms. It is valuable for the clinician to warn the child or adolescent and the parents about the dangerous disinhibiting effects of alcohol and other drugs.

The clinician treating the suicidal child or adolescent during the days after an attempt should be available to the patient and family, have experience managing suicidal crises, and have support available for him or herself.

Once a therapeutic alliance is established and the child or adolescent has attended the first treatment sessions, the child or adolescent is more likely to continue treatment. Length of the treatment is individual, but 3–6 months should be a rule, with successively fewer contacts up to one or two years, sometimes longer.

Long-term treatment management

Psychotherapy

Psychotherapy, an important component of treatment for the mental disorders associated with suicidal behaviour, should be tailored to the particular needs of the patient. Cognitive behavioural therapy, interpersonal therapy, dialectical behavioural therapy, psychodynamic therapy, and family therapy are all options.[23,25–29]

Psychopharmacology

Any medication prescribed to the suicidal child or adolescent must be carefully monitored by a third party and any change of behaviour or side-effects should be reported immediately.[22]

Lithium

Lithium greatly reduces the rate of both suicides and suicide attempts in adults with bipolar disorder. Discontinuing lithium treatment in bipolar patients is associated with an increase in suicide morbidity and mortality. Clinical guidelines on the optimum treatment strategies for bipolar adolescents have been established.

Antidepressants

Tricyclic antidepressants should not be prescribed for the suicidal child or adolescent as a first line of treatment. They are potentially lethal, because of the small difference between therapeutic and toxic levels of the drug, and they have not been proved effective in children or adolescents.

Selective serotonin reuptake inhibitors (SSRIs) reduce suicidal ideation and suicide attempts in non-depressed adults with cluster-B (borderline, antisocial, histrionic, narcissistic) personality disorders. They are safe in children and adolescents, have low lethality, and are effective in treating depression in non-suicidal adolescents. Further research is needed to determine whether SSRIs influence suicidal behaviour or ideation in children and adolescents. Since SSRIs may have a disinhibiting effect (especially in patients with SSRI-induced akathisia—subjective restlessness accompanied by observed different kinds of movement) and increase suicidal ideation in a small number of adults who were not previously suicidal, children and adolescents prescribed SSRIs must be carefully monitored to ensure that any new suicidal ideation or akathisia is noted. Finally, it should be noted that the decrease in youth suicide rates may parallel the increased use of SSRI medications in this age group.

Anxiolytics

Other medications that may increase disinhibition or impulsivity, such as the benzodiazepines and phenobarbital, should be prescribed with caution in children and adolescents.

Prevention of suicidal behaviour

Prevention strategies for preventing suicidal behaviours can be effective, which has been shown in a randomized controlled trial (RCT). In this

RCT, an awareness-based programme entitled the Youth Mental Health Awareness Programme was shown to be effective in preventing suicide attempts and severe suicidal ideation.[30]

Case Study

John was a 17-year-old boy who was admitted to an adolescent unit after swallowing 20 pills of fluoxetine, which he had been taking for depression. He reported being depressed for as long as he could remember. As a child he had been obese and was frequently the object of ridicule from his schoolmates. In addition he suffered from a learning disability, which greatly distressed his parents who had hoped that this intelligent child would be a source of pride to them. This was especially a blow to his father, who was a computer technician and was frustrated by his own failure to become an engineer.

At an early age John developed symptoms of oppositional disorder. He was disobedient at school and would talk back to his parents at home. He got into frequent fights with his younger brother, who suffered from attention deficit disorder and also had a short temper. As he approached puberty, John's conduct began to get worse. He started to steal and to lie and to write graffiti all over his school and also to vandalize property. He began to smoke heavily and would often play truant from school. He managed to lose weight and became an attractive youngster; however, he still regarded himself as ugly and had a poor self-image. Several attempts at psychological treatment failed, owing to his lack of compliance.

At about the age of 13 he began to drink alcohol and smoke marijuana. In addition he would also get 'high' on solvents. At the age of 14 he began to write poetry and songs, all of which were pervaded by themes of death and suicide. He would listen for hours to music, especially heavy metal and 'trash'. He identified with Kurt Cobain's suicide and also with the suicide of a friend at school. The final trigger for his suicide attempt was a break-up with his girlfriend.

On examination he was dishevelled, with long hair and many ear-rings, and he was defiant and angry and very obviously depressed. The main theme of his thought was hatred towards his parents, especially his father. He dismissed his mother as 'irrelevant'.

The unit diagnoses were 'double' depression (dysthymia and recurrent major depressive disorder), conduct disorder, substance abuse, attention deficit disorder, and developmental reading disorders. In addition, he was thought to have a borderline personality disorder.

Surprisingly, he made good progress on the unit and developed a close relationship with his therapist, a psychiatric resident. However, when the resident had to leave the unit and go to another rotation, John became very angry and upset and decided to discharge himself. Attempts at rehabilitation were at first promising but his drug habit got worse and he started to use hallucinogens in order to self-medicate his depression. He then asked to return to the inpatient unit. Once again there was a period of progress until one day while at home on leave he had an argument with his mother and then another argument with his girlfriend. He took a large dose of lysergic acid diethylamide (LSD) and threw himself out of a fifth storey window of his home.

This case illustrates many of the risk factors that are relevant to adolescent suicide—the presence of mental illness, alcohol and drug abuse, conduct disorder, and poor communication within the family. In addition, the presence of a personality disorder and lack of compliance with therapy may be due to disappointment made this case all the more difficult to treat.

References

1 **World Health Organization (WHO)**. Preventing suicide: a global imperative. Geneva; 2014.

2 **Brunner R, Kaess M, Parzer P, Carli V, Hoven CW, . . . Wasserman D**. Life-time prevalence and psychosocial correlates of adolescent direct self-injurious behaviour: a comparative study of findings in 11 European countries. J Child Psych Psychiat 2014 Apr;**55**(4):337–348.

3 **Carli V, Wasserman C, Hoven CW, Chiesa F, Guffanti G, . . . Wasserman D**. A newly identified group of adolescents at 'invisible' risk for psychopathology and suicidal behaviour: findings from the SEYLE study. World Psychiatry. 2014 Feb;**13**(1):78–86.

4 **Shaffer D, Gould MS, Fisher P, Trautman P, Moreau D, Kleinmann M, et al**. Psychiatric diagnosis in child and adolescent suicide. Arch Gen Psychiatry. 1996;**53**:339–348.

5 **Evans E, Hawton K, Rodham K**. Factors associated with suicidal phenomena in adolescents: a systematic review of population-based studies. Clin Psych Rev. 2004;**24**:957–979.

6 **Page A, Morrell S, Hobbs C, Carter G, Dudley M, Duflou J, et al**. Suicide in young adults: psychiatric and socio-economic factors from a case-control study. BMC Psychiatry. 2014;**14**(1):68.

7 **Balázs J, Miklósi M, Keresztény A, Hoven CW, Carli V, . . . Wasserman D**. Adolescent subthreshold depression: psychopathology, functional impairment and increased suicide risk. J Chil Psych Psychiat. 2013 Jun;**54**(6):670–677.

8 **Sarchiapone M, Mandelli L, Carli V, Iosue M, Wasserman C, . . . Wasserman D**. Hours of sleep among adolescents and its association with anxiety, emotional problems and suicidal ideation. J Sleep Med. 2014 Feb;**15**(2):248–254.

9 **Costello EJ, Copeland W, Angold A**. Trends in psychopathology across the adolescent years: what changes when children become adolescents, and when adolescents become adults? J Child Psychol. 2011;**52**(10):1015–1025.

10 **Kessler RC, Birnbaum H, Shahly V, Bromet E, Hwang I, McLaughlin K, et al**. Age differences in the prevalence and co-morbidity of DSM-IV major depressive episodes: results from the WHO World Mental Health Survey Initiative. Depress Anxiety. 2010;**27**:351–364.

11 **Goldstein TR, Ha W, Axelson DA, Goldstein BI, Liao F, Gill MK, et al**. Predictors of prospectively examined suicide attempts among youth with bipolar disorder. Arch Gen Psychiatry. 2012;**69**(11):1113–1122.

12 Kelleher I, Lynch F, Harley M, Molloy C, Roddy S, Fitzpatrick C, et al. Psychotic symptoms in adolescence index risk for suicidal behavior: findings from 2 population-based case-control clinical interview studies. Arch Gen Psychiatry. 2012;**69**:1277–1283.

13 Kokkevi A, Richardson C, Olszewski D, Matias J, Monshouwer K, Bjarnason T. Multiple substance use and self-reported suicide attempts by adolescents in 16 European countries. Eur Child Adolesc Psychiatry. 2012;**21**(8):443–450.

14 Guillaume S, et al. Characteristics of suicide attempts in anorexia and bulimia nervosa: a case-control study. PloS One. 2011;**6**(8):e23578.

15 Gvion Y, Apter A. Aggression, impulsivity and suicide behavior: a review of the literature. Arch Suicide Res. 2011;**15**(2):93–112.

16 Kaess M, Durkee T, Brunner R, Carli V, Parzer P, . . . Wasserman D. Pathological Internet use among European adolescents: psychopathology and self-destructive behaviours. Eur Child Adolesc Psychiatry. 2014;**23**:1093–1102.

17 Daniel SS, Goldston DB, Erkanli A, Franklin JC, Mayfield AM. Trait anger, anger expression, and suicide attempts among adolescents and young adults: a prospective study. J Clin Child Adolesc Psychol. Sep 2009;**38**(5):661–671.

18 Ohring R, Apter A, Ratzoni G, Weizman R, Tyano S, Plutchik R. State and trait anxiety in adolescent suicide attempters. J Am Acad Child Adolesc Psychiatry. 1996;**35**:154–157.

19 Freud S. Beyond the pleasure principle. Penguin UK; 2003.

20 Menninger KA. Man against himself. New York, NY: Harcourt, Brace and Company; 1938.

21 Apter A, Bleich A, King RA, Kron S, Fluch A, Kotler M, et al. Death without warning? A clinical postmortem study of suicide in 43 Israeli adolescent males. Arch Gen Psychiatry. 1993;**50**:138–142.

22 Wasserman DZ, Rihmer Z, Rujescu D, Sarchiapone M, Sokolowski M, . . . Carli V. The European psychiatric association (EPA) guidance on suicide treatment and prevention. Eur Psychiatry. 2012;**27**(2):129–141.

23 Kernberg P. Psychological interventions for the suicidal adolescent. Am Journal Psychotherapy. 1994;**48**:52–63.

24 Brent DA. The aftercare of adolescents with deliberate self-harm. J Child Psychol Psychiatr Allied Disciplines. 1997;**38**:277–286.

25 Kruesi MJ, Grossman J, Pennington JM, Woodward PJ, Duda D, Hirsch JG. Suicide and violence prevention: parent education in the emergency department. J Am Acad Child Adolesc Psychiatry. 1999;**38**:250–255.

26 Mufson L, Weissman MM, Moreau D, Garfinkel R. Efficacy of interpersonal psychotherapy for depressed adolescents. Arch Gen Psychiatry. 1999;**56**(6):573–579.

27 Rathus JH, Miller AL. Dialectical behavior therapy adapted for suicidal adolescents. Suicide Life Threat Behav 2002;**32**(2):146–157.

28 Diamond GS, Reis BF, Diamond GM, Siqueland L, Issacs L. Attachment-based family therapy for depressed adolescents: a treatment development study. J Am Acad Child Adolesc Psychiatry. 2002;**41**(10):1190–1196.

29 Eskin M. Problem solving therapy in the clinical practice. Newnes; 2012.

30 Wasserman D, Hoven CW, Wasserman C, Wall M, Eisenberg R, . . . Wasserman D. School-based suicide prevention programmes: the SEYLE cluster-randomised, controlled trial. Lancet. 2015;**385**:1536–1544.

Chapter 21

Older adults and suicide

Siobhan T O'Dwyer and Diego De Leo

Prevalence of suicidal behaviours

As the population ages, the rate of suicide in older adults is becoming a cause for concern. Older adults have high rates of death by suicide and, in many nations, have higher rates of suicide than any other age group.[1] Among older adults, the suicide rate is also consistently higher in men than in women.

There are, however, some populations where older adults do not have high rates of suicide. Suicide in older people has been reported to be almost non-existent in the indigenous peoples of Australia, New Zealand, Canada, the US, and the Arctic Circle.[2,3] This is explained by the younger average age of these populations (a result of the social, economic, and health consequences of colonization), and by the fact that older people in these communities have meaningful and respected roles as the keepers of knowledge and tradition.[2] Suicide rates in older adults are also very low in predominantly Islamic countries of the Middle East, including Bahrain, Egypt, Kuwait, Iran, and Syria,[4] where religious beliefs prohibit suicide and cultural factors prevent the reporting of deaths by suicide in order to protect surviving families.

Methods of suicide vary across countries and by gender. In England and Wales, for example, the most common methods for older men and women are hanging and poisoning, respectively.[5] In the US, the most common method for older men is firearm, while for older women it is poisoning.[6] In Singapore the most common method for older adults is jumping from a height (~73% of older suicides), consistent with the fact that the vast majority of Singaporeans live in high-rise accommodation.[7] Despite cultural and gender differences in methods, the heightened lethality of the methods chosen by older adults is seen across the world and reflected in the fact that the ratio of attempted suicides to suicides is markedly lower in older adults than in other age groups.[8,9]

In recent years, the rate of suicide in older adults in the UK, Europe, and the US has declined.[1,5,10] Although this is positive, it does not diminish the fact that older adults remain a high (if not the highest) risk group for suicide and should certainly not be taken to mean preventative activities are not required.

Risk factors

A range of factors has been associated with suicide in older adults; they span psychological, physical, social, and economic domains.

Psychiatric disorders

Psychiatric disorders, particularly depression and anxiety, are consistently identified as risk factors for suicide in older adults. Psychiatric illness is present in more than two-thirds of older suicides and the odds of an older adult having an Axis I diagnosis are markedly higher for suicides than matched controls.[11] Abuse or inappropriate use of prescription medications, particularly painkillers and those used to treat psychiatric disorders, can also place older adults at increased risk of suicide and Canadian research has found that the risk is heightened by multiple prescriptions and increases with medication strength.[12,13] Alcohol abuse may also be a risk factor for suicide in older adults, particularly when it co-occurs with psychiatric illness, but the evidence in older suicides is quite limited.[14]

Personality traits

Certain personality traits, as well as personality disorders, are associated with increased suicide risk for older adults. In particular, conscientiousness and anankastic personality traits have been found to be more common in older suicides than controls.[15,16]

Physical health problems

Physical health problems are significantly more common in older suicides than younger ones. Furthermore, the risk increases with multiple comorbidities. Compared with older people with no identified illness, older people with three illnesses have a threefold increase in suicide risk, while those with five illnesses have a fivefold increase in risk.[12] The specific conditions that appear to confer greater risk for older adults include stroke, heart disease, cancer (particularly metastatic disease), chronic lung disease, and conditions which cause severe pain. For older men, prostate cancer is also a risk factor, particularly in the first year after diagnosis.[17]

Hospitalization and contact with health services

In the weeks and months preceding suicide, older adults are more likely to have seen a doctor than younger suicides and matched controls. In the US, one in four older suicides saw their doctor within one week of their suicide.[18] In Canada, older suicides were almost twice as likely to have seen a doctor in the week before their death (compared with controls) and, of those who saw a doctor in the preceding month, three-quarters had three or more visits.[12] While general medical contact prior to suicide is high in older adults, specific contact with mental health professionals is low. In Taiwan, for example, older suicides were less likely to have used a mental health service than younger suicides in both the month and the year before suicide.[19] Taken together, this evidence suggests that when older adults reach out for help, the services they receive are inadequate.

Hospitalization is also a risk factor for suicide in older adults. In Finland, for example, approximately 30% of older suicides between 1988 and 2003 occurred within one month of discharge from hospital.[20] Interestingly, among older suicides in Finland, approximately 80% of diagnoses given during the last hospitalization were non-psychiatric. There was also a gender effect, with older Finnish women more likely to have suicided in the first month after hospitalization than older men. In Denmark, however, the risk conferred by hospitalization is strongest for older men. Danish men over 80 who were hospitalized with medical illnesses had the highest suicide rate of all age groups, while the risk of suicide in men over 80 with three or more medical illnesses requiring hospitalization was triple that of those with no comorbidity.[21] This evidence suggests that the post-discharge period should be a focus of attention for suicide-prevention activities for older adults, particularly those with multiple illnesses, and a range of health professionals (including pharmacists, community nurses, and case managers) could all play a role.

Socio-economic status

A range of socio-economic factors can influence suicide risk in older adults. Low education, financial problems, and difficulties with work or retirement, for example, have all been identified as risk factors. Although socio-economic factors are not—usually—easy to modify, they do serve as useful markers for identifying older adults who might be at risk or who could benefit from additional support, particularly when other risk factors are present.

Social isolation and loss

Isolation and a lack of social interaction are also risk factors for suicide in older adults, even after accounting for the influence of mood disorders and occupational status. Family conflict and bereavement can also contribute to social isolation in older adults, particularly older men. The loss of a partner confers an eightfold increase in suicide risk for older men in the first year after the loss and this risk is maintained in subsequent years.[22] For older women who are bereaved, the risk increases fivefold in the first year, but decreases in subsequent years.[22] Outreach services and programmes that offer social support may be crucial for suicide prevention in older adults and recently bereaved people would be an ideal target for these services.

Long-term care

Placement into residential or long-term care may also expose older adults to an increased risk of suicide. A US study of suicides between 1990 and 2005 found that while the rate of suicide among community-dwelling older adults declined over the 16 years, there was no change in the rate for those in long-term care.[23] Mezuk and colleagues argue that this is because 'whatever protective factors are acting on community-dwelling elderly people . . . are not reaching those in long-term care'.[23]

While the evidence on risk factors highlights the multidimensional nature of suicide risk in older adults and suggests a number of avenues for preventative action, it is important to note that the majority of data come from Western studies and are rarely broken down by ethnicity or other demographic factors. As a result, our understanding of the risk factors for suicide among sub-groups of older adults, or those in developing nations, is limited.

Emerging issues

SARS

In 2003, the Severe Acute Respiratory Syndrome (SARS) epidemic hit Hong Kong, claiming 300 lives. Older adults were disproportionately affected by the syndrome and, at the time of the epidemic, there was also a significant increase in suicides among older adults in Hong Kong. The rate of suicide among older adults in 2003 was the highest during the period 1993 to 2004 and the peak in older adult suicide rates coincided with the height of the epidemic. A study of 22 older adult suicides, in which the SARS epidemic was specifically identified as a contributing factor in suicide notes and informant reports, identified three common factors: being disconnected, feeling like a burden, and fear of contracting SARS.[24] Although only one of the suicide cases had actually contracted SARS, fear of the syndrome was so extreme in some cases that it triggered or worsened psychiatric symptoms. Disconnection was the result of forced or voluntary quarantine measures, which left older adults socially isolated and unable to engage in usual activities, while those with chronic conditions, pain, or disability had expressed concern about being a burden on their families during an already difficult time. When future epidemics strike there is a need to ensure that: the redirection of public health resources is not to the detriment of mental health services; outreach services are provided to older adults who may be isolated by quarantine measures or misinformed about the relative risks of contracting the illness; and resources are available to help older people reconnect with their community after the epidemic has passed.[24]

Dementia

Dementia is the term used to describe the syndrome caused by a range of degenerative conditions including Alzheimer's disease. There is no cure and most people with dementia experience a progressive loss of functioning across domains including cognition, communication, mood, behaviour, and basic activities of daily living. Despite the poor prognosis for most people diagnosed with dementia, there is no consistent evidence that people with dementia have higher rates of suicide than the general population.[25] The exception is for those with Huntington's disease, who have a risk of suicide three times greater than the general population, a fact that is generally linked to the familial nature of the disease.[25] People with dementia do, however, experience suicidal ideation and self-harm, which has led some to suggest that advancing dementia may inhibit the ability to plan and execute a suicidal act. This is consistent with evidence that has found suicide risk in people with dementia to be highest in the period immediately after diagnosis and in those of younger age.[25,26] Where suicide does occur in people with dementia, risk factors include mental illness (particularly depression), insight, younger age, recent diagnosis, expression of suicidal intent, history of self-harm, and substance abuse.[25,26] As Haw et al.[25] note, however, the existing evidence on suicide and dementia has significant methodological limitations and much remains to be understood.

Homicide-suicide

Homicide-suicide is defined as a homicide that is followed, within one week, by the suicide of the perpetrator. Although homicide-suicide is a relatively rare phenomenon, recent research suggests that older adults are disproportionately represented among both perpetrators and victims of domestic homicide-suicides and that cases of domestic homicide by people aged over 65 are more likely to end in the suicide of the perpetrator than not.[27,28] Although the small number of homicide-suicides limits research results, the existing evidence shows that the vast majority of homicide-suicide cases are committed by men, against a female spouse, using a firearm.[28,29] In the case of older, spousal homicide-suicides, as many as 40% of perpetrators are providing care for a spouse with a long-term illness or disability,[28] and some research has suggested that more than 70% of older homicide-suicides may have suicide as their primary motive.[30] Other risk factors include a history of domestic violence, relationship breakdown, alcohol abuse, and mental illness.[27-29] Although there is debate about the conceptual similarities between suicides and homicide-suicides, the recommendations for prevention are largely the same and include: better identification of at-risk older adults (both potential perpetrators and potential victims) in primary- and community-care settings; better treatment of physical and mental health risk factors in older adults; and means restriction.[27,28,30]

Suicide prevention

Given the high rates of suicide in older adults, there is a clear need for evidence-based prevention activities and the literature on risk factors highlights some obvious targets for this work. Despite this, there are only a small number of trials of interventions designed to prevent suicide in this group.

A systematic review of papers published between 1966 and 2009 found only 11 distinct interventions that aimed to reduce suicidality in older adults and were empirically evaluated.[31] Five of the studies were classified as 'Indicated' programmes—that is, programmes that target people who are already experiencing suicidal thoughts or displaying suicidal behaviours. Four were classified as 'Selective'—that is, targeting people who are considered high risk, but have not yet experienced suicidal thoughts or behaviours. One study incorporated 'Indicated', 'Selective', and 'Universal' (targeting an entire population or community) activities. The interventions were delivered in primary care, in clinical settings, and by telephone. The majority of the studies (9 out of 11) addressed risk factors, such as depression and social isolation, and six of the nine resulted in reductions in suicidal ideation among participants or reductions in suicide rates in the participating community. Two studies failed to include specific measures of suicidality, despite the interventions being designed to prevent suicide. Only two studies took a strengths-based approach, focusing on improving protective factors rather than reducing risk factors and both reported positive effects on suicidal ideation. In the review article, Lapierre et al.[31] recommended that future interventions should: focus on the detection, treatment, and management of mood disorders; include family members and friends; consider all contacts with older adults (e.g., home visits, nursing care, case management) as an opportunity for suicide prevention; address the impact of physical risk factors such as pain, poor sleep, and chronic disease on suicide risk; and be multifaceted. They also highlighted the need for research on means restriction specifically targeting older adults, media guidelines on how to report suicide, and online interventions.[31]

Since that review was conducted, three additional studies have been published—one concerning an indicated intervention, and two a selective one. Chan and colleagues[32] reported a two-year follow-up of a multi-faceted suicide-prevention programme, known as the Elderly Suicide Prevention Programme (ESPP), for older adults in Hong Kong. ESPP included treatment of depression, gatekeeper training, aftercare of suicide attempters, and care management including multidisciplinary care planning and review meetings. It was implemented at both the primary care and tertiary care (psychiatric service) levels and included only older adults who had made a suicide attempt. At a two-year follow-up there were significantly higher rates of completed suicide among the comparison group (an historical cohort receiving standard psychogeriatric care), than in the prevention programme group. Although antidepressants prescription rates were comparable across the two groups, the rate of dropouts from services was significantly higher in the comparison group, suggesting that continuity of care may have been a key aspect of the ESPP intervention.[32]

Almeida et al.[33] conducted the Depression and Early Prevention of Suicide in General Practice (DEPS-GP) study, a cluster-randomized trial of more than 300 physicians and more than 21,000 patients in Australia. Physicians in the intervention group received a three-part intervention including printed educational materials (about assessing and diagnosing depression, and identifying and managing suicide risk), personalized feedback on an audit of 20 patients (including the number of patients in their practice with depression or suicidal ideation, and the specific symptoms reported by those patients), and regular newsletters (including information on signs and symptoms, screening tips, and case studies). Over a 24-month follow-up, older adults whose physicians were allocated to the intervention group were significantly less likely to report self-harm behaviour (defined as any of: suicide ideation, suicide attempt, or intentional self-injury). Interestingly, older adults who reported no self-harm behaviour at baseline and were seen by a physician in the intervention group had lower odds of reported self-harm behaviour during follow-up than those treated by a control physician, but the intervention had no effect on those who reported self-harm behaviour at baseline. Also, the intervention had no significant effects on symptoms of depression. Almeida et al. noted that there were no differences between intervention and control patients in terms of antidepressants use, contact with mental health professionals, or other support, which suggests that physicians' attitudes towards, and willingness to discuss, issues related to suicide may have been the crucial factor in the success of this intervention. This study is also notable because it addresses the absence of research on training for physicians identified in Lapierre et al's[31] review, a gap which is particularly concerning when considered in light of research that suggests that physicians are less willing to treat suicidal ideation in older adults.[34]

Bartsch et al.[35] evaluated Senior Reach Gatekeeper Referral programmes delivered in Colorado and Mid-Kansas (US). The programmes had three components—training, referral, and treatment. In the training component, traditional (e.g., physicians, service providers) and non-traditional (e.g., bus drivers, retail staff) community partners were trained to identify and refer older adults in the community experiencing risk factors such as poor health, isolation, and abuse. Older adults identified by these partners were referred to a telephone outreach or call centre for assessment and referral to community services or clinicians. In the treatment phase, older adults were offered mental health treatment, case management, crisis intervention, and advocacy. Data on suicidal ideation were collected at baseline and discharge from the programme (or six months after baseline, whichever came first). In both programmes there was a significant decrease in the percentage of clients with suicidal ideation (from 79.4% to 54.2% in Colorado, and from 78.9% to 49.2% for Mid-Kansas) and there was no difference between those referred by traditional partners and those referred by non-traditional partners, which suggests that the responsibility for suicide prevention need not rest solely on physicians or health professionals, but rather can be shared across all sections of the community.

Across all the studies conducted to date, only a handful have examined the effects by gender and, where they have, the programmes have generally been found to be more effective for women. There is also an absence of programmes targeting older people in residential/long-term care, older people from specific ethnic or cultural groups, and older people in developing nations.

While much remains to be done for truly evidence-based suicide prevention for older adults, an international expert panel has provided a key list of considerations to guide future efforts.[36] When taken together, the items on the list clearly highlight the importance of taking an holistic approach to suicide prevention in older adults that: encompasses indicated, selective, and universal prevention activities; shares the responsibility for suicide prevention across policymakers, researchers, health professionals, community-service providers, family carers, and individuals; takes a positive approach to ageing in which decline and distress are not considered inevitable features of ageing; and, recognizes that older adults are a heterogeneous group for which a 'one-size-fits-all' approach' is unlikely to be effective.

Case Study

At the time of his suicide attempt Mr B, aged 77 years, had been a widower for three months. He suffered from a functional disability as a result of the amputation of one leg for an incurable vascular problem. His two daughters both lived in distant cities.

After their mother's death, the daughters had begun devoting a halfday each week to looking after their father. They also arranged for some cleaning and cooking to be carried out by home help hired through private agencies. In cooperation with the family doctor, after Mr B's serious suicide attempt, they requested urgent installation of the 'Tele-Help/Tele-Check' service in his home.

Mr B attempted suicide by dropping a radio in the bath in an effort to electrocute himself. After three weeks in hospital, he was discharged with a prescription for 100 mg sertraline daily and the recommendation that a social worker visit him at home at least once a week.

Mr B had no previous history of psychiatric disorders. A retired blue-collar worker, he had no friends or particular hobbies and spent most of his time watching television. He used to play cards with his wife. He was opposed to the idea of connection to the 'Tele-Help/Tele-Check' service, fearing complete abandonment by his daughters.

In the first month of being connected, he made two emergency calls to the service. In both cases, he expressed strong suicidal ideation. Now that he has been connected to the service for nearly two years, Mr B receives an average of three check calls a week from the Tele-Help operator, with whom he has established highly effective and supportive communication.

References

1 **World Health Organization**. World suicide report—preventing suicide: a global imperative. Geneva; 2014.

2 **Hunter E, Harvey D**. Indigenous suicide in Australia, New Zealand, Canada and the United States. Emerg Med. 2002;**14**:14–23.

3 **Broderstad AR, Eliassen B-M, Melhus M**. Prevalence of self-reported suicidal thoughts in SLiCA. The survey of living conditions in the Artic (SLiCA). Glob Health Action. 2011;**4**:10226.

4 **Pritchard C, Amanullah S**. An analysis of suicide and undetermined deaths in 17 predominantly Islamic countries contrasted with the UK. Psychol Med. 2007;**37**:421–430.

5 **Shah A, Buckley L**. The current status of methods used by the elderly for suicides in England and Wales. J Inj Violence Res. 2011;**3**(2):68–73.

6 **Karch D**. Sex differences in suicide incident characteristics and circumstances among older adults: surveillance data from the National Violent Death Reporting System—17 US States, 2007–2009. Int J Environ Res Public Health 2011; **8**:3479–3495.

7 **Chia B-H, Chia A, Ng W-Y, Tai B-C**. Suicide methods in Singapore (2000–2004): type and associations. Suicide Life Threat Behav 2011;**41**(5):574–583.

8 **De Leo D, Padoani W, Scocco P, Lie D, Bille-Brahe U, Arensman E, et al.** Attempted and completed suicide in older subjects: results from the WHO/EURO multicentre study of suicidal behaviour. Int J Geriatr Psychiatry 2001;**16**:300–310.

9 **Dombrovski AY, Szanto K, Duberstein P, Conner KR, Houck PR, Conwell Y**. Sex differences in correlates of suicide attempt lethality in late life. Am J Geriatr Psychiatry 2008;**16**:905–913.

10 **Innamorati M, Tamburello A, Lester D, Amore M, Girardi P, Tatarelli R, et al.** Inequalities in suicide rates in the European Union's elderly: trends and impact

of macro-socioeconomic factors between 1980 and 2006. Can J Psychiatry 2010;**55**(4):229–238.

11 **Conwell Y, Van Orden K, Caine ED.** Suicide in older adults. Psychiatr Clin North Am 2011;**34**(2):451–468.

12 **Juurlink DN, Herrmann N, Szalai JP, Kopp A, Redelmeier DA.** Medical illness and the risk of suicide in the elderly. Arch Intern Med 2004;**164**:1179–1184.

13 **Voaklander DC, Rowe BH, Dryden DM, Pahal J, Saar P, Kelly KD.** Medical illness, medication use and suicide in seniors: a population-based case-control study. J Epidemiol Community Health. 2008;**62**:138–146.

14 **Blow FC, Brockmann, LM, Barry KL.** Role of alcohol in late-life suicide. Alcohol Clin Exp Res 2004;**28**(5):48S–56S.

15 **Useda JD, Duberstein PR, Conner KR, Beckman A, Franus N, Tu X, et al.** Personality differences in attempted suicide versus suicide in adults 50 years of age or older. J Consult Clin Psychol. 2007;**75**(1):126–133.

16 **Harwood D, Hawton K, Hope T, Jacoby R.** Psychiatric disorders and personality factors associated with suicide in older people: a descriptive and case-control study. Int J Geriatr Psychiatry 2001;**16**:155–165.

17 **Fall K, Fang F, Mucci LA, et al.** Immediate risk for cardiovascular events and suicide following a prostate cancer diagnosis: prospective cohort study. PLoS Med. 2009;**6**(12):e1000197.

18 **Miller M, Mogun H, Azrael D, Hempstead K, Solomon DH.** Cancer and the risk of suicide in older Americans. J Clin Oncol 2008;**26**(29):4720–4724.

19 **Lee H-S, Lin H-C, Liu T-C, Lin S-Y.** Contact of mental and nonmental health care providers prior to suicide in Taiwan: a population-based study. Can J Psychiatry 2008;**53**(6):377–383.

20 **Karvonen K, Hakko H, Koponen H, Meyer-Rochow VB, Rasanen P.** Suicides among older persons in Finland and time since hospitalization discharge. Psych Serv. 2009;**60**(3):390–393.

21 **Erlangsen A, Vach W, Jeune B.** The effect of hospitalization with medical illnesses on the suicide risk in the oldest old: a population-based register study. J Am Geriatr Soc 2005;**53**:771–776.

22 **Erlangsen A, Jeune B, Bille-Brahe U, Vaupel JW.** Loss of partner and suicide risks among oldest old: a population-based register study. Age and Ageing. 2004;**33**:378–383.

23 **Mezuk B, Prescott MR, Tardiff K, Vhalov D, Galea S.** Suicide in older adults in long-term care: 1990–2005. J Am Geriatr Soc 2008;**56**:2107–2111.

24 **Yip PS, Cheung YT, Chau PH, Law YW.** The impact of epidemic outbreak: the case of Severe Acute Respiratory Syndrome (SARS) and suicide among older adults in Hong Kong. Crisis. 2010;**31**(2):86–92.

25 **Haw C, Harwood D, Hawton K.** Dementia and suicidal behavior: a review of the literature. Int Psychogeriatr 2009;**21**(3):4400–4453.

26 Seyfried LS, Kales HC, Ignacio RV, Conwell Y, Valenstein, M. Predictors of suicide in patients with dementia. Alzheimers Dement 2011;7(6):567–573.

27 Bell CC, McBride DF. Commentary: homicide-suicide in older adults—cultural and contextual perspectives. J Am Acad Psychiatry Law 2010;38:312–317.

28 Malphurs JE, Cohen D. A statewide case-control study of spousal homicide-suicide in older persons. Am J Geriatr Psychiatry 2005;13(3):211–217.

29 Bourget D, Gagne P, Whitehurst L. Domestic homicide and homicide-suicide: the older offender. J Am Acad Psychiatry Law 2010;38(3):305–311.

30 Salari S. Patterns of intimate partner homicide suicide in later life: strategies for prevention. Clin Interv Aging 2007;2(3):441–452.

31 Lapierre S, Erlangsen A, Waern M, De Leo D, Oyama H, Scocco P, et al. A systematic review of elderly suicide prevention programs. Crisis. 2011;32(2):88–98.

32 Chan SS, Leung VP, Tsoh J, Li SW, Yu CS, Yu GK, et al. Outcomes of a two-tiered multifaceted elderly suicide prevention program in Hong Kong Chinese community. Am J Geriatr Psychiatry 2011;19(2):185–196.

33 Almeida OP, Pirkis J, Kerse N, Sim M, Flicker L, Draper B, et al. A randomized trial to reduce the prevalence of depression and self-harm behavior in older primary care patients. Ann Fam Med 2012;10(4):347–356.

34 Uncapher H, Arean PA. Physicians are less willing to treat suicidal ideation in older patients. J Am Geriatr Soc 2000;48(2):188–192.

35 Bartsch DA, Rodgers VK, Strong D. Outcomes of Senior Reach gatekeeper referrals: comparison of the Spokane Gatekeeper Program, Colorado Senior Reach, and Mid-Kansas Senior Outreach. Care Manag J 2013;14(1):11–20.

36 Erlangsen A, Nordentoft M, Conwell Y, Waern M, De Leo D, Lindner R, et al. Key considerations for preventing suicide in older adults: consensus opinions of an expert panel. Crisis. 2011;32(2):106–109.

Suicide risk assessment

Chapter 22

Suicide risk assessment

Danuta Wasserman

Systematic clinical assessment of suicide risk

Suicide risk assessment is the most difficult kind of assessment in psychiatric practice, since it is about life and death and arouses fear in doctors themselves. Doctors need not—and cannot—assume responsibility for the life of a suicidal patient but, on the other hand, they must put their knowledge into practice in an optimal way with the goal of preventing a threatening suicide.[1–3]

Many suicidal patients, like other psychiatric patients, hesitate to consult a psychiatrist for as long as possible. Not infrequently, they finally do so after repeated urging from family members, friends, or colleagues. It is, therefore, essential to give such patients ample time and attention. Assessment of suicide risk touches on patients' most pressing problems, including their reflections on life and death. It includes the causes of their suicidality and their future prospects. It also encompasses what suicidal patients have themselves done to solve their problems, and on their expectations.[4–6]

Suicide risk assessment should take place on several levels and relate to the patient, his or her families, and social networks, and also to the availability of treatment, rehabilitation, and prevention resources in the community. Assessing risk involves factors that exacerbate and factors that hinder the development of the suicidal process, such as:

+ suicidal intention;
+ previous psychiatric disorders and suicidal behaviour;
+ suicide in the family or acquaintances (suicide models); and
+ the patient's suicidal communication.

Assessment of the nature of family, friends and networks support is vital. If, for example, there are no acute negative life events present and the family is supportive, suicide risk does not necessarily arise.[3]

In addition to a clinical interview, one can use the instruments suggested in Chapter 25, which form part of various appraisal scales, to evaluate suicide risk. The questions posed must feel natural both to the patient and to the doctor.

The suicidal process

Suicide risk is a crescendo phenomenon. Movement from sporadic thoughts of death to more frequent suicide wishes or from diffuse suicide plans to schemes that include detailed choices of method and place in the near future indicate there is a rising scale of suicide risk in the suicidal process (see also Chapter 3). Advanced suicide plans or actual attempts with a high intentionality and pronounced anxiety as well as with active methods, indicate high suicide risk. People who have easily aroused feelings of hopelessness, suicidal ideation, and a history of previous suicide attempts, and also those who have models in the form of family members or acquaintances who have attempted or committed suicide, make up a clear group in terms of long-term risk of suicidal behaviour.

In some cases, the above-described crescendo phenomenon can be repeated during the suicidal patient's life (a cyclical course); for example, a suicide attempt can be performed by a young female or male at the age of 15 or 16 and be repeated when they are 24 or 30, or later on in their lives. Therefore, it is important to explore the individual patient's suicidal processes.

In assessing suicide risk, one must ask questions and explore the answers to questions such as: What does life mean to this person? Is there anything that appeals to him or her? What is about to happen in the patient's life, over the next 24 hours or the month ahead? If he or she invariably looks on the dark side and has no plans for the future or supportive resources—family, friends, or work—the risk of suicide is high.

Suicidal communication

Suicidal communication may range from no hint of suicidal intent or just the occasional expression of suicidal intent in upsetting situations—sometimes under the influence of alcohol, and indicating little or no risk of suicide—to suicidal statements of intent with a blend of seriousness and denial that distinctly alarms other people and indicates medium to high risk. Repeated, clear verbal expression of serious suicidal thoughts and suicide plans without being under the influence of alcohol or a quarrel with a partner indicates a high suicide risk.

Relationships

Suicide risk is low if the patient has good relationships with relatives or friends who are ready to help in times of need. Such relationships imply prospects of successfully working through the kinds of problems that trigger the suicidal situation.[7] On the other hand, suicide risk is elevated if the patient's relationships are characterized by ambiguous communication, ambivalence, and aggressiveness, and if close relatives and friends have long since given up hope of cohabiting or socializing with him or her. In this situation, it is important to assess whether the family and closest friends can serve as support for the suicidal person in the treatment, or whether the family or social network itself needs support or treatment. Albeit it takes a considerable effort from the psychiatrist to motivate a suicidal person to involve family or significant others in the treatment plan, however, it is an important measure to be taken.

Sometimes, risk is difficult to assess if there are frequent separations from and reconciliations with one and the same partner, or if there are relationships that undergo constant ups and downs, with growing social problems. If, in such a situation, relationships are definitively broken off, suicide risk is high.

Psychosocial situation

Male, elderly, divorced, single, or unemployed people with excessive alcohol use or alcohol use disorder, mental illness, or personality disorder and who experience adverse life events are at high risk of suicide if they have previously experienced serious suicide plans or attempted suicide.

Mental illnesses and personality disorders

A renewed bout of depression, Bipolar Disorder, or other psychosis when negative life events are present and the suicidal person has begun resorting to alcohol may push him or her rapidly from a group characterized by low or medium to high suicide risk into a very high-risk group. If this happens, immediate intervention by the family and the health-care services is required.

However, when a patient is reluctant to undergo treatment, even very experienced health-care staff may unfortunately shy away from compulsory treatment or hospitalization due to an exaggerated fear of violating the patient's integrity.

Patients who can cope with their life situation without exposing themselves to undue stress and strain and who can manage the treatment of their basic illnesses while receiving support from their partners, family or friends do not necessarily have a high suicide risk, although more or less intense suicidal ideation is constantly present. For these people, especially those with dysthymic and protracted chronic depression suicidal ideation is one way of relating to life.

It is sometimes difficult to assess suicide risk in patients with dysthymia or brain damage whose suicidal process is chronic. It can also be difficult to assess suicide risk in immature, impulsive, or violent young people with a prepondency to act out their fantasies.

In chapters 6–12, more details can be found about the mental illnesses and personality types that contribute to suicide risk in the event of an unfavourable social situation and of definitive, sudden losses and narcissistic injuries.

Substance misuse

Misuse of alcohol or narcotics in conjunction with other psychiatric morbidity, risk of social exclusion and definitive, sudden losses or narcissistic injuries imply a high suicide risk (see Chapter 7). The risk is often reduced by immediate hospitalization and by starting rehabilitation and treatment of the substance use disorder and the underlying psychiatric morbidity simultaneously.

Somatic illness

Somatic illnesses and situations that place people in the risk zone for suicide are described in Chapter 13. The risk of suicide may be high in people suffering from disabling, painful, or terminal illnesses who simultaneously develop depression and experience sudden losses or narcissistic injuries in the absence of good support from the family and adequate pain relief and proper nursing. Illnesses in organs of symbolic importance to the individual, such as breasts to a woman or genital organs to both sexes, may contribute to an elevated suicide risk when other risk factors are also present.

Suicide risk assessment after suicide attempts

In a regressed state (after attempting suicide) suicidal patients' psychological defence mechanisms are weakened. When they regain consciousness after attempting suicide, patients are usually in a state of profound despair and feel ashamed, although they are also often highly relieved to be alive still and wish to be helped. It is, therefore, much easier at this time to explore their affective state and problems. But in a few hours patients may rapidly 'close up' again and deny their need of help. It is, therefore, essential to try to fit the suicide risk assessment into a therapeutic 'window of opportunity', when patients have neither regressed too far nor once again lost contact with their desperation and nor distanced themselves from the need for professional help and lost motivation for treatment.

Many people repeat their suicide attempts, or commit suicide, very soon after being discharged from hospital. This is partly due to poor treatment compliance, which in turn could be the result of poorly 'timed' suicide risk assessment.[3] The doctor should ensure not only that the patient is given the name of the person responsible for follow-up and an appointment for an initial return visit but also that contact with the patient has taken place.

Suicide risk assessment before temporary discharge

Striking the right balance between keeping suicidal patients in hospital too long and discharging them too early is not easy. Temporary discharge—a day or weekend out—may be a good test of the suicidal patient's ability to cope with reality. Before every temporary discharge, the doctor needs to get in touch with the patient's relatives and to be in a position to judge whether there are supportive factors in the patient's surroundings or whether the problems are still so severe as to entail a risk of suicide.

Assessment for the purpose of discharge, whether temporary or permanent, is paramount since several surveys from various countries show that many patients take their lives shortly after leaving psychiatric hospital.[8,9]

Previous psychiatric care and the patient's attitude towards care

Suicide risk is high if a patient has previously been admitted to inpatient psychiatric care for mental illness or a suicide attempt[9] and has an ambivalent or even hostile attitude towards care services. The same is true if such a patient has declined or broken off treatment or failed to understand the purpose of undergoing treatment at all. Suicide risk is also exacerbated when psychiatric patients relapse (recurrent disease) due to psychological distress or a critical change in their life, and when they feel at the same time that no one understands them, or they experience paranoid ideation and think that they are being persecuted.

It is sometimes difficult to assess suicide risk in patients who show rapid swings between a positive and perhaps a flattering attitude towards staff and a negative attitude, with open hostility and rejection of the care offered. Elevated suicide risk is indicated by previous psychiatric care without mutual trust between the patient and the staff who provided the care and by swings between negative and positive attitudes to the doctor in charge and care services in general. If, on the other hand, the patient has shown appreciation of care received previously and has expressed confidence in the staff providing the treatment, and has the same attitude in the current situation, suicide risk is low.

Respect for suicidal patients' wishes

Few people commit suicide after mature and balanced consideration. Most patients show distinct psychiatric conditions or psychological distress and are too regressive in their conceptual world with its restricted cognition ('tunnel vision') to be capable of exerting responsibility for themselves at the moment when suicidal ideation is very strong and suicide plans are in the forefront of their minds. Therefore, it is important not only to emphasize patients' responsibility for their own lives, but also to be prepared to assume professional responsibility and to initiate supportive measures and sometimes to impose restrictions, including involving compulsory institutional care.

It is important for doctors to have a sense of commitment to their patients and to speak frankly to them and their families. It is also essential for the doctor to point out that, as a professional, he or she is aware that the desire to commit suicide is often ambivalent in nature and, in most cases, disappears when the problems fade away and the psychiatric illness is treated.

Assuming professional responsibility

When assessing suicide risk, it is vital for doctors to be aware of their own psychological functioning and of how far they themselves fear suicidal fantasies, death, weakness, and abandonment. This awareness may be helpful, not only in attempts to convince patients of the value of life, but also in listening to patients' arguments about their reasons for choosing death. Suicidal patients should, in the assessment of suicide risk, be allowed to describe and contemplate their own problems with respect to life, death and suicide, without being made to feel guilty or ashamed. A patient should not feel that such matters are taboo in his or her talks with doctors who assess suicide risk. This kind of open attitude on the doctor's part often relieves the patient's tension and may even reduce suicide risk.

Reducing and gauging risk of suicide

In assessing suicide risk, the doctor must be prepared to take steps that immediately reduce the suicide risk.[3,10] These steps are often of a psychiatric, psychological, and psychosocial nature, including (in certain cases) immediate commitment to hospital. It is important to remember that suicide risk is always changing: today it is different from yesterday and tomorrow it will be different from today. It is, therefore, vital to monitor patients and their families in order to be able to assess the development of the suicidal process again, in a clinically sensitive way. Various scales may then be helpful, especially those designed for self-appraisal, which can arouse the patient's curiosity and bring an element of activity into the treatment. Patients can see concrete results by being able, for example, to monitor their own scores and thus feeling as if they are taking their destiny into their own hands. These scales may also be useful for patients who have a poor communicative capacity or are reluctant to confide in the doctor or care staff.

After completion of suicide risk assessment

Suicide risk assessment should culminate in a conclusion as to whether the risk is low, high, or difficult to assess. The presence of warning signs and acute triggers judged in the context of the presence of chronic risk factors for suicidal behaviours, and the absence of protective factors buffering acute suicidal risk, constitute the basis for the clinical assessment. In the concluding discussion with the doctor, patients should be asked whether there are any other matters that the doctor has omitted to ask about, whether the patient received answers to their questions, and whether the family can be contacted.

Once a suicide risk assessment has been completed, it is vital to take active steps to transfer the patient to the relevant facilities to receive the further care that is deemed appropriate. The relatives, when the patient's consent is given, should be informed of the procedure and whom to contact if they need to. Similarly, they should be told whom to contact if the patient breaks off treatment.[3]

References

1 Fowler JC. Suicide risk assessment in clinical practice: pragmatic guidelines for imperfect assessments. Psychotherapy (Chicago, IL). 2012;**49**(1):81–90.

2 Schechter M, Maltsberger JT. The clinical interview as a method in suicide risk assessment. In: Wasserman D, Wasserman C, editors. The Oxford Textbook of Suicidology and Suicide Prevention: a global perspective. Oxford: Oxford University Press; 2009. p. 319–327.

3 Wasserman D, Rihmer Z, Rujescu D, Sarchiapone M, Sokolowski M, Titelman D, et al. The European Psychiatric Association (EPA) guidance on suicide treatment and prevention. European Psychiatry. 2012;**27**(2):129–141.

4 Harriss L, Hawton K, Zahl D. Value of measuring suicidal intent in the assessment of people attending hospital following self-poisoning or self-injury. Br J Psychiatry. 2005;**186**:60–66.

5 Silverman MM, Berman AL. Suicide risk assessment and risk formulation Part I: a focus on suicide ideation in assessing suicide risk. Suicide Life Threat Behav 2014;**44**(4):420–431.

6 Hendin H. Recognizing a suicide crisis in psychiatric patients. In: Wasserman D, Wasserman C, editors. The Oxford Textbook of Suicidology and Suicide Prevention: a global perspective. Oxford: Oxford University Press; 2009. p. 327–334.

7 Joiner Jr. TE. Why people die by suicide. Cambridge, MA: Harvard University Press; 2005.

8 Hunt IM, Bickley H, Windfuhr K, Shaw J, Appleby L, Kapur N. Suicide in recently admitted psychiatric in-patients: a case-control study. J Affect Disord. 2013;**144**(1–2):123–128.

9 Large M, Sharma S, Cannon E. Risk factors for suicide within a year of discharge from psychiatric hospital: a systematic meta-analysis. Aust NZ J Psychiat. 2011;**45**:619–628.

10 Simon RI. Suicide risk assessment: gateway to treatment and management. In: Simon RI and Hales RE, eds. American Psychiatric Publishing textbook of suicide assessment and management (2nd edn). Washington, DC: American Psychiatric Publishing; 2012: 3–28.

Chapter 23

The suicidal patient–doctor relationship

Danuta Wasserman

Introduction

The relationship that develops between the patient and the doctor in the course of the suicide risk assessment has a crucial bearing on the quality of the assessment and on the motivational process for suggested care, which if successful gives long-term gains in the treatment of mental disorders and mental health problems.[1–3] The process that arises in every interpersonal relationship is known as 'transference'. In transference, the previous perceptions, experiences, and unconscious wishes of those involved come to the fore and their usual relationship patterns and conflicts are reactivated. Conflicts and ways of relating to others can be staged in an unconscious or only partially conscious way. In psychiatric terminology, the patient's reaction is known as 'transference' and the doctor's or therapist's response as 'countertransference'.[4,5]

The suicidal patient's transference

Many suicidal patients complicate all their relationships, including that with the doctor, whom they may see as a saviour or an enemy. The patient may expect love and appreciation but also disparagement. The expectation of receiving help immediately, or that help will never be forthcoming, may also characterize the assessment situation. A suicidal patient's expectations may be expressed in various ways.

Many suicidal patients do not seek help or cooperate well. Some patients show a hostile, silent, and rejecting attitude towards the doctor in the assessment situation. Others may be provocative or 'act superior'. These reactions may occur because earlier perceptions of rejection and disapproval and memories of narcissistic injury, of being ignored or feeling like an outsider have arisen in the patient's mind. Leaving or rejecting others seems preferable to being left.[5]

Some suicidal patients may be entirely indifferent to whether they live or die. Others may have exaggerated expectations that the doctor can offer quick and easy solutions to their problems and these patients can be easily disappointed.

Interaction between the suicidal patient's and doctor's ambivalence

Suicidal patients are highly ambivalent. They swing from wanting to die to wanting to live and between despair and hope.[6] Sometimes during the short assessment, only the positive side of the ambivalence is manifested and the negative side can be missed altogether. A suicidal person's ambivalence may interact with the ambivalence of the doctor performing the assessment. This is expressed in the doctor's perception of the patient's strength and not their need for care, or the patient's weakness, in which case there is a risk of the doctor exerting too much control over the patient. Sometimes, a doctor's ambivalence towards a suicidal patient may result in the doctor misjudging or completely missing suicide risk, owing to a kind of unconscious consensus arising between the patient, who is reluctant to display his or her vulnerability, and the doctor, who is unwilling to recognize the patient's suicidality.[5]

Patients may hide their needs

In a structured and soothing assessment situation, suicidal people may temporarily calm down and cease to show their desperation or to communicate their profound suicidal ideation or suicide plans, however marked they may be. This may be because of a sense of shame or a temporary feeling that all is well.

Many suicidal people are reluctant to show their vulnerability and try to manage without the help of others, hiding their feelings of uncertainty and inferiority.[7] Not infrequently, this kind of attitude develops in childhood. As children, these patients were very often obliged to cope on their own without being capable of doing so.

In a desperate situation, despite strong reflections about suicide and an acute need for the help they seek, they may repress their suicidality.[8,9] Consequently, unless exploratory questions are asked, suicidality is not detected if the doctor is neither inclined nor trained to recognize it.

The doctor's countertransference

Doctors are unavoidably influenced by their patients' transference and projections. Like all human beings, doctors have various personality traits, characters, and psychological conflicts. They assess suicide risk and the need for admission, nursing, and treatment, not only according to their professional knowledge but also according to their individual values and attitudes to life, death, and suicide.

Many employees in the health-care services choose their occupation to master fear of death, dependence, and helplessness. Suicidal patients' self-destructive behaviour runs counter to the instinct of self-preservation and the desire to cure and alleviate, that are so strongly felt in most health-care staff. Partly as a result of this, doctors may, in a verbal or non-verbal way, both consciously and unconsciously, show disapproval of patients who have attempted suicide or have plans to commit suicide.

Most doctors feel empathy and exhibit interest when performing assessment of suicide risk, and establish a sound relationship with a suicidal patient. However, there are also doctors who may be extremely worried and see suicide risk everywhere. They 'persecute' patients in an insensitive way with questions about suicidal ideation and suicide attempts. Instead of winning patients' confidence and motivating them to undergo treatment, they frighten them away.

Other doctors may be indifferent, uncommitted, unobservant, and passive in their approach. Others may have an exaggerated sense of helplessness and think that there is nothing they can do. Not infrequently, doctors who are of a depressive disposition can adopt such an attitude and even become suicidal themselves. Others may feel questioned in their professional role and conclude that they are bad at their job when their narcissistic feeling is threatened.

Sometimes, a doctor may have a strong desire to be rid of the patient, whom they perceive as provocative and frustrating to deal with. In some cases, doctors may even show dismissive and negative attitudes and reject the patient. This kind of attitude may be a manifestation of the doctor's unresolved, underlying aggressive conflicts.[4,5,7,10]

Role assigned to the doctor

The role assigned to doctors and therapists by the patient, and the patient's reactions to them, do not only involve repetition of the patient's old conflicts or patterns. These reactions also depend on the current emotional attitude of the doctor who meets them, which may precipitate the patient's transference reaction.

Doctors' own mental conflicts influence their feelings towards a suicidal person and may impede the assessment of suicide risk. Awareness of one's 'blind spots' prevents misinterpretations. Doctors and therapists who have a good knowledge of their own psychological functioning (fostered by training, regular supervision, and teamwork) may be able to use their own personality as an asset in the assessment and treatment process and to manage the trying emotions experienced by both their patients and themselves.[11]

Difficulties in suicide risk assessment

Assessing suicide risk is difficult because suicidal people are full of inconsistencies and contradictions. Their thoughts often flit back and forth from one subject, feeling, or argument, to another.

Suicidal patients' denial of reality and their ambivalence, not only about life and death but also about any form of treatment, may be hard for the assessing clinician to deal with. The same applies to aggressive and manipulative reactions, which are not uncommon in suicidal patients. Being alternately idealized and disparaged, subjected to various provocations and tested to see how much one 'cares', and how much effort one is inclined to make may be very trying for a clinician performing a suicide risk assessment and when treating a suicidal patient. To experience patient suicide is common in clinical practice. Even if the majority of clinicians are able to cope with the trauma of losing a patient by suicide, the creation of formal and informal professional networks, which help with the debriefing of emotions and increase awareness of the impact of patient suicide on a professional, should be stimulated.[12]

Specific training of mental health professionals that work with suicidal patients is also now seen as being beneficial to both doctor and patient. It helps health-care staff to be confident in their own abilities and aware of patients' needs. This, in turn, helps the patient, who will be met by professionals who can deal with conflict in a conducive way and can promote compliance to treatment clearly and calmly.[13–16]

In assessing suicide risk and during the treatment, it is essential to be aware of suicidal patients' characteristics—their vulnerability, their exaggerated tendency to take offence, their shame and sense of guilt, their marked emotional liability, and their tendency to respond with a rejecting attitude as soon as they have the slightest perception that one does not care about them. Doctors need to be trained in showing empathy, giving comfort and reacting in a friendly way, since this greatly assists the implementation of adequate suicide risk assessment and recognizing a suicide crisis.[17,18]

Through friendly dialogue, one can help suicidal people to verbalize perceptions that they have difficulty in pinning down and turning into words. This is the basis of interpersonal communication and the best way to help in integration of fragmented thoughts and emotions. It is also vital to assess what kind of needs have been frustrated, as when they are not addressed, they will fuel suicidal ideation and suicide plans.

References

1 Moore PJ, Sickel AE, Malat J, Williams D, Jackson J, Adler NE. Psychosocial factors in medical and psychological treatment avoidance: the role of the doctor–patient relationship. J Health Psychol. 2004 May;9(3):421–433.

2 Nolan P, Badger F. Aspects of the relationship between doctors and depressed patients that enhance satisfaction with primary care. J Psychiatr Ment Health Nurs. 2005 Apr;12(2):146–153.

3 Shea SC. The interpersonal art of suicide assessment: interviewing techniques for uncovering suicidal intent, ideation, and actions. In: Simon RI, Hales RE, eds. The American Psychiatric Publishing textbook of suicide assessment and management (2nd edn). Washington, DC: American Psychiatric Publishing; 2012:29–56.

4 Maltsberger JT, Buie DH. Countertransference hate in the treatment of suicidal patients. Arch Gen Psychiatry. 1974;**30**:625–633.

5 Wolk-Wasserman D. Some problems connected with the treatment of suicide attempt patients: transference and countertransference aspects. Crisis. 1987;**8**:69–82.

6 Brown GK, Steer RA, Henriques GR, Beck AT. The internal struggle between the wish to die and the wish to live: a risk factor for suicide. Am J Psychiatry. 2005 Oct;**162**(10):1977–1979.

7 Henseler H. Narzisstische Krisen. *Zur Psychodynamik des Selbstmords.* [Narcissistic crises. On the psychodynamics of suicide.] Hamburg: Rowholt Taschenbuch Verlag; 1974.

8 Hendin H, Maltsberger JT, Lipschitz A, Haas AP, Kyle J. Recognizing and responding to a suicide crisis. Suicide Life Threat Behav. 2001 Summer;**31**(2):115–128.

9 Hendin H, Maltzberger JT, Haas AP, Szanto K, Rabinowicz H. Desperation and other affective states in suicidal patients. Suicide Life Threat Behav. 2004 Winter;**34**(4):386–394.

10 Hendin H, Haas AP, Maltsberger JT, Koestner B, Szanto K. Problems in psychotherapy with suicidal patients. Am J Psychiatry. 2006 Jan;**163**(1):67–72.

11 Schechter M, Maltzberger JT. The clinical interview as a method in suicide risk assessment. In: Wasserman D, Wasserman C, eds. Oxford textbook of suicidology and suicide prevention: a global perspective. Oxford: Oxford University Press; 2009: 319–325.

12 Ruskin R, Sakinofsky I, Bagby RM, Dickens S, Sousa G. Impact of patient suicide on psychiatrists and psychiatric trainees. Acad Psychiatry. 2004 Summer;**28**(2):104–110.

13 McNiel DE, Fordwood SR, Weaver CM, Chamberlain JR, Hall SE, Binder RL. Effects of training on suicide risk assessment. Psychiatr Serv. 2008;**59**(12):1462–1465.

14 Schmitz WM, Jr., Allen MH, Feldman BN, Gutin NJ, Jahn DR, Kleespies PM, et al. Preventing suicide through improved training in suicide risk assessment and care: an American Association of Suicidology Task Force report addressing serious gaps in U.S. mental health training. Suicide Life Threat Behav. 2012;**42**(3):292–304.

15 Cramer RJ, Johnson SM, McLaughlin J, Rausch EM, Conroy MA. Suicide risk assessment training for psychology doctoral programs: core competencies and a framework for training. Train Educ Prof Psychol. 2013;**7**(1):1–11.

16 Wu CY, Lin YY, Yeh MC, Huang LH, Chen SJ, Liao SC, et al. Effectiveness of interactive discussion group in suicide risk assessment among general nurses in Taiwan: a randomized controlled trial. Nurse Educ Today. 2014;**34**(11):1388–1394.

17 Ramberg IL, Wasserman D. Benefits of implementing an academic training of trainers program to promote knowledge and clarity in work with psychiatric suicidal patients. Arch Suicide Res. 2004;**8**(4):331–343.

18 Hendin H. Recognising suicidal crisis in psychiatric patients. In: Wasserman D, Wasserman C, eds.: Oxford textbook of suicidology and suicide prevention: a global perspective. Oxford: Oxford University Press; 2009(**43**):327–331.

Chapter 24

Heuristics and biases in suicide risk assessment

Gergö Hadlaczky

Introduction

Research investigating the effects of heuristics and biases on specific-ally suicide risk assessments is non-existent, despite the large body of research of these effects on other fields where human decision-making is central. Heuristics are cognitive processes that allow us to come to quicker conclusions. The advantage of such mental short-cuts, or rules of thumb, is that we can sometimes solve complex problems without a substantial increase in cognitive resources. But at other times heur-istics can lead to significant errors in decision-making. The second term 'bias' regards the partiality of judgements. Impartial judgements may lead to errors in decision-making when the partiality is caused by fac-tors that are unrelated to the judgement. For instance, one study investi-gated psychiatrists' information-search and decision-making behaviour during patient assessments.[1] The majority of psychiatrists, in this study, searched primarily for information that would *confirm* their initial diag-nosis. This often led to that the initial diagnosis remained uncorrected, and consequently, the incidence of misdiagnosis was significantly more frequent (70%), compared with psychiatrists who searched for informa-tion that would question their initial diagnosis (27% misdiagnosis). In this example of the so-called *confirmation bias*, search strategies were guided by satisfying the participants' subjective hopes of having made the right diagnosis to begin with, rather than being guided by finding the most appropriate diagnosis, objectively.

Suicide risk assessment is difficult task because the outcome we are trying to predict is the result of a complex and ambiguous interaction between various psychopathologies, personality traits or states, genetic factors, socio-economic risk-factors, etc.[2] This is exacerbated by the fact that suicidal patients often have a strong motivation to conceal their suicidal ideation as well as other information that may be valuable in assessment.[3] Thus, clinicians must often face equivocal and inconclusive information.

The clinician can direct the conversation and explore relevant topics with greater control over how relevant information is extracted. Consciously or unconsciously the clinician also takes part of the various types of 'latent' information; e.g., the demeanour, expression, or body language of the patient. However, clinical interviews are highly subjective, based on the specific clinicians' past experiences, knowledge as well as other external and situational factors that may 'bother' the clinician at the time of the interview (i.e., being just before a lunch break). As such, the clinical interview is a potential gold mine in terms of information, but the quality of the assessment is highly exposed to threats from various cognitive biases. This is especially the case during uncertainty, time pressure, and high cognitive effort, during which the effects of cognitive biases loom large.[4-6]

Based on a large list of cognitive biases and heuristics that have been investigated in the field of judgement and decision-making since the 1970s,[7] Croskerry[8,9] identified around 30 that may affect physicians. In an attempt to address how biases might more specifically affect psychiatrists' judgement, Crumlish and Kelly[10] reviewed ten different heuristics that might occur in the psychiatric practice (some of which are already mentioned by Croskerry[8]). In this chapter, an attempt is made to describe those that may be specifically relevant to suicide risk assessment. These biases are described in Table 24.1 and those considered to be most specific to suicide risk assessment are described in more detail below. Recommendations to minimize the negative effects of these biases are also described.

Anchoring

Anchoring occurs when a judgement or decision is influenced by the first piece of information presented.[7] This initial piece of information is called an anchor, to which all subsequent information is adjusted.

Table 24.1 Examples of heuristics and biases that may affect suicide risk assessment

Bias*	Description
Anchoring:	The first piece of (relevant or irrelevant) information acquired has disproportionately large influence on judgements. The initial impression of the patient (e.g., calm and relaxed) may bias following impressions (agitated) and thus disrupt the suicide assessment process.
Representativeness:	The tendency to assign events to a prototypical event, which results in outliers to be missed. If the clinician has a prototypical image of a 'high suicide risk patient', s/he is likely to underestimate the suicide risk in patients that do not fit this profile.
Confirmation bias:	Searching for, and accepting information that confirms our beliefs, while ignoring information that refute it.
Availability:	Examples that quickly come to mind are considered to be more likely to occur, those that are less available are considered less likely to occur. A clinician that recently experienced a patient-suicide is likely to overestimate the suicide risk in subsequent patients; clinicians that have not seen suicidal patients in a long time may underestimate the suicide risk.
Overconfidence bias:	Individuals are far more confident in their abilities than is justified by the facts, especially experts and specialists. Overconfidence bias may result in superficial assessments of the patients' suicide risk, based on incomplete information, intuition, hunches.
Sunk cost:	Even in the face of direct evidence, we are less likely to abandon a theory if we have substantially invested in it. If a patient has been assessed as having a 'low suicide risk' after thorough time consuming clinical investigation, it becomes difficult to change this assessment to 'high suicide risk', even in the face of clear evidence.
Base-rate neglect:	Base-rate neglect is the tendency to overlook background frequencies when making a probability judgements.
Aggregate bias:	The belief that aggregated data from a large population (e.g., evidence-based guidelines or psychometric tools) does not apply to specific patients. Clinicians may assume that their patients are atypical, and thus incompatible with guidelines and decide not to follow them.
Outcome bias:	The tendency to assess preferred outcomes to be more likely than negative outcomes. This may result in the grave underestimation of suicide risk.
Fundamental attribution error:	The tendency to attribute judgements about individuals to their character, rather than their situation. Clinicians may blame their patient for their suicide attempt, instead of considering that it was the result of factors which the patient cannot control (illness or stressful life events, etc.)

(Continued)

Table 24.1 (continued) Examples of heuristics and biases that may affect suicide risk assessment

Bias*	Description
Visceral bias:	Emotions between clinician and patient (transference and countertransference), may irrationally influence the assessment of suicide risk.
Diagnosis momentum:	The tendency to assume that previous physicians' diagnosis of a patient is correct. It becomes increasingly difficult to refute the initial diagnosis with the number of clinicians that have accepted it. This is most problematic if the first diagnosis was merely a suggested possibility.
Gambler's fallacy:	The belief that when something occurs more frequently than what is expected by chance, it will continue at a rate lower than chance to balance out. This bias could lead to the underestimation of the suicide risk of a patient, if several preceding patients also had a high suicide risk.
Multiple alternatives bias:	Multiple options may increase the difficulty in making a decision, which in turn may result in reverting to the status quo choice, even when this is not optimal.
Order effects:	The order of how information is presented influences how well we remember it. The first and last piece of information that was presented will be recalled more easily, and thus have a greater impact on the clinicians judgement of suicide risk.
Vertical line failure:	Thinking inside the box due to repetitive and routine working ways. This may lead to inflexible thinking and the neglect of alternate possibilities to suicide risk assessment.

*Biases source data from Croskerry[8,9] and Crumlish & Kelly,[10] that are considered, in this chapter, to be specifically relevant for suicide risk assessment.

Anchoring is an extremely powerful and well-documented bias, especially if the anchor is contextually relevant. In terms of suicide risk assessment, anchoring might present itself in clinicians overreliance on the first impression of information given by patients. If, in the early phases of the clinical interview, the patient provides responses and a façade contrary to the clinicians expectation of a suicidal patient, the impression might taint information gained in subsequent parts of the clinical interview, and perhaps even information gained through administered questionnaires. This could lead to a bias where the assessment of suicide risk made by the clinician is lower than the actual risk.

One method of minimizing the negative effects of this bias may be the administration of standardized and validated questionnaires for suicide risk assessment *before* the start of the clinical interview. Although biological and psychometric tools may not give as much information as the clinical interview, their strength is their objectivity: the resulting assessments are unbiased and consistent. The clinician should take part of the results before conducting the interview. This way, the assessment provided by the questionnaire will serve as the 'anchor' to which further information, gained throughout the clinical interview, is adjusted. This process can reduce potential biases stemming from subjective first impressions of the patient.

Representativeness

The representativeness heuristic refers to the influence of internal representation of an event, on the judgement of that event's likelihood.[7] A patient that reflects the clinician's stereotype image of a suicidal person is more likely to receive a high suicide risk assessment. Perhaps more importantly, patients that do *not* represent this stereotype are more likely to be judged non-suicidal. This is problematic because the assessment is based on the clinician's subjective internal representation of what suicidal patients are like. This may differ amongst clinicians, but more importantly, the population of individuals with severe suicide risk are usually highly heterogenous and not likely to fit any specific stereotype.

One suggestion for reducing this bias is through the use of self-reflection. Once the suicide risk assessment has been made, clinicians could reflect over how well the patient's stereotype corresponds to their risk assessment. If there is a high congruence—i.e., the patient does not seem like the 'type of person who would attempt suicide' and the risk assessment is low—there may be good reason to consider that the assessment is the result of representativeness bias. In this case it may be beneficial for the clinician to review the notes taken during the interview.

Confirmation bias

Confirmation bias the tendency to look for information that supports an initial assumption or judgement and disregard any contradictory information.[11] The previously mentioned study by Mendel et al.[1] illustrates how confirmation bias adversely affects the diagnosis of those psychiatrists who only sought after information that would support their preliminary diagnosis.

Similarly, in suicide risk assessment, confirmation bias, especially coupled with anchoring and representativeness, may result in extremely biased judgements. If a patient puts on a façade, and gives a first impression to the clinician that is perceived as non-suicidal, the clinician is likely to search for information confirming the low suicide risk while ignoring information suggesting high risk. This could lead to an artificially deflated risk assessment.

After an interview, clinicians are advised to write down a number of specific questions, to which certain answers provided by the patient may lead to the falsification of their original assessment. By doing so, even if the questions are not used, the clinician develops a frame of mind that may be less susceptible to confirmation bias.

Availability

The availability heuristic is the tendency to base probability judgements how easily examples of events are recalled.[6] Often, this can be a helpful heuristic, especially among experienced clinicians who will have had encountered the symptoms of a common disease frequently and thus that disease will easily be matched with the associated symptoms, when encountered. However, the availability heuristic can also be misleading because the ease with which information is recalled will not always correspond to its probability. This is relevant in suicide risk assessment with regards to previous experiences and reports of suicides, or suicidality. Clinicians that have recently experienced a suicide or were exposed to highly publicized reports of one, are more likely to overestimate the suicide risk of patients. On the other hand, clinicians that have not been exposed these types of experiences, are more likely to underestimate suicide risk in patients.

It may help clinicians to reflect on the effect of recent experiences (or the lack thereof) on their risk assessment, directly after it is completed. For example: could I be underestimating the suicide risk of this patient because I have never had a patient that died in suicide? Or could I be overestimating this risk, because of the tragic death of my patient last week?

Base-rate neglect

Base-rate neglect is the tendency to overlook background frequencies when making a probability judgement.[12] For example, imagine that a patient is tested positive on a suicide risk scale with 99% accuracy and the prevalence of suicide is 10 in 100,000. What percent probability would you assign to the suicide risk? Most individuals disregard base-rates (i.e., the prevalence) when faced with the question above, and consider the probability to be higher than the correct answer,[13] which in this case is 1%. However, if the result on the same scale was positive but the patient was diagnosed with schizophrenia, the probability of suicide would be increased severely, because the prevalence of suicide in schizophrenics is much higher (estimated to be 5%). Base-rates are an extremely useful source of information and should be used as a point of departure in suicide risk assessment. It is advised to periodically carry out literature searches regarding the prevalence of suicide in patient groups that often frequent the clinic (i.e., prevalence of suicide in schizophrenics, depressed males, individuals in certain age groups, ethnic backgrounds, etc.). A list of results from this data may alleviate unnecessary strain on the memory of the clinician.

Overconfidence bias

People exhibit overconfidence bias when they estimate their ability to successfully carry out a task to a greater extent than is justified by the facts. It has been shown that physicians often demonstrate over-confidence in medical decisions, which may result in, e.g., incorrect treatment.[14] Similarly, in suicide risk assessment some clinicians might exhibit unduly overconfidence in their ability to predict suicide.[15] During evaluation of a patient, an overconfident clinician might rely too heavily on his or her ability to predict the risk of suicide and miss out on relevant information, or coupled with confirmation bias, ignore relevant counter-indicative information. The biggest challenge in minimizing the suicide risks associated with this bias is that the overconfident clinician seldom considers him or herself to be overconfident, and is thus unlikely to seek help for this problem. The aim of mentioning this bias in this chapter is preventative; namely, to reduce prospective effects on those clinicians that are not yet a victim of the overconfidence bias.

Sunk cost

Sunk cost is the inability to forgo a judgement or a decision that we are heavily invested in.

Clinicians that have spent a significant amount of effort and time in a clinical evaluation of a patient might feel reluctant to change their assessment about the patient's risk of suicide, if the transformational information arrives too late in the interview process. Once the time and effort has already been 'spent', there is often a reluctance to 'start afresh' when other explanatory alternatives present themselves, because it is perceived as if the time and effort were invested in vain.[16]

One practical (but not always possible) recommendation for this problem is to postpone the final verdict of the suicide risk assessment, and during the period of postponement take the safest precautionary measures. It is also recommended in clinical practice that suicide risk assessment should be done at two different interviews. The time and effort that has been spent on a task is judged to be much greater directly after the completion of the task (especially in a state of exhaustion), than say, one day later. Individuals should be less likely to fall victim to the sunk cost fallacy on the day following the risk assessment.

Discussion

Clinical interviews provide a treasure trove of information about the patient in suicide risk assessment. However, a number of heuristics and biases described above are challenging this assessment method. The first step towards improving the negative effects of heuristics and biases is by being aware of them.[17] As a second step, clinicians may learn specific strategies and techniques which allow for the reduction of these biases,[8,9,18–20] thereby increasing the accuracy of suicide risk assessment. The overarching theme of these strategies is the application of meta-cognition (thinking about thinking). This involves becoming aware of how our judgements and decisions are formed and how they affect the reasoning process. Stepping back from the issue and taking a moment to reflect on the thinking process, as well as implementing some more specific cognitive strategies, allows for improved judgements.

Practical strategies may also be useful, such as the application and analysis of accurate psychometric scales (especially *before* the clinical interview) and the frequent use of relevant base-rates. The use of these may help minimize errors related to a number of heuristics and biases (such as anchoring heuristic and confirmation bias). Implementing environmental safeguards with the aim of creating optimal conditions for judgement and decision-making may also be useful. This may involve reducing cognitive load by decreasing reliance on memory through the use of, e.g., checklists during the clinical interview, and incorporating more breaks in the schedule in order to reduce cognitive depletion.

References

1 Mendel R, Traut-Mattausch E, Jonas E, et al. Confirmation bias: why psychiatrists stick to wrong preliminary diagnoses. Psychol Med. 2011;**41**(12):2651–2659.

2 Wasserman D. A stress-vulnerability model and the development of the suicidal process. In: Wasserman D, eds. Suicide: an unnecessary death. London: Martin Dunitz; 2001: 13–28.

3 Busch KA, Fawcett J, Jacobs DG. Clinical correlates of inpatient suicide. J Clin Psychiatry. 2003;**64**(1):14–19.

4 Finucane ML, Alhakami A, Slovic P, Johnson SM. The affect heuristic in judgments of risks and benefits. J Behav Decis Mak. 2000;**13**(1):1–17.

5 **Gilbert DT**. Inferential correction. In: Gilovich T, Griffin D, Kahneman D, eds. Heuristics and biases: the psychology of intuitive judgment. New York, NY: Cambridge University Press; 2002.

6 **Tversky A, Kahneman D**. Availability: a heuristic for judging frequency and probability. Cog Psychol. 1973;**4**:207–232.

7 **Tversky A, Kahneman D**. Judgment under uncertainty: heuristics and biases. Science. 1974;**185**(4157):1124–1131.

8 **Croskerry P**. The importance of cognitive errors in diagnosis and strategies to minimize them. Acad Med 2003;**78**(8):775–780.

9 **Croskerry P**. Cognitive forcing strategies in clinical decision-making. Ann Emerg Med. 2003;**41**(1):110–120.

10 **Crumlish N, Kelly BD**. How psychiatrists think. Adv Psychiatr Treat. 2009;**15**(1):72–79.

11 **Nickerson RS**. Confirmation bias: a ubiquitous phenomenon in many guises. Rev Gen Psychol. 1998;**2**(2):175–220.

12 **Koehler J**. The base-rate fallacy reconsidered: descriptive, normative, and methodological challenges. Behav Brain Sci. 1996;**19**:1–17.

13 **Axelsson S**. The base-rate fallacy and the difficulty of intrusion detection. ACM Transactions on Information and System Security. 2000;**3**(3):186–205.

14 **Stiegler MP, Neelankavil JP, Canales C, Dhillon A**. Cognitive errors detected in anaesthesiology: a literature review and pilot study. Bri J Anaesth. 2012;**108**(2):229–235.

15 **Pokorny AD**. Suicide prediction revisited. Suicide Life Threat Behav 1983;**23**(1):1–10.

16 **Bornstein BH, Chapman GB**. Learning lessons from sunk costs. J Exp Psychol Appl. 1995;**1**(4):251–269.

17 **Croskerry P**. Achieving quality in clinical decision-making: cognitive strategies and detection of bias. Acad Emerg Med. 2002;**9**(11):1184–1204.

18 **Carroll A**. How to make good-enough risk decisions. Adv PsychiatrTreat. 2009;**15**(3):192–198.

19 **Croskerry P, Singhal G, Mamede S**. Cognitive debiasing 2: impediments to and strategies for change. BMJ Quality & Safety. 2013;**22** (Suppl 2):bmjqs–2012.

20 **Graber ML, Kissam S, Payne VL, et al**. Cognitive interventions to reduce diagnostic error: a narrative review. BMJ Quality & Safety. 2012;**21**(7):535–557.

Chapter 25

Psychometric scales in suicide risk assessment

Per Bech, Lis R Olsen,
and Göran Högberg

Introduction

The relationship between suicidal thoughts or ideations and planned suicide acts has been described by the Suicidal Ladder,[1] in which the suicide item in the Hamilton Depression Scale[2] (Table 25.1) was included.

The fifth edition of the Diagnostic and Statistical Manual of Mental Disorders (DSM-5),[3] in contrast to the DSM-IV, includes 'suicide risk' in the index of the manual covering 25 different disorders. In the Glossary section, DSM-5 differentiates between suicide (the act of intentionally causing one's own death), and suicide attempt (an attempt to end one's own life, which may lead to one's death). However, throughout the DSM-5 when describing 'suicide risk' for each disorder, it is difficult to understand the dialectic between a suicide attempt versus a planned suicide. Even when describing suicide risk in major depression, the DSM-5 states that suicidal behaviour exists at all times during a major depressive episode (obviously because this is a criterion of a depressive episode). However, it is mentioned that risk of completed suicide is seen for 'male sex, being single or living alone, and having prominent feelings of hopelessness' (which is actually an element of depressed mood in the Hamilton Depression Rating Scale (Table 25.1)).

The psychometric approach has been to identify short scales in the measurement of the suicidal process. As stated by Ottosson,[4] the suicidal process can be measured with a reasonable degree of accuracy provided a good therapist–patient relationship has been established and the most informative questions have been used. Based on the

Table 25.1 Suicide item in the Hamilton Depression Rating Scale/Questionnaire (Suicidal ladder)

Score	Item
0 :	No suicidal thoughts (*I have not had any thoughts that life is not worth living*)
1 :	The patient feels that life is not worthwhile, but he or she expresses no wish to die (*I feel that life is not really worth living anymore*)
2 :	The patient wishes to die, but has no plans for taking own life (*I wish I were dead, but I haven't made any plans for this*)
3 :	Vague, but still active plans to take own life (*I have had vague thoughts about killing myself*)
4 :	Has serious plans to take own life (*I have serious plans to kill myself*)

Reproduced from *Acta Psychiatrica Scandinavica*, 73(S326), Bech P, Kastrup M, Rafaelsen OJ, 'Mini-compendium of rating scales for states of anxiety, depression, mania, and schizophrenia with corresponding DSM-III syndromes', pp. 7–37, copyright (1986), with permission from John Wiley and Sons Ltd.

psychology of personal constructs, the suicidal person is accepted as a researcher at the same level as the therapist, because nobody knows better than the patient what it is like to feel that life is not worth living. From the psychometric perspective we have selected scales in which the questions are formulated in a language representing the complaints people have in their conversations in the community about the everyday stressors and strains of modern living. Such questionnaires as the Eysenck Personality Questionnaire (EPQ-R)[5] or the WHO-5 Well-being Index (WHO-5)[2] are examples of scales in this respect.

Selection of psychometric scales specifically measuring suicidal risk

Although the DSM-5 considered including a dimensional approach for measuring the severity of mental disorders, including suicidal behaviour, this was not realized in the final publication. When dealing with the domains in DSM-5—i.e., attempted suicide, and suicidal ideas—the following scales listed below are helpful.

The Suicide Intent Scale

The Suicide Intent Scale (SIS) was developed by Beck et al.[6] to measure the suicide attempter's wish to die at the time of the attempt. In a follow-up study by Beck et al.,[7] the SIS was found without validity in prediction of committed suicide among individuals who have attempted suicide. In other words, the SIS is a scale that measures the severity of a suicide attempt but is without predictive validity for committed suicide.

The Scale for Suicidal Ideation (SSI-C)

This scale was developed by Beck et al.[8] to measure the severity of suicidal thoughts and impulses. Like the Hamilton Depression Scale (HAM-D), it is an interview-rated scale. It contains 19 items, each of which can be scored from 0 to 2, implying that theoretically scores can range from 0 (no suicidal ideation) to 38 (extreme suicidal ideation). The very high coefficient alpha (0.89) indicates that many of the items have the same level of information; i.e., can substitute each other. The items are so redundant that we recommend using the global evaluation as found in the HAM-D of suicidal thoughts and impulses (Table 25.1).

Figure 25.1 shows the psychometric properties of the SSI-C by a triangle in which (A) is the internal validity, (B) the inter-rater reliability, and (C) the external validity. The term validity has to do with the two major aspects: internal versus external. Internal validity

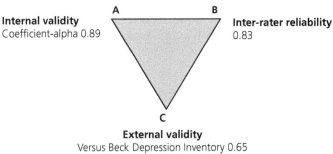

Fig. 25.1 Psychometric properties of the Beck Scale for Suicide Intent (SSI)

Adapted from Wasserman D., Suicide: An unnecessary death, Figure 18.1, Copyright (2001), with permission from Martin Dunitz/Informa.

expresses to what extent the scale is a measurement of the dimension being examined. Traditionally, Cronbach's alpha is used as an indicator of internal validity. An alpha coefficient of 0.80 or higher indicates that the scale has acceptable internal validity. External validity expresses the correlation of the scale with another criterion. Concurrent validity is an analysis of the correlation of the scale with another scale, and predictive validity is to what extent a cut-off score on the scale can predict an event taking place in the future—e.g., a suicidal act.

Inter-rater correlation is the extent to which clinicians agree when using the scale in an interview with the same group of patients. The intra-class coefficient is here used to express the degree of consensus. An intra-class coefficient of 0.70 is an indicator of acceptable agreement between clinicians.

As shown in Fig. 25.1, the external validity of the SSI-C is evaluated by an association between depression scales such as the Beck Depression Inventory (BDI) or the HAM-D, as indicated by Beck et al.[7]

The Beck Hopelessness Scale

This scale was developed by Beck et al.[6] and it is still one of the most frequently used self-reported questionnaires in this field.

The extremely high coefficient alpha (0.93) signifies that many of the items are redundant. Using factor analysis, Aish and Wasserman[9] have actually found that the variance of the items is covered by one single item: 'My future seems dark to me'. Hopelessness is part of the HAM-D measuring depressed mood (Table 25.2).

The SAD PERSON Scale

This scale was originally developed by Patterson et al.[10] but was modified by Hockberger and Rothstein,[11] and standardized by Goldberg and Murray[12] (Table 25.3). This scale actually covers the risk factors specified in DSM-5 under major depression (male sex, being single or living alone, and being hopeless). However, we still need follow-up studies evaluating the predictive validity of this scale with regards to committed suicide.

Table 25.2 Depressed mood item in the Hamilton Depression Rating Scale/ Questionnaire

Score	Item
0 :	Neutral mood (*I have been in my usual good mood*)
1 :	It is doubtful whether the patient is more despondent or sad than usual (e.g., the patient indicates vaguely that he or she is more depressed than usual) (*I have felt a little more sad than usual*)
2 :	The patient more clearly is concerned by unpleasant experiences, although he or she is still without hopelessness (*I have been clearly more sad than usual, but haven't felt hopeless*)
3 :	The patient shows clear non-verbal signs of depression and/or is at times overpowered by hopelessness (*I have been so gloomy that I briefly have felt overpowered by hopelessness*)
4 :	The patient's remarks on despondency and hopelessness or the non-verbal signs dominate the interview and the patient cannot be distracted from them (I have been so low in my moods that everything seems dark and hopeless)

Reproduced from *Acta Psychiatrica Scandinavica*, 73(S326), Bech P, Kastrup M, Rafaelsen OJ, 'Mini-compendium of rating scales for states of anxiety, depression, mania, and schizophrenia with corresponding DSM-III syndromes', pp. 7–37, copyright (1986), with permission from John Wiley and Sons Ltd.

The role of internalized hostility (interpersonal sensitivity, anxiety, self-depreciation)

The EPQ-R has neuroticism as the major personality trait; this includes interpersonal sensitivity (being easily hurt), anxiety (nervousness, worrying, tension), and self-depreciation (guilt feelings).

Obviously, a high negative correlation is seen between neuroticism and well-being, this is illustrated by Rogers et al.[13] using the WHO-5 well-being index.

Neuroticism is also considered to be a predictor of partial response in trials of antidepressants where these patients are characterized

Table 25.3 The SAD PERSONS Scale for assessing the risk of suicide

Acronym and Domain (if present score 1)		Score
Sex: Male	(0–1)	
Age: Younger than 20 or older than 45 years	(0–1)	
Depression	(0–1)	
Previous attempts	(0–1)	
Ethanol abuse	(0–1)	
Rational thinking loss; e.g., organic brain syndrome, affective disorders, schizophrenia	(0–1)	
Social support lacking	(0–1)	
Organized plan for suicide	(0–1)	
No spouse or not living with relation	(0–1)	
Sickness, poor physical health	(0–1)	
Total score	(0–10)	

Standardization: total score 0–2, low risk; 3–4, moderate risk (close monitoring as outpatient, consider admission); 5–6, high risk (admission is advised); 7–10, very high risk of suicide (admission required).

Source data from Psychosomatics, 24(4), Patterson W.M., Dohn H.H., Bird J. and Patterson G.A., Evaluation of suicidal patients: the SAD PERSONS scale, p. 343-5, 348-9, Copyright (1983), with permission from Elsevier; The Journal of emergency medicine, 6(2), Hockberger R.S. and Rothstein R.J., Assessment of suicide potential by nonpsychiatrists using the SAD PERSONS score, p. 99-107, Copyright (1988), with permission from Elsevier; Goldberg D and Murray R, The Maudsley Handbook of Practical Psychiatry, Fifth Edition, Copyright (2006), with permission from Oxford University Press.

by such symptoms as anxiety-related symptoms and concentration problems.[14] In a matched case-control study of suicide, Fang et al.[15] showed that high neuroticism but low extraversion is a risk marker of suicide.

The role of externalized hostility (impulsivity or risk-taking behaviour)

The EPQ-R[5] was revised as regards the dimension of psychoticism because the first version had overlapping items of impulsivity and extraversion. In this revised version the association between extraversion and sociability was maintained, whereas a new item of impulsivity or risk-taking behaviour was adopted. It is the risk-taking behaviour that predisposes to suicide. The hidden bipolarity in depression has the dark side of hypomanic states as a risk of suicide. The Eysenck impulsivity dimension includes such items as: being an impulsive person, preferring drugs with dangerous effects, preferring to follow own rules rather than the official ones, being more easy-going about right and wrong than most people.

WHO-5 as a screening tool in the suicidal process

In the theory of human needs and homeostasis, hedonic need should be seen as a global index of such elements as achievement (striving), aggression, autonomy, harm-avoidance, and succour (seeking support).[2] The WHO-5 was developed as such a global measure of general psychological well-being (Table 25.4). When measuring quality of life or general well-being it is important to avoid symptom-related language and to use only positively phrased questions.

In a comparison of the most frequently used well-being scales from a clinical-judgement perspective, Hall et al.[16] identified the WHO-5 to be the most valid. A psychometric validation analysis of the WHO-5, using both non-parametric and parametric item response models, found the scale to be uni-dimensional; i.e., acceptable scalability for the total scale score as a sufficient measure of well-being.

The standardization of the WHO-5 in screening for depression has supported our own cut-off scores.[2] A WHO-5 score ≤ 50 indicates decreased well-being and is the threshold for mild depression. A WHO-5 score of ≤ 30 is the threshold for moderate depression, and a WHO-5 score of ≤ 20 is the threshold for severe depression.

When correlating the WHO-5 with the Major Depression Inventory (MDI) item 'How much of the time in the past two weeks have you felt that life wasn't worth living?' (from 0 = 'at no time', to 5 = 'all the time'), a Spearman coefficient of –0.38 was obtained.[17] A correlation between the WHO-5 and the BDI gave a coefficient of -0.73. Using item 15 in the Hopkins Symptom Checklist (SCL-90): 'How much were you over the past week bothered by thoughts of ending your life', the correlation coefficient to the WHO-5 was –0.27. Using item 59: 'How much were you bothered by thoughts of death and dying?', the correlation coefficient to the WHO-5 was –0.32.

Table 25.4 WHO (Five) Well-Being Index

Over the last two weeks	All of the time	Most of the time	More than half of the time	Less than half of the time	Some of the time	At no time
1 I have felt cheerful and in good spirits	5	4	3	2	1	0
2 I have felt calm and relaxed	5	4	3	2	1	0
3 I have felt active and vigorous	5	4	3	2	1	0
4 I woke up feeling fresh and rested	5	4	3	2	1	0
5 My daily life has been filled with things that interest me	5	4	3	2	1	0

Please indicate for each of the five statements which is closest to how you have been feeling over the last two weeks. Notice that higher numbers mean better well-being.

Example: If you have felt cheerful and in good spirits more than half of the time during the last two weeks, put a tick in the box with the number 3 in the upper right corner.

Reproduced from Bech P, *Clinical Psychometrics*, copyright (2012), with permission from John Wiley and Sons.

The here-and-now assessment of suicide risk: the Columbia Suicide Severity Rating scale (C-SSRS)

The Columbia Suicide Severity Rating Scale (C-SSRS), introduced in 2008,[18] relies on previous studies in which suicidal ideation and suicidal behaviour were shown to be of importance for predicting future outcome. Instead of conceiving these as uni-dimensional constructs it aims at separating suicidal ideation from suicidal behaviour and does so in four sub-scales; two on ideation and two on behaviour.

The first ideation subscale, 'severity of ideation', follows the principle of the HAM-D suicide item with items going from low to more serious ideation (suicidal ladder). These items are: (i) wish to be dead; (ii) non-specific active suicidal thoughts, (iii) suicidal thoughts with methods; (iv) suicidal intent; and (v) suicidal intent with a plan.

The second ideation subscale quantifies the ideation according to frequency, duration, controllability, deterrents, and reason for ideation. This scale asks about several aspects of the concept of suicidal thoughts which might be useful in targeting treatment and evaluating subsequent response.

The reasons for suicidal ideation range from getting attention, revenge or a reaction from others, on to a wish to completely end or stop the pain; the measures in-between being on a continuum of these extremes.

It can be argued that this list entails a risk of cultural bias. Reasons such as shame or a wish to be reunited with a deceased loved person might occur in other settings. The C-SSRS is quite new and ensuing research might modify some aspects of the scale.

In the first behaviour subscale the groups are the following: (i) actual attempts; (ii) non-suicidal self-injurious behaviour; (iii) interrupted attempts; (iv) aborted attempts; and (v) preparatory acts or behaviour.

The second behaviour subscale classifies actual and potential lethality of the suicide attempt.

A special feature of the C-SSRS is the precise definition of an actual suicide attempt: 'Was there any part of you which wanted to die?'

The C-SSRS is intended to support both research and clinical practice and can be administered in different versions for different time frames. The baseline version assesses the worst-point ever ideation; this being evaluated as a strong predictor of subsequent suicide. This is in accordance with Beck et al.[8]

The C-SSRS is a semi-structured clinical interview, but has also become available as a fully structured electronic scale as the electronic eC-SSRS,[19] based on interactive use of touch-tone telephones.

An ongoing area of debate is the validity of the retrospective method regarding prospectively measured mental health variables. Recent reports have shown that the retrospective method used in C-SSRS predicted later suicide attempts in an adolescent setting (Posner 2011) as well as in a mixed adult clinical population.[20] In a study by Kerr et al.[21] it was found that in severely delinquent girls, re-evaluated 7–12 years later, there was a fair agreement between participants' report of suicide attempts at baseline and follow-up. However, the association was weak as regards interrupted and aborted attempts and preparatory act.

The psychometric properties of the C-SSRS are shown in Fig. 25.2. The high Cronbach alpha was established by Posner et al.,[18] who also found a concurrent validity of 0.63 with the item of suicidal ideation in the BDI. The inter-observer reliability (Kappa) of 0.81–0.91 was reported by Kerr et al.[21]

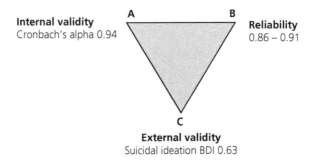

Fig. 25.2 Psychometric properties of the Columbia-Suicide Severity Rating Scale

Combining scales to assess suicide risk

An attempt has been made to combine scales measuring stressors (life events) and personality traits (including neuroticism, impulsivity, or hostility) by use of a statistical model resulting in different weights (positive versus negative) in discriminating between persons without and with a history of suicide attempts.[22] This attempt to transform positively and negatively weighted items into a one-dimensional sub-space of an originally two-dimensional scale selection has previously been criticized by Eysenck when classifying depressed patients.[23] However, this preliminary step in combining suicide risk items seems interesting but should be replicated in other samples and in different settings.

Conclusion

Completed suicide is a rare event and cannot easily be predicted by scales only, as suicide attempts and completed suicides are often committed in a special mental state with strong internal agony and agitation. This very state of inner turmoil may not be present when using scales in the everyday clinical setting. It is extremely important in the evaluation of suicidality to establish empathetic contact with the patient to capture the underlying strong emotional states when present. This gives a role to the experience of the clinician; at times described as a clinical intuition. By use of the short psychometric scales described in this chapter the intuition of the clinician might be activated, when the scale conveys the mental pain of the patient and translates it into scores and words, ranking them on the suicidal ladder.

References

1 **Bech P, Awata S**. Measurement of suicidal behaviour with psychometric scales. In: Wasserman D, Wasserman C, editors. Oxford textbook of suicidology. Oxford: Oxford University Press; 2007:305–311.

2 **Bech P**. Clinical psychometrics. Oxford: Wiley Blackwell; 2012.

3 **American Psychiatric Association**. Diagnostic and statistical manual of mental disorders, fifth edition (DSM-5). 5th edn. Washington, DC: American Psychiatric Association; 2013.

4 **Ottosson J**. Prevention of suicide. In: Stromgren E, editor. Origin, prevention and treatment of affective disorders. London: Academic Press; 1979: 256–268.

5 **Eysenck SBG, Eysenck HJ, Barrett P**. A revised version of the psychoticism scale. Person individ D. 1985;**6**(1):21–29.

6 **Beck AT, Schuyler D, Herman J**. Development of suicidal intent scales. In: Beck AT, Resnik HLP, Lettieri DJ, editors. The prediction of suicide. Maryland: Charles Press; 1974: 45–56.

7 **Beck AT, Schuyler D, Herman I**. The Suicide Intent Scale (SIS). In: Rush AJ, editor. Handbook of psychiatric measures. Washington, DC: American Psychiatric Association; 2008: 244–245.

8 **Beck AT, Kovacs M, Weissman A**. Assessment of suicidal intention: the Scale for Suicide Ideation. J Consult Clin Psychol. 1979 Apr;**47**(2):343–352.

9 **Aish AM, Wasserman D, Renberg ES**. Does Beck's Hopelessness Scale really measure several components? Psychol Med. 2001 Feb;**31**(2):367–372.

10 **Patterson WM, Dohn HH, Bird J, Patterson GA**. Evaluation of suicidal patients: the SAD PERSONS scale. Psychosomatics. 1983 Apr;**24**(4):343–345, 348–349.

11 **Hockberger RS, Rothstein RJ**. Assessment of suicide potential by nonpsychiatrists using the SAD PERSONS score. J Emerg Med. 1988 Mar–Apr;**6**(2):99–107.

12 **Goldberg D, Murray R**. The Maudsley handbook of practical psychiatry. Oxford: Oxford University Press; 2006.

13 **Rogers ME, Creed PA, Searle J**. Person and environmental factors associated with well-being in medical students. Pers Indiv Differ 2012 3;**52**(4):472–477.

14 **Fawcett J, Scheftner WA, Fogg L, Clark DC, Young MA, Hedeker D, et al.** Time-related predictors of suicide in major affective disorder. Am J Psychiatry. 1990 Sep;**147**(9):1189–1194.

15 **Fang L, Heisel MJ, Duberstein PR, Zhang J**. Combined effects of neuroticism and extraversion: findings from a matched case control study of suicide in rural China. J Nerv Ment Dis. 2012 Jul;**200**(7):598–602.

16 Hall T, Krahn GL, Horner-Johnson W, Lamb G. Examining functional content in widely used health-related Quality of Life scales. Rehabil Psychol. 2011 May 2011;**56**(2):94–99.

17 Ellervik C, Kvetny J, Christensen KS, Vestergaard M, Bech P. Prevalence of depression, quality of life and antidepressant treatment in the Danish General Suburban Population Study. Nord J Psychiatry. 2014;**01**(29):1–6.

18 Posner K, Brown GK, Stanley B, Brent DA, Yershova KV, Oquendo MA, et al. The Columbia-Suicide Severity Rating Scale: initial validity and internal consistency findings from three multisite studies with adolescents and adults. Am J Psychiatry. 2011 Dec;**168**(12):1266–1277.

19 Mundt JC, Greist JH, Gelenberg AJ, Katzelnick DJ, Jefferson JW, Modell JG. Feasibility and validation of a computer-automated Columbia-Suicide Severity Rating Scale using interactive voice response technology. J Psychiatr Res. 2010 Dec;**44**(16):1224–1228.

20 Mundt JC, Greist JH, Jefferson JW, Federico M, Mann JJ, Posner K. Prediction of suicidal behavior in clinical research by lifetime suicidal ideation and behavior ascertained by the electronic Columbia-Suicide Severity Rating Scale. J Clin Psychiatry. 2013 Sep;**74**(9):887–893.

21 Kerr DC, Gibson B, Leve LD, Degarmo DS. Young adult follow-up of adolescent girls in juvenile justice using the Columbia Suicide Severity Rating Scale. Suicide Life Threat Behav. 2014 Apr: **44**(2);129–133.

22 Blasco-Fontecilla H, Delgado-Gomez D, Ruiz-Hernandez D, Aguado D, Baca-Garcia E, Lopez-Castroman J. Combining scales to assess suicide risk. J Psychiatr Res. 2012 Oct;**46**(10):1272–1277.

23 Eysenck HJ. The classification of depressive illnesses. Br J Psychiatry. 1970 Sep;**117**(538):241–250.

Chapter 26

Strategies in suicide prevention

Danuta Wasserman

Attitudes towards the suicide-prone person

Suicide is preventable, but different groups of suicidal people require different strategies. Risk factors, risk situations, and treatment options have been described in previous chapters. However, it is not enough to convey this knowledge without, at the same time, shedding light on the strong feelings aroused by suicide. These may range from compassion and guilt to fear of, and turning one's back on, people who attempt or commit suicide because the act openly challenges the instinct of self-preservation, which (in most people) is strong.

Many young people and people who have not experienced suicidal thoughts or mental ill-health tend to interpret suicide as an act that expresses both control over one's life situation and freedom. The truth is, however, that most suicidal acts arise in situations in which life is unbearable and everything is perceived as being out of reach of the individual's control. In this kind of situation, philosophical statements about suicide being a human right can seem derisive and uncaring to a person on the brink of suicide, and distressing to the devoted health professional. For a person who lacks knowledge of suicidology, this kind of 'philosophical' attitude may serve as a pretext for not intervening when someone is suicidal, on the grounds that the individual's integrity and right of self-determination should be respected. This kind of view may also make health-care staff passive, with devastating consequences for suicidal patients and their relatives.

Taboos as psychological defence mechanisms

The strong taboo on suicide that still exists and the distress it arouses and has aroused throughout history make it difficult to approach the problem of suicide in an open and scientific way. To this day, suicide is associated with shame, uneasiness, and guilt. As a result, suicides are concealed and the view is reinforced of suicide as being predestined and impossible to prevent or treat.

The guilt that we may feel, both individually and collectively, because there are people among us who have no wish to live, contributes to our deafness to suicidal communication and our desire to ward off the knowledge that this communication is in the majority of cases a conscious or unconscious cry for help. Suicidal communication usually brings to the fore in the recipient uncomfortable thoughts about death and the meaning of the life. Keeping at bay problems that evoke strong negative feelings and reflections is a normal psychological defence mechanism. In the bustle of everyday life, the main wish of most people is probably to avoid dealing with it. As professionals, however, we must strive for awareness of the issues raised by suicide and how they affect our work.

Suicide-prevention programmes

In 2014, the World Health Organization (WHO)[1] drafted a strategic document for working with suicide prevention, and there are currently several national programmes for suicide prevention in existence. The WHO has previously published a series of documents on how to prevent suicide in psychiatric and general-practice settings, in schools, prisons, and in survivors of suicide, as well as documents on how to report suicide in the media. WHO resources include:[2]

- Preventing Suicide: a resource for general physicians;
- Preventing Suicide: a resource for media professionals;
- Preventing Suicide: a resource for teachers and other school staff;
- Preventing Suicide: a resource for primary health-care workers;
- Preventing Suicide: a resource for jails and prisons;
- Preventing Suicide: a resource for prison officers;
- Preventing Suicide: how to start a survivors' group;
- Preventing Suicide: a resource for counsellors;
- Preventing Suicide: a resource at work;

- Preventing Suicide: a resource for police, firefighters and other first line responders;
- Preventing Suicide: a resource for suicide case registration; and
- Preventing Suicide: a resource for non-fatal suicidal behaviour case registration.

Strategies in suicide prevention

In suicide-prevention work, strategies can be pursued through the health-care services or directed at the general population (Fig. 26.1). Although various psychiatric treatments[3–5] have had the best-documented effects on suicide prevention, the emphasis of work needs to shift to an earlier stage of the suicidal process to public health-oriented interventions, and it is advisable that both sets of strategies go hand in hand, for maximum overall impact.

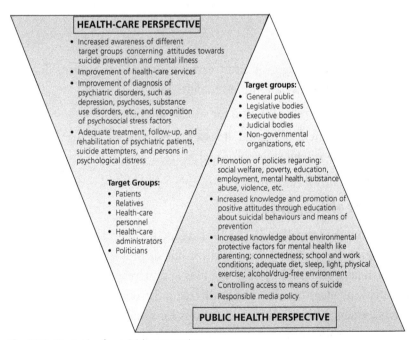

Fig. 26.1 Strategies for suicide prevention
Adapted from Wasserman D., Suicide: An unnecessary death, Figure 23.1, Copyright (2001), with permission from Martin Dunitz/Informa.

Health-care approach

When suicide-prevention efforts are initiated in the population by means of information campaigns, many new individuals or groups in need of help are found. Psychiatric staff may become discontented if they lack the knowledge and resources to provide satisfactory care for those who seek help. Such dissatisfaction may have an adverse impact on suicidal people who, being very fragile, sensitive, and thin-skinned, may feel rejected if they meet frustrated staff. Poor care increases the risk of suicidal acts, since it is not only people's propensity to seek and accept help that determines whether their suicidal process can be arrested or whether it culminates in attempted or completed suicide. The course of the suicidal process also depends on the capacity of others, including care staff, to recognize suicidal people's needs and give them adequate treatment.

Therefore, the work in suicide-preventive activities in many countries focuses on a risk group-oriented, three-pronged strategy to facilitate the successive development of population-oriented suicide prevention. The strategy consists of:

- identifying risk groups;
- improving the diagnosis and treatment of suicidal patients, including those who have attempted suicide; and
- offering better rehabilitation for suicide attempters.

Adequate treatment of mental illnesses in psychiatric settings has hitherto been one of the most thoroughly tried-and-tested strategies for reducing suicide risk.[3–5]

Public health approach

The objective of the 2014 WHO World Suicide Report 'Preventing suicide: a global imperative' is to prioritize suicide prevention on the global public health and public policy agendas and increase overall awareness of suicide as a legitimate public health issue. Through this report, WHO offers evidence-based recommendations for reducing mortality due to suicide and calls on partners to step up their advocacy and prevention efforts. The WHO uses the socio-ecological model as a framework for suicide prevention comprising societal, community, interpersonal, and individual levels (Fig. 26.2). The objectives are to encourage and support

RISK FACTORS FOR SUICIDE

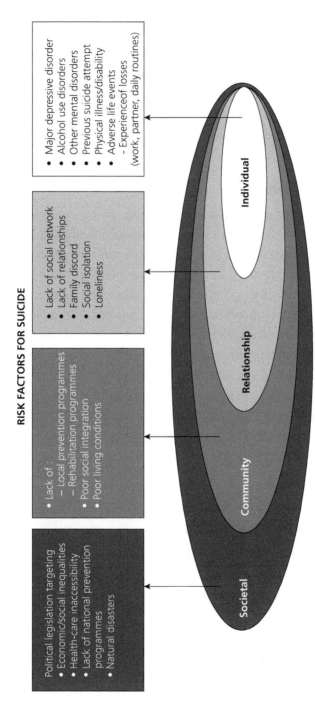

- Major depressive disorder
- Alcohol use disorders
- Other mental disorders
- Previous suicide attempt
- Physical illness/disability
- Adverse life events
  - Experience of losses (work, partner, daily routines)

- Lack of social network
- Lack of relationships
- Family discord
- Social isolation
- Loneliness

- Lack of :
  - Local prevention programmes
  - Rehabilitation programmes
- Poor social integration
- Poor living conditions

- Political legislation targeting
- Economic/social inequalities
- Health-care inaccessibility
- Lack of national prevention programmes
- Natural disasters

Individual

Relationship

Community

Societal

Fig. 26.2 The social-ecological model as a framework for suicide prevention: risk factors for suicide

countries to develop and strengthen comprehensive suicide-prevention strategies in a multisectorial public health approach.[1,6,7]

For a national suicide-prevention strategy, it is essential that governments assume their role of leadership, as they can bring together a multitude of stakeholders who may not otherwise collaborate. Governments are also in a unique position to develop and strengthen surveillance and to provide and disseminate data that are necessary for an informed action.

Psychosocial support

Modern society is evolving along paths that give individuals greater responsibility for their own lives and personal development through expanded access to knowledge, mediated in part by the explosive growth of information technology. At the same time, many people are increasingly isolated and lack support in their immediate surroundings. Numerous people are in the throes of existential crisis and, in their loneliness, may find life pointless and see suicide as the only possible way out.

Population-oriented suicide prevention focuses on building up supportive networks and strengthening the life skills that protect people in difficult situations and also on providing close-range support to counteract the isolation felt by susceptible people. The back-up for vulnerable people who need support from others to cope with stress because they lack a network of family and friends is needed in some cases throughout the whole life. This support works best if it is socially and culturally adapted to the recipients' needs.

Public attitudes and knowledge

Changes in attitudes towards people close to suicide and more knowledge about prevention of suicide and mental ill-health are further objectives. In many countries, population-oriented efforts concentrate on children and adolescents because it can be difficult to influence adults and the elderly to change their attitudes, whereas the young are relatively flexible. In an initiative to develop evidence-based methods for promoting mental health and reducing suicidal behaviours among youth, the EU funded a project called 'Saving and Empowering Young Lives in Europe' (SEYLE), which was performed in 168 randomly assigned schools with 11,110 school-based adolescents recruited from 10 European countries. In this randomized controlled trial, results showed that the universal school-based intervention 'Youth Aware of Mental Health' (YAM, http://www.y-a-m.org)[8] significantly reduced the incidence of severe suicidal ideation and suicide attempts by half.[8]

Programmes aimed at increasing knowledge of mental health and ill-health and of health-promoting measures attempt to eliminate the fears and misunderstandings that surround suicide. However, there is a degree of risk that poorly devised information inputs may provoke suicidal acts, especially among adolescents and certain sensitive people. Being suggestible, these people may imitate a suicidal behaviour that has taken place in their immediate surroundings or one that has received coverage in the mass media.

It is not wrong to speak and write about suicide, but it must be done in the right way, without glorifying or romanticizing the act or dismissing it as incomprehensible (see WHO resources for media professionals[2]). The difficulties in life that have contributed to suicidal peoples' decisions to take their own lives should be described honestly, without circumvention. Simultaneously, specific and practical examples and options for extricating oneself from a suicidal dilemma should be given. Hushing up the problem, showing ambivalence, and turning a blind eye to the subject only strengthen prejudices and reinforce ignorance, thereby leaving suicidal people to cope unaided.

Environmental measures

Population-oriented suicide prevention also includes environmental measures, such as restriction of access to dangerous means of committing suicide (e.g., weapons, toxic pharmaceuticals, and pesticides)—see Chapter 34.

Various types of policy regarding employment, leisure, planning of residential areas, and availability of alcohol as well as legislation concerning health-care and medical services and weapon ownership, are other typical examples of public health measures. Improvement of the work environment, especially for health-care providers, and counteracting stress and burn-out that may lead to suicide are further public health strategies that are used in several countries.

Networks

National and international networks comprising researchers, professional, and lay members are another category of population-oriented inputs. In Sweden, nationwide suicide prevention has been coordinated since 1993 by the National Centre for Suicide Research and Prevention of Mental Ill-Health (NASP), together with the Public Health Agency of Sweden since 2015. These regional efforts, which are adapted to local traditions and conditions, are implemented through regional networks that involve both professionals and lay people on a voluntary basis.

Research

In several countries, databases are being compiled to permit monitoring and identification of trends and patterns of completed and sometimes attempted suicide, their socio-demographic and psychiatric characteristics, as well as the kinds of treatment provided.

References

1 **World Health Organization (WHO).** World Suicide Report: Preventing suicide: a global imperative. Geneva; 2014. ISBN 978 92 4 156477 9.

2 **World Health Organization (WHO).** Preventing suicide: a resource series. Geneva; 2000. Available at: http://www.who.int/mental_health/resources/preventingsuicide/en/

3 **Wasserman D, Rihmer Z, Rujescu D, Sarchiapone M, Sokolowski M, Titelman D, et al.** The European Psychiatric Association (EPA) guidance on suicide treatment and prevention. Eur Psychiatry. 2012;**27**(2):129–141.

4 **American Psychiatric Association (APA).** Practice guideline for the assessment and treatment of patients with suicidal behaviors. Am J Psychiatry. 2003;**160**(11 Suppl):1–60.

5 **National Institute for Health and Clinical Excellence (NICE).** Self-harm: longer-term management. NICE clinical guideline CG133. 2011.

6 **Anderson M and Jenkins R.** The role of the state and legislation in suicide prevention: the five continents perspective. In: Wasserman D, Wasserman C, eds. The Oxford textbook of suicidology and suicide prevention: a global perspective. Oxford: Oxford University Press; 2009:373–380.

7 **Saxena S, Funk M, Chisholm D**. World Health Assembly adopts Comprehensive Mental Health Action Plan 2013–2020. Lancet. 2013;**381**(9882):1970–1971.

8 **Wasserman D, Hoven CW, Wasserman C, Wall M, Eisenberg R, Hadlaczky G, et al**. School-based suicide prevention programmes: the SEYLE cluster-randomised, controlled trial. Lancet 2015;**385**(9977):1536–1544.

Section VII

Suicide prevention

VIIA Health-care perspective
VIIB Public health perspective

VIIA

Health-care perspective

Pharmacological treatment of underlying psychiatric disorders in suicidal patients

Hans-Jürgen Möller

Introduction

In general, the treatment and prevention of suicide demands a complex approach of different psychosocial and psychopharmacological interventions.[1] Often, the combination of both can create more than one treatment possibility. Recent studies and reviews have demonstrated a positive interaction between psychotherapy and psychopharmacotherapy in several diagnoses, such as anxiety disorders, depression, and personality disorders. The combination of psychopharmacological interventions with psychotherapy should always be considered as part of a complex treatment strategy.

Besides counselling and other psychotherapeutic approaches (see Chapter 28), psychopharmacological treatment is necessary for many suicidal patients, especially if the suicidal crisis occurs in the context of a psychiatric disorder. Pharmacological or other neurobiological interventions (e.g., electroconvulsive therapy) in people at risk of committing suicide are usually aimed either at actual prevention of suicide by mostly sedative–anxiolytic medications or at specific treatment of a psychiatric disorder that may be the underlying cause. To date there is no specific psychopharmacological/neurobiological treatment for suicidality per se, only interventions that focus on the underlying psychopathological syndrome or disorder.

Although 5-hydroxyindoleacetic acid levels in cerebrospinal fluid have repeatedly been found to be lower in suicidal patients and patients who have attempted/committed suicide than in controls, which indicates deficiencies in the serotonergic transmitter system, the resulting consequences for treatment have not yet been sufficiently investigated. The hypothesis that serotonergic antidepressants might be more favourable than other treatments for depressed patients with suicidality cannot be corroborated.[2] Conversely, it was previously assumed that serotonergic antidepressants, like the selective serotonin reuptake inhibitors (SSRIs), might have a specific risk of increasing suicidality in (subgroups of) depressed patients.[3] This has now finally proven not to be the case.[4]

Altogether, the low potential risk of antidepressants to induce suicidality, related especially to younger age, personality conditions like borderline personality disorder, specific genetic dispositions,[5] etc., can be controlled relatively well under careful clinical management[6] and should be balanced against the important positive effects.[7]

Suicidality and suicidal behaviour mostly occur in the following constellations:

+ Acute suicidality due to psychosocial stress conditions.
+ Acute or chronic suicidality as a symptom or result of a relevant psychiatric disorder.
+ Combination of both of the above constellations.

This chapter describes psychopharmacological approaches to the above conditions.

Abnormal reactions to common psychosocial stressors

When suicidality results from abnormal reactions to common psychosocial stressors such as problems at work or in the family or partnership, psychopharmacological interventions are mainly aimed at sedation, anxiolysis, sleep induction, or suppression of disturbing vegetative symptoms. Benzodiazepines (or in cases of predominant sleep disturbances the modern non-benzodiazepine hypnotics) are, in general, the treatment of first choice. The selection of the specific compounds and dose varies according to the individual case. The aim should be to induce not only sedation but also affective–emotional distancing. Some doctors tend to be very restrictive in prescribing benzodiazepines—even in these conditions—because they are afraid of the risk of dependency; this risk is in fact relatively low, especially as regards a real dependency with dose escalations beyond the licensed dose and not a low-dose dependency, which occurs more often.[8] They prefer to use sedating antidepressants, such as doxepine, or low doses of sedating neuroleptics as surrogates. However, given the extraordinarily good tolerability of benzodiazepines and the high compliance of patients with these drugs, the risk–benefit assessment should favour the benzodiazepines in these special conditions, especially given the fact that, in general, only short-term medication is needed.

The treatment with benzodiazepines should carefully follow the guidelines, especially concerning the following points: only short-term medication, lowest dose possible, slow down-titration. An inadequate psychopharmacological regime can carry a high risk of continued suicidality and, therefore, undertreatment with benzodiazepines should be avoided.[8] The non-psychopharmacological treatment approach, sometimes suggested on the basis of psychodynamic theories, is not sufficient if there is a clear syndrome-related indication for acute psychopharmacological treatment—e.g., emotional instability, severe anxiety, depressive mood, sleep disturbances, or other psychiatric syndromes of relevant intensity.

In cases of longer-lasting depressive reactions, antidepressants should be considered as well. Modern antidepressants with better tolerability than the tricyclic antidepressants should preferably be chosen.

Anxiety disorders

Interestingly, anxiety disorders have a somewhat similar risk for suicidal behaviour as depression, probably among other reasons because of the highly prevalent comorbidity with major depression. The World Federation of Societies of Biological Psychiatry (WFSBP) has published guidelines for treatment of anxiety disorders.[9] In addition to psychotherapeutic procedures, antidepressants are often prescribed. For most anxiety disorders, including obsessive–compulsive disorders, SSRIs are the preferred choice for acute and maintenance treatment. In case of insufficient response, benzodiazepines or pregabalin might be alternatives, but in case of benzodiazepines the risk of dependency has to be carefully considered, as discussed above. If suicidality occurs during extremely severe episodes of, e.g., general anxiety disorder, monotherapy is often not sufficient to overcome the critical situation as quickly as possible. Short-term administration of benzodiazepines may be necessary in addition.

Unipolar and bipolar depression

Being tired of life or longing for death are symptoms that occur almost regularly in depression, especially in moderate or severe cases. Furthermore, a large number of patients who are thinking about suicidal acts attempt suicide or even die from suicide. When selecting an antidepressant for suicidal depressive patients with a major depressive episode, compounds with a sedative profile (e.g., amitriptyline, doxepin, mianserin, mirtazapine) should be favoured; drugs that increase drive, such as monoamine oxidase (MAO) inhibitors or desipramine, may increase the risk of suicide.[3] Another aspect of drug selection is that the antidepressant should be safe in overdose, which is proven especially for SSRIs. However, SSRIs are also known to increase drive or cause agitation; therefore, such signs should be carefully monitored and if necessary reduced by sedative compounds. If a tricyclic antidepressant is chosen, the smallest dose should be prescribed to avoid the risk of lethal intoxication in case of suicidal overdose. Most tricyclic antidepressants have a high risk of fatal outcome if dosages of 1000 mg or more are taken.

SSRIs are nowadays widely used as a first-line treatment for depression, particularly for outpatients, mainly because of their better tolerability and compliance.[10] It should be remembered that SSRIs have no sedative potential and in some cases even cause agitation. The degree of sedation achieved even by a sedative antidepressant in a highly excited, suicidal depressive patient is sometimes insufficient, and it may be necessary to co-prescribe a benzodiazepine or a sedative neuroleptic. The dose depends on the patient's nervousness and agitation and individual reaction, and it should be chosen so that the inner restlessness and agitation wear off as completely as possible and significant sedation and promotion of nocturnal sleep are achieved. Since the benzodiazepines seem unfavourable in patients with a history of addiction, a sedative neuroleptic in a small dose may be chosen for these patients. In the case of delusional depression, a full antipsychotic treatment with neuroleptics is recommended, in addition to the antidepressant treatment.

In cases of depression with suicidality that are extremely difficult to treat by other means, electroconvulsive therapy[10] should also be considered, especially because of the rapid onset of action in comparison with antidepressants. Electroconvulsive therapy is also an important option in patients who are opposed to antidepressant treatment.

Although there were intensive discussions in recent years as to whether antidepressants are sufficiently beneficial in the treatment of depression, especially also considering suicidality/suicidal behaviour, empirical clinical studies as well as ecological studies gave predominantly positive results.[4,7,11]

In the case of acute bipolar depression, guidelines for psychopharmacological treatment have changed considerably in the last decade,[12] particularly the rule to avoid antidepressants as much as possible because of the risk of inducing manic or mixed episodes. Besides this unwanted effect, which destabilizes the bipolar disorder, it should be underlined that both conditions are associated with a risk of suicide attempts or even suicide, probably more than the pure depressive episode in the context of bipolar disorder. When the discussion about the potential negative effect of SSRIs on suicidality arose, the hypothesis was brought forward that some of the unwanted events of suicidal behaviour were a result of undetected switches into mild hypomania or mixed states.

Unipolar and bipolar depression are usually recurrent. Thus, in patients who have had two or more recurrent episodes, treatment is required to prevent relapse after acute and maintenance treatment. Antidepressants or lithium are recommended for preventing relapse in unipolar depression.[10]

In bipolar depression mood stabilizers, such as anticonvulsants or some second-generation antipsychotics like quetiapine or olanzapine and especially lithium, are the maintenance treatment choices.[13] Of great interest is the increasingly confirmed result that prophylactic treatment with lithium reduces the well-known excess mortality of patients with unipolar or bipolar depression (e.g., the lifetime risk of suicide is about 15% for unipolar depression and 20% for bipolar disorder) to within the normal range. This effect is apparently not only due to the reduction of depressive/manic relapses and related suicidal behaviour, but also seems to be the consequence of a direct effect on suicidal behaviour itself. Whether other mood stabilizers have the same benefit is still under discussion.

Attention should be paid to two additional problems when antidepressants are given to suicidal patients with depression. First, immediate antidepressant therapy is contraindicated in cases of intoxication with psychotropic substances (e.g., in an attempted suicide). In case of need, the fading period of intoxication should be bridged with low-potency neuroleptics. Second, an increase in drive or normalization of reduced drive often occurs during antidepressant treatment before brightening of mood (so-called drive-mood dissociation). This may require a temporary prescription or a dose increase of a concomitant sedative medication until mood starts to brighten, in order to counteract the increased risk of acting on suicidal impulses.

Schizophrenia

In case of suicidality in the context of an acute schizophrenic episode, the predominant task is to treat the psychosis in the best ways possible and in a sufficient number of ways.[14] Suicidality associated with a schizophrenic psychosis often requires medication in addition to the standard treatment of the schizophrenic symptoms, especially in cases of severe anxiety or excitation. Sedating antipsychotics are mostly used in these cases, owing to their additional antipsychotic effects, or benzodiazepines are administered. If higher doses of a sedating antipsychotic are initially required to achieve adequate sedation, special attention must be paid to the risk of acute hypotension with a tendency to collapse, particularly directly after standing up.

A different approach is required for suicidal schizophrenia patients who have depressive or negative symptoms. If depressive symptoms with suicidality exist as part of a post-psychotic depression, for example, or negative symptoms in the context of a deficit syndrome, pharmaco-therapy should generally follow the guidelines for the treatment of these conditions.[14,15] This means that additional treatment with antidepressants in the case of post-psychotic depression and treatment with special second-generation antipsychotics in the case of negative symptoms is favourable; in the case of negative symptoms as part of a deficit syndrome, treatment should probably be combined with an SSRI. If the suicidal symptoms are part of a depressive syndrome due to a side-effect of neuroleptic treatment (pharmacogenic depression or akinetic depression), especially during treatment with high potency first-generation antipsychotics, the neuroleptic dose should be reduced, if possible, or an anti-Parkinson's drug such as biperiden administered in addition.

Schizophrenia, in most cases, needs maintenance therapy with anti-psychotics.[15] Besides other aspects the risk to induce pharmacogenic depression and related suicidality should be considered in the decision for the most appropriate medication. The antipsychotic clozapine has some proven efficacy in reducing suicidality.

Personality disorders

Personality disorders are frequently associated with chronic, repetitive suicidality. At special risk are histrionic and borderline patients. In general, the efficacy of psychopharmacological treatment of personality disorders is not well established.[16] In borderline cases, especially, the occasional risk of paradoxical reactions to benzodiazepines or tricyclic antidepressants should be taken into consideration.[17] In most cases, only treatment of the acute critical condition is recommended. Benzodiazepines, antidepressants with a sedative–anxiolytic profile, or low-potency neuroleptics in small dosages can be administered as a short-term intervention. It should be taken into account that these suggestions are based on clinical experience but not on clinical trials. Long-term treatment with benzodiazepines should normally be avoided because of the risk of abuse.

There are only a few studies dealing with the question as to whether a medium-term psychopharmacological approach might be useful in the prevention of further suicide attempts in patients with a history of repeated suicide attempts. The studies that have been performed have mostly investigated comorbidity with personality disorders of the impulsive, histrionic, and borderline type.[18]

References

1 **Wassermann D, Rihmer Z, Rujescu D, Sarchiapone M, Sokolowski M,** . . . **Carli V.** The European Psychiatric Association (EPA) guidance on suicide treatment and prevention. Eur Psychiatry. 2012;**27**:129–1941.

2 **Möller H-J, Steinmeyer EM.** Are serotonergic reuptake inhibitors more potent in reducing suicidality? An empirical study on paroxetine. Eur Neuropsychopharmacol. 1994;**4**:55–59.

3 **Möller H-J, Baldwin D, Goodwin G, Kasper S, Okasha A, Stein DJ, et al.** Do SSRIs or antidepressants in general increase suicidality? WPA Section on Pharmacopsychiatry consensus statement. Eur Arch Psychiatry Clin Neurosci. 2008;**258**:3–23.

4 **Möller H-J, Bitter I, Bobes J, Fountoulakis K, Höschl C, Kasper S.** EPA position statement on the value of antidepressants in the treatment of unipolar depression. Eur Psychiatry. 2012;**27**:114–128.

5 **Musil R, Zill P, Seemüller F, Bondy B, Meyer S,** . . . **Riedel M.** Genetics of emergent suicidality during antidepressant treatment—data from a naturalistic study on a large sample of inpatients with major depressive episode. Eur Neuropsychopharmacol. 2013;**23**:663–674.

6 **Seemüller F, Riedel M, Obermeier M, Bauer M, Adli M,** . . . **Möller HJ.** Outcomes of 1014 naturalistically treated in-patients with major depressive episode. Eur Neuropsychopharmacol. 2010 May;**20**(5):346–355.

7 **Möller H-J.** Evidence for beneficial effects of antidepressants in depressive patients: a systematic review. Eur Arch Psychiatry Clin Neurosci. 2006;**256**:329–343.

8 **Möller HJ.** Effectiveness and safety of benzodiazepines. J Clin Psychopharmacol. 1999;**19**(Suppl2):2–11.

9 **Bandelow B, Zohar J, Hollander E, Kasper S, Möller H-J.** World Federation of Societies of Biological Psychiatry (WFSBP) guidelines for the pharmacological treatment of anxiety, obsessive–compulsive and post-traumatic stress disorders—first revision. World J Biol Psychiatry. 2008;**9**:248–312.

10 **Bauer M, Pfennig A, Severus E, Whybrow PC, Angst J, Möller H-J.** World Federation of Societies of Biological Psychiatry (WFSBP) guidelines for biological treatment of unipolar depressive disorders, part 1: update 2013 on the acute and continuation treatment of unipolar depressive disorders. World J Biological Psychiatry. 2013;**14**:334–385.

11 **Baldessarini RJ, Tondo L, Strobom IM, Fawcett J, Licinio J,** . . . **Tohen M.** Ecological studies of antidepressant treatment and suicidal risks. Harv Rev Psychiatry. 2007 Jul–Aug;**15**(4):133–145.

12 Grunze H, Vieta E, Goodwin GM, Bowden C, Licht RW, . . . Kasper S. The World Federation of Societies of Biological Psychiatry (WFSBP) guidelines for the biological treatment of bipolar disorders: update 2010 on the treatment of acute bipolar depression. World J Biol Psychiatry. 2010 Mar;11(2):81–109.

13 Grunze H, Vieta E, Goodwin GM, Bowden C, Licht RW, . . . Kasper S. The World Federation of Societies of Biological Psychiatry (WFSBP) guidelines for the biological treatment of bipolar disorders: update 2012 on the long-term treatment of bipolar disorder. World J Biol Psychiatry 2013 Apr;14(3):154–219.

14 Hasan A, Falkai P, Wobrock T, Liebermann J, Glenthoj B, . . . Möller H-J. World Federation of Biological Psychiatry (WFSBP) guidelines for biological treatment of schizophrenia, part 1: update 2012 on the acute treatment of schizophrenia and the management of treatment resistance. World J Biol Psychiatry 2012;13:318–378.

15 Hasan A, Falkai P, Wobrock T, Liebermann J, Glenthoj B, . . . Möller HJ. World Federation of Societies of Biological Psychiatry (WFSBP) guidelines for biological treatment of schizophrenia, part 2: update 2012 on the long-term treatment of schizophrenia and management of antipsychotic-induced side effects. World J Biol Psychiatry. 2013;14:2–44.

16 Herpertz S, Zanarini M, Schulz CS, Siever L, Lieb K, Möller H-J. World Federation of Societies of Biological Psychiatry (WFSBP) guidelines for biological treatment of personality disorders. World J Biol Psychiatry. 2007;257:402–412.

17 Möller H-J. Provocation of aggressive and autoaggressive behavior by psychoactive drugs. Eur Neuropsychopharmacol. 1994;4:232–234.

18 Montgomery SA, Montgomery DB, Green M, Bullock T, Baldwin D. Pharmacotherapy in the prevention of suicidal behavior. J Clin Psychopharmacol. 1992 Apr;12(2 Suppl):27S–31S.

Chapter 28

Psychological treatments for suicidal individuals

Megan Chesin, Andriy Yur'yev,
and Barbara Stanley

Introduction

Recognition of suicidal thoughts or behaviour as a modifiable target for psychosocial treatment began in earnest in the 1950s with the
pioneering work of Dr Edwin Shneidman. Schneidman showed that,
contrary to popular belief at the time, suicidal individuals were, in
many cases, neither treatment resistant nor help-rejecting. However,
not much was done to develop suicide-specific treatments until four
decades later. In the early 1990s, the first comprehensive treatment
targeting suicide prevention among high suicide risk patients with
borderline personality disorder, dialectical behaviour therapy (DBT[1]),
was developed. Today, some longer-term psychological treatments to
prevent suicide meet current standards for evidence-based practice.
These treatments are almost exclusively based on the principles and
techniques of cognitive and behavioural therapies. Adaptations for
suicidal individuals include targeting warning signs of suicidal crises
as well as motivational and skills deficits common to suicidal patients.
There is variety as to where, when, and how psychological treatments
to prevent suicide are delivered. Suicide prevention is targeted during crisis intervention on hotlines, during brief suicide-prevention
efforts in acute care settings, and through longer-term inpatient or
outpatient treatment provided by mental health clinicians. The purpose of this chapter is to outline longer-term and brief (one-session)
psychological treatments to prevent suicidal behaviour as well as to
summarize empirical support for such treatments.

Longer-term interventions

Currently, two longer-term (ten sessions or more) psychological treatments to prevent suicide have the largest evidence base. These two approaches are:

1 cognitive behavioural therapy (CBT) for suicide or suicide attempt prevention;[2] and

2 dialectical behaviour therapy (DBT[1]).

CBT for suicide prevention

In CBT approaches, therapy is guided by an understanding of the specific factors involved in the development and maintenance of the pathology. Thus, in CBT-based treatment of the suicidal patient, treatment is guided by specific understanding of the combination of factors that contribute to the development and maintenance of the suicidal state. Chain analysis or detailed analysis of the events, behaviours, feelings, thoughts, and sensations surrounding the last suicide event in combination with standard intake assessment procedures are employed to identify individual treatment targets.

According to the well-accepted stress-diathesis model of suicidal behaviour, suicidal behaviour occurs when an individual predisposed to suicidal behaviour (e.g., by family history of suicidal behaviour, childhood maltreatment, biological vulnerability in serotonergic system, maladaptive cognitive style including problem-solving deficits) is triggered by an acute stressor (e.g., by interpersonal conflict, depressive episode, financial problems).[3] In cognitive conceptualizations of suicidal behaviour, resulting maladaptive tendencies towards hopelessness, attentional biases towards suicide-relevant stimuli or cues, and attentional fixation on suicide as the only solution are thought to be particularly salient in maintaining suicide risk.[4] Given the central role of cognitive factors in the development and maintenance of suicidal behaviour in cognitive theories of suicidal behaviour, CBT adapted to prevent suicide includes problem-solving skills training as well as training in thought monitoring and cognitive restructuring. As patients realize their self-efficacy in solving problems (the ultimate goal of problem-solving skills training in CBT), hopelessness may be reduced.

Other components of CBT-based approaches to prevent suicide include safety planning and psycho-education on signs and symptoms of suicidal behaviour and lethal means restriction, as well as skills training in behavioural activation, emotion regulation, distress tolerance, assertiveness, and social skills. Motivation is enhanced through discussions of reasons for living and development of a hope kit (i.e., a collection of objects that represent reasons for living; e.g., photos of loved ones, motivational phrases).

Relapse prevention is particularly important in CBT for suicide prevention and thus, at the end of treatment, in adaptations of CBT for suicide prevention, multiple sessions focused on skills generalization and coping ahead for suicidal crisis are provided. In some CBT-based approaches, booster sessions may also be offered after the acute phase of treatment has ended. In these sessions, skills generalization, motivation, and safety monitoring are continued foci. Additionally, particularly when suicidal adolescents are the target population, family members may be included in treatment. Figure 28.1 provides an overview of the structure and content of treatment sessions in CBT-Suicide Prevention (CBT-SP),[5] a manualized CBT-based treatment to prevent suicide in adolescent suicide attempters.

It should be noted that, though not a specific focus of CBT-based treatment for suicide prevention, formation of a good therapeutic alliance enables therapy and is necessary, but not sufficient, for it to be conducted properly.

The evidence base for CBT-based approaches to prevent suicide

In randomized controlled trials (RCTs) comparing CBT-based approaches to treatment as usual (TAU), CBT-based approaches have been shown to be effective in reducing suicide behaviour risk, broadly defined to include hopelessness, suicidal thoughts, and suicide attempts, among high suicide-behaviour risk groups and to be feasible with and acceptable to the target population (e.g.,[6]). Two trials are particularly noteworthy for their rigour. Brown et al.[7] showed suicide attempters presenting to the emergency department who received ten sessions of

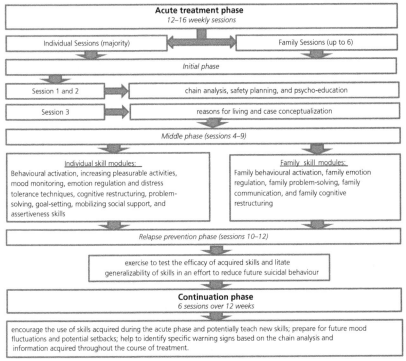

Fig. 28.1 Structure and content of treatment sessions in CBT for suicide prevention

cognitive therapy (CT) for suicide prevention were half as likely to re-attempt suicide as attempters receiving enhanced TAU. Importantly, significant reductions in suicide attempt risk and depression were maintained over 18 months follow-up. Meanwhile, in an open trial of CBT-SP, CBT-SP was associated with relatively low rates of suicide re-attempt and suicide-related events (e.g., hospitalizations for suicidal thoughts) among depressed adolescents who had a recent history of suicide attempt. Feasibility and acceptability were also high with nearly three-quarters of the sample completing at least 12 sessions of CBT-SP and nearly all CBT-SP recipients indicating the intervention was helpful.[8]

Dialectical Behaviour Therapy

DBT[1] was designed to increase safety among patients who engaged in non-suicidal self-injury and suicidal behaviour, and manualized for the treatment of borderline personality disorder (BPD). DBT is a more intensive and complex therapy than CBT approaches to suicide prevention detailed, though many CBT principles and procedures are employed in it. In DBT, emotion dysregulation is considered to be the key difficulty for chronically suicidal BPD patients. Emotion dysregulation is posited to arise from the interaction between an individual difficulty in understanding, expressing, and managing emotions and an invalidating environment, prototypically a childhood environment characterized by abuse and/or neglect. BPD, and the characteristic emotion dysregulation, manifests as severe behavioural, interpersonal, and cognitive dysfunction and often includes suicidal behaviour.

Similar to CBT, DBT is focused on behaviour and mood monitoring, skills acquisition and generalization, and development and maintenance of motivation for change. Treatment techniques include chain analysis, solution generation and analysis, and psycho-education and skills training. In DBT, compared with CBT, the therapeutic relationship is considered a more central mechanism for affecting behaviour change, with the therapist often employing his or her response to patient behaviour to reinforce adaptive behaviour and to try to reduce maladaptive behaviours. Another significant difference between CBT and DBT is the inclusion of acceptance and dialectic strategies in DBT. Acceptance-based protocols and strategies include validating patient pain and those pieces of patient perspective and behaviour that are valid or make sense given, for example, the patient's prior experiences or normative behaviour. In dialectical strategies, such as gaining commitment for a small amount of change (e.g., staying safe for one night) and then asking for a great deal of change (e.g., staying safe for the duration of treatment) or balancing acceptance of where the patient is with the need for behaviour change, opposite techniques or positions are combined to produce a more complete understanding of behaviour, commitment to behaviour change, or a more effective solution for affecting it. Finally, where CBT is a protocols-driven approach, DBT is a principles-driven approach. Thus, treatment, especially individual sessions, are less proscribed in DBT.

Standard DBT lasts one year and includes both individual and group skills-training sessions. In DBT, individual treatment is structured around a hierarchy whereby suicidal behaviour and non-suicidal self-injury (NSSI) are addressed first when present. Behaviours that interfere with successful therapy and maintenance of a good working therapeutic relationship are the next priority, and quality-of-life interfering behaviours; e.g., severe problems with relationships and substance abuse, and skills acquisition are lower priority targets. Other components of standard DBT include telephone-based skills coaching between sessions, to encourage skills generalization and help maintain patient safety, and therapist consultation meetings, to increase therapist adherence and motivation.[1]

The evidence base for DBT

There is good evidence that DBT reduces suicide attempts and service utilization for suicide-related concerns relative to TAU and even treatment by experts. Findings from ten RCTs conducted by eight different groups consistently show that DBT is a more efficacious treatment for NSSI and suicidal behaviour among adults with BPD than TAU, treatment by experts, and supportive psychotherapy. In a meta-analysis of five of the above RCTs, Panos et al.[9] found DBT to be moderately more effective in reducing suicidal behaviour and NSSI than active control treatments, including TAU, supportive psychotherapy, and manualized psychodynamic or client-centred therapy. Importantly, some trials show decreases in self-injury and suicidal behaviour among patients receiving DBT are maintained in the months to years following treatment (e.g.,[10]). DBT has also been adapted to treat suicidal adolescents, with a family-skills training component added and the duration of the treatment shortened. Findings from a controlled trial of DBT for suicidal adolescents were promising and showed adolescents receiving DBT realized greater reductions in suicidal ideation and were hospitalized less often during treatment than adolescents who received supportive-psychodynamic treatment.[11] However, DBT has a number of disadvantages, including significant costs associated with implementation of the intensive treatment.[12] Further, improvements in terms of secondary outcomes, such as remittance rates of mood, anxiety, and eating disorder among suicidal DBT patients, have been disappointing, with DBT often showing no relative advantage to TAU or other treatments.

Other approaches with demonstrated efficacy or effectiveness in reducing suicide risk

Collaborative assessment and management of suicidality (CAMS)

CAMS is an atheoretical, multi-pronged, therapeutic framework to reduce suicide risk that draws on therapeutic techniques from multiple interventions.[13] In CAMS, treatment starts with a structured and detailed assessment of individual risk factors for suicidal behaviour. To aid in this endeavour, a suicide status form (SSF) is completed collaboratively by the therapist and patient during the initial treatment sessions. Next, thorough understanding of the patient's suicidality is used to identify the most relevant interventions. Such interventions may include development and use of individualized coping cards, identification of social supports or social-skills training. It will certainly include development of a crisis response plan and lethal means restriction, as well as time and effort devoted to increasing motivation and adherence to treatment. Suicide risk assessment, preferably using well-validated suicide risk assessment tools, is ongoing throughout treatment. Non-specific factors are also targeted, including development of a strong therapeutic alliance between the patient and therapist, and maintenance of empathy and non-judgement towards suicidal behaviour on the part of the therapist. The suicidal patient is expected to be an active participant and collaborator in the assessment of his/her own suicidality and the creation of the treatment plan in CAMS. CAMS ends when a patient reports no active suicidal ideation and has not engaged in suicidal behaviour for three consecutive sessions. Studies show that CAMS lasts for approximately 10–12 sessions in practice. In multiple uncontrolled studies, CAMS treatment has been associated with reductions in suicidal thinking. For example, findings from an RCT comparing CAMS to TAU showed greater reductions in suicidal ideation among those receiving CAMS and that these reductions in suicidal ideation were maintained at 12-months follow-up. Further, treatment satisfaction and retention were greater among CAMS recipients.[13]

Interpersonal psychotherapy (IPT)

Heisel et al.[14] adapted IPT for older adults at suicide risk by incorporating structured safety monitoring into each of the 16 sessions, encouraging patients to engage in between-session phone contact with therapists when suicide-related concerns were present, and by targeting factors, especially interpersonal factors, associated with increased suicidal ideation. In the pilot, uncontrolled trial, adapted IPT was associated with decreased suicidal ideation. Feasibility, tolerability, and acceptability were also high.[14] Support for continuing to adapt and test IPT to prevent suicide also comes from studies showing standard IPT-reduced suicidal ideation among depressed patients and a brief (four-session) interpersonal psychodynamic therapy, compared with TAU, reduced the recurrence of self-injury and suicidal ideation among self-injuring patients (e.g.,[15]).

Psychodynamic approaches

Three psychodynamic approaches to treating BPD are efficacious for reducing suicidal behaviour among BPD patients: transference-focused psychotherapy, mentalization-based treatment, and sequential brief Adlerian psychodynamic psychotherapy. Though a detailed description of these treatments is beyond the scope of this chapter, briefly, these treatments are alike in their time-limited nature (40–78 weeks in duration), their foci on current maladaptive interpersonal dynamics and difficulties in emotion regulation and interpersonal functioning, and their reliance on the treatment relationship as a main mechanism of change. All are supported by RCTs in which the psychodynamic approach was found to be superior to active treatment in reducing suicidal behaviour among BPD patients.[16]

The combination of psychotherapy and psychopharmacotherapy in the treatment of suicidality

In practice, suicidal individuals often receive both pharmacotherapy and psychotherapy. A thorough review of the evidence base of the anti-suicide properties of different medications is beyond the scope of this chapter. Psychopharmacological agents with known anti-suicide effects include lithium, clozapine, and selective serotonin reuptake inhibitors (SSRIs).[17] To further refine treatment recommendations, studies comparing medication plus therapy to evidence-based practices are needed as is rigorous study of when and for whom medication may be contraindicated; i.e., may increase risk for suicide.

Brief interventions

Longer-term psychological treatment, alone or in combination with psychopharmacological treatment, can reduce suicide risk among patients. Unfortunately, many individuals at risk for suicide do not engage or maintain in longer-term treatment. For instance, 40–50% of suicidal individuals who present to and are discharged directly from the emergency department (ED) will not attend any follow-up outpatient mental health-care appointments. Further, only 30–40% of suicidal patients stabilized and then referred to outpatient mental health treatment after ED presentation are compliant with longer-term treatment.[18]

Broadly, brief psychosocial suicide-prevention interventions with at least some empirical support can be divided into four types: CBT-based interventions, contact interventions, those that combine the two, and manual-assisted CT (MACT). Brief CBT-based suicide-prevention interventions require one face-to-face session and can be delivered by professionals or trained paraprofessionals. Such interventions include: psycho-education about suicide behaviour warning signs and risk factors, crisis and treatment resources, and/or means restriction. They sometimes include individualized crisis planning. Enhancing motivation for ongoing treatment may also be targeted. When the patient is an adolescent, adult involvement in the brief intervention is encouraged. Such CBT-based interventions have been shown to increase lethal-means restriction and treatment engagement in the months following ED discharge.[19]

Meanwhile, contact interventions involve periodic post-discharge written contact by hospital staff. Typically, letters or texts provide well-wishes and contact information for hospital services should the former patient need care. Findings from an initial RCT testing contact interventions were very promising and showed that those who received the contact intervention were significantly less likely to suicide over a two-year follow-up than those who had not. Others, meanwhile, have found contact interventions only improve safety among the subset of suicidal individuals who engage in repeated self-harm.[20]

Combined interventions

Given the promising findings for brief CBT-based and contact interventions, three combined interventions have been developed and tested. These interventions, as detailed in Table 28.1, provide a brief intervention pre-discharge and then semi-structured follow-up contact

Table 28.1 Combined brief CBT-based and contact interventions

Intervention	Pre-Discharge Component	Post-Discharge Component	Evidence
Youth Nominated Support Team-Version II (YST-II)	Training of youth-nominated adults in means restriction, suicide warning signs and crisis resources.	Weekly supportive contact by youth-nominated adults.	No differences in suicidal ideation between adolescents randomized to YST-II in addition to TAU and those who only received TAU.
Brief Intervention and Contact (BIC)	Psycho-education on risk and protective factors for suicidal behaviour as well as mental health and crisis resources.	Nine clinician-administered phone calls over 18 months consisting of a mood and safety check.	In a multinational RCT, significant reductions in suicide rates at 18-months follow-up among BIC compared with TAU participants.
Safety Planning Intervention + Structured Follow-up (SPI-SFU)	Completion of individualized crisis survival plan (i.e., Safety Plan) listing warning signs, distractions, social supports, professional and personal resources who can provide assistance in crisis and means restriction.	Clinician-administered phone calls during transition to outpatient treatment. Calls consist of mood and safety checks, discussion of Safety Plan, and review of progress towards engaging in outpatient treatment.	Findings from an RCT show suicidal veterans receiving SPI-SFU were significantly less likely to make an attempt within six months after treatment compared with those receiving TAU. On interview, key participant and staff informants perceived SPI-SFU as helpful in increasing safety and follow-up treatment engagement among patients at risk for suicidal behaviour.

post-discharge. Though data are limited, such combined interventions seem to improve safety among adults.

Taken together, CBT-based brief interventions, contact interventions, or their combination may increase safety. Importantly, such interventions provide contact and resources to suicidal individuals who may not otherwise know of or have such support. Definitive conclusions regarding the utility of contact interventions and targeted, brief CBT-based interventions for reducing suicidal behaviour and increasing treatment engagement among discharging patients awaits further study. Feasibility and acceptability must also continue to be tested. Limited staff time and training on suicide assessment and prevention, unless addressed, may preclude wide-spread dissemination of such interventions.

Manual-Assisted Cognitive Therapy (MACT)

MACT is a bibliotherapeutic approach to suicide prevention, which is augmented by up to six individual therapy sessions. The content of MACT self-help books is based on CBT and DBT, and includes guided chain analysis of the most recent incident of self-injury, problem-solving and distress tolerance skills training, and relapse prevention planning. In a small pilot study, adult patients who had a history of recent, repetitive self-harm (suicide intent unknown) who received MACT, compared with TAU, trended to have less frequent self-harm episodes and reduced depression with treatment. On average, MACT patients participated in only 2.7 sessions of individual therapy and 30% completed only bibliotherapy. Further, patients reported they found bibliotherapy to be the most helpful component of the intervention. Findings from a larger, follow-up RCT, however, were not as promising and showed no difference between patients receiving TAU and MACT in self-injury outcomes.[21]

Directions for future research: considerations for developing and testing treatments to prevent suicidal behaviour

Developing and testing treatments to prevent suicidal behaviour is laden with ethical and methodological difficulties, including difficulties systematically capturing suicide-related events and assigning high suicide risk individuals to a standard treatment or waiting list control condition, or conversely, to receive experimental treatment. Thus, determining and comparing the effectiveness of treatments to prevent suicide is difficult. Limits to the current literature include a lack of specificity regarding for whom among the diverse group of suicidal individuals evidence-based treatments work. For example, slightly more than half of suicide victims complete on their first attempt.[22] The most rigorous studies of psychosocial treatments to prevent suicide have only included individuals who have a history of suicide attempt. Thus, whether DBT and CT, for instance, are effective for reducing suicide risk among high suicide risk groups who do not have a history of suicide attempt (e.g., older, white males) is unknown and a direction for future study. Similarly, whether current evidence-based psychological treatments work to prevent suicide among patients who have schizophrenia spectrum disorders is unclear, with the majority of studies included in a systematic review of ten RCTs comparing the addition of psychological treatment with TAU for reducing suicidal behaviour among schizophrenic patients showing no additional benefit (in terms of reduced suicidal ideation or behaviour) with the addition of psychological treatment.[23] Additional treatment development work is needed to effectively adapt psychosocial treatment to prevent suicidal behaviour among psychotic patients.

Another direction for future research is developing and testing group-based treatments for suicidal behaviour given the cost-effectiveness of the group modality. To date, we know of only two group-therapy approaches to suicide prevention that have been manualized and tested: developmental group psychotherapy[24] and a one-session DBT skills-based group treatment.[25] Only DGP has been rigorously tested with mixed result, with one RCT showing DGP compared with TAU participants were less likely to re-engage in self-injurious behaviour (suicide intent unknown) for six months during and after treatment, and another RCT showing no such benefit for DGP participants.[26] Preliminary pilot data from an open trial of the one-session DBT skills-based treatment is promising and shows reductions in suicidal ideation and increased coping skill use with treatment among participants.[25]

Clinical implications

Given what is known about suicide behaviour risk and prevention, effective management and treatment of suicidal individuals likely involves:

- consistent monitoring of suicide risk;
- a focus on the present;
- targeting of factors known to be involved in the experience and maintenance of suicidal urges and behaviours, including emotion dysregulation, problem-solving, and other skills deficits; and
- targeting of particular specific and idiosyncratic manifestations of the generally identified maintaining factors.

Currently, only CBT and DBT are manualized treatments to prevent suicide with significant empirical support. There are, however, numerous reasons, including brief treatment options, to be optimistic about the prospects for engaging and treating acutely suicidal people.

References

1 **Linehan MM.** Cognitive-behavioral treatment of borderline personality disorder. New York, NY: Guilford; 1993.

2 **Brown GK, Have TT, Henriques GR, Xie SX, Hollander JE, Beck AT.** Cognitive therapy for the prevention of suicide attempts: a randomized controlled trial. JAMA 2005;**294**:563–570.

3 **Mann JJ, Waternaux C, Haas GL, Malone KM.** Toward a clinical model of suicidal behavior in psychiatric patients. Am J Psychiatry. 1999;**156**:181–189.

4 **Wenzel A, Beck AT.** A cognitive model of suicidal behavior: theory and treatment. Appl Prev Psychol 2008;**12**(4):189–201.

5 **Stanley B, Brown G, Brent DA, Wells K, Poling K, Curry J, et al.** Cognitive-behavioral therapy for suicide prevention (CBT-SP): treatment model, feasibility, and acceptability. J Am Acad Child Adolesc Psychiatry 2009;**48**(10):1005–1013.

6 **Hvid M, Vangborg K, Sorensen HJ, Nielsen IK, Stenborg JM, Wang AG.** Preventing repetition of attempted suicide—II. The Amager project, a randomized controlled trial. Nord J Psychiatry. 2011;**65**(5):292–298. Epub 2010/12/22.

7 **Brown GK, Ten Have T, Henriques GR, Xie SX, Hollander JE, Beck AT.** Cognitive therapy for the prevention of suicide attempts. JAMA. 2005;**294**(5):563–570.

8 **Brent DA, Greenhill LL, Compton S, Emslie G, Wells K, Walkup JT, et al.** The Treatment of Adolescent Suicide Attempters study (TASA): predictors of suicidal events in an open treatment trial. J Am Acad Child Adolesc Psychiatry 2009;**48**(10):987–996.

9 Panos PT, Jackson JW, Hasan O, Panos A. meta-analysis and systematic review assessing the efficacy of dialectical behaviour therapy (DBT). Res Soc Work 2013.

10 Linehan MM, Comtois K, Murray AM, et al. Two-year randomized controlled trial and follow-up of dialectical behavior therapy vs therapy by experts for suicidal behaviors and borderline personality disorder. Arch Gen Psychiatry 2006;**63**(7):757–766.

11 Rathus JH, Miller AL. Dialectical behavior therapy adapted for suicidal adolescents. Suicide Life Threat Behav 2002;**32**(2):146–157.

12 Pasieczny N, Connor J. The effectiveness of dialectical behaviour therapy in routine public mental health settings: an Australian controlled trial. Behav Res Ther 2011;**49**(1):4–10.

13 Jobes DA. Managing suicidal risk: a collaborative approach. New York, NY: Guilford; 2006.

14 Heisel MJ, Duberstein PR, Talbot NL, King DA, Tu XM. Adapting interpersonal psychotherapy for older adults at risk for suicide: preliminary findings. Prof Psychol Res Pr. 2009;**40**(2):156–164.

15 Szanto K, Mulsant BH, Houck P, Dew MA, Reynolds CF. Occurrence and course of suicidality during short-term treatment of late-life depression. Arch Gen Psychiatry. 2003;**60**(6):610–617.

16 Amianto F, Ferrero A, Pierò A, Cairo E, Rocca G, Simonelli B, et al. Supervised team management, with or without structured psychotherapy, in heavy users of a mental health service with borderline personality disorder: a two-year follow-up preliminary randomized study. BMC Psychiatry. 2011;**11**(1):1–14.

17 Cipriani A, Hawton K, Stockton S, Geddes JR. Lithium in the prevention of suicide in mood disorders: updated systematic review and meta-analysis. BMJ. 2013;346.

18 Lizardi D, Stanley B. Treatment engagement: A neglected aspect in the psychiatric care of suicidal patients. Psych Serv. 2010;**61**:1183–1191.

19 Kruesi MJ, Grossman J, Pennington JM, Woodward PJ, Duda D, Hirsch JG. Suicide and violence prevention: parent education in the emergency department. J Am Acad Child Adolesc Psychiatry 1999;**38**(3):250–255.

20 Beautrais AL, Gibb SJ, Faulkner A, Fergusson DM, Mulder RT. Postcard intervention for repeat self-harm: randomised controlled trial. Br J Psychiatry. 2010;**197**(1):55–60.

21 Tyrer P, Thompson S, Schmidt U, Jones V, Knapp M, Davidson K, et al. Randomized controlled trial of brief cognitive behaviour therapy versus treatment as usual in recurrent deliberate self-harm: the POPMACT study. Psychol Med. 2003;**33**(6):969–976.

22 Isometsä ET, Lönnqvist JK. Suicide attempts preceding completed suicide. Br J Psychiatry 1998;**173**(6):531–535.

23 Donker T, Calear A, Grant J, van Spijker B, Fenton K, Hehir K, et al. Suicide prevention in schizophrenia spectrum disorders and psychosis: a systematic review. BMC Psychology. 2013;**1**(1):6.

24 **Wood, A.**, Trainor, G., Rothwell, J., Moore, A. N. N., & Harrington, R. (2001). Randomized trial of group therapy for repeated deliberate selfharm in adolescents. J Am Acad Child Adolesc Psychiatry, 40(11), 1246–1253.

25 **Ward-Ciesielski EF.** An open pilot feasibility study of a brief dialectical behavior therapy skills-based intervention for suicidal individuals. Suicide Life Threat Behav 2013;**43**(3):324–335.

26 **Hazell PL, Martin G, McGill K, Kay T, Wood A, Trainor G, et al.** Group therapy for repeated deliberate self-harm in adolescents: failure of replication of a randomized trial. J Am Acad Child Adolesc Psychiatry 2009;**48**(6):662–670.

Chapter 29

Education of general practitioners in depression and suicide prevention

Wolfgang Rutz and Zoltán Rihmer

The Gotland study

The Gotland study, with its successes and shortcomings, illustrates the potential and limitations of medical and psychiatric services—in terms of how well they treat and monitor psychiatric morbidity as the immediate cause of most suicides, by fulfilling their obligatory duties.

The Swedish island of Gotland, with a population of some 60,000, is an epidemiological laboratory. Despite their apparently high quality of life and the beautiful surroundings, the inhabitants of Gotland have undergone dramatic social transition when in the 1970s the number of people employed in agriculture, forest culture, and fishing industries decreased dramatically by about 80%. In the early eighties, the island was one of the 'black spots' for suicidality in Sweden with suicide rates being the highest in Sweden, well above urban rates. One feature was the high and very often violent suicidality, often in females. The prescription rate in Gotland for antidepressants on the other hand was among the lowest in Sweden, compensated by high over-prescriptions of sedative, anxiolytic, and hypnotic drugs.

In this alarming situation, strong initiatives for a training campaign were taken by the island's general practitioners (GPs), who were eager to help their patients but felt helpless and incompetent. To help the GPs tackle the island's depression and suicide problems, the local psychiatric department and the Swedish Committee for Prevention and Treatment of Depressions (PTD Committee), consisting of leading academics and clinicians in the field of depression, jointly initiated a training programme on depression in primary health-care.

This comprehensive, structured programme comprised two courses of two days each and was offered to all GPs on Gotland over a two-year period with unstructured but continuous supervising and supportive contacts in-between. It covered most aspects of early diagnosis and monitoring of depressive disorders. All but one GP participated.

The study was implemented as a training programme in the early 1980s, evaluated until the early 1990s, and followed up with mainten-ance training until 1998. Detecting and treating depressive conditions as the principal feature of the suicidal process was the aim of the Gotland study. The programme was given in a somewhat luxurious hotel envir-onment deemed conducive to learning. It lasted two consecutive days and the night in-between and afforded time and scope for interaction, discussion, and sharing of personal clinical and private experience, as well as lectures, video presentations, role playing, and case discussions. The participants were able to influence the programme after the first year by pointing out what topics they were missing and they were given all the teaching material in written form printed in two books for use in training their own teams.

The problem of depression and its detection and monitoring was pre-sented in an integrative and synoptic way. Becoming depressed and suicidal, and also recovery was described as a multifactorial and multi-dimensional process. Accordingly, multidisciplinary and multimodal methods of intervention and help were said to be required, demon-strated, and taught. The sometimes crucial, life-saving, and inevitable first aid by psychopharmacological treatment was explained, as was the need for psychotherapeutic follow-up and support in a process-related way to guarantee a positive long-term outcome.

Psychotherapy and pharmacotherapy were presented as complemen-tary and process-related approaches rather than as alternative strategies, according to the maxim that 'there is a time for everything'.

The distinction between 'endogenous' and 'exogenous' aetiology was consequently avoided, as were the fictitious contradictions between the psychodynamic, psychosocial, and biological approaches. Instead, a stress-vulnerability model was used. The need for integrative thinking was, therefore, emphasized in terms of multifactoriality and the need for process-related action. This 'holistic' approach also resulted in efforts to describe depression not as a distinct nosological entity associated with various comorbidities but, rather, as a state connected with anxiety, drug abuse, alcoholism, and temporary personality changes. Various types of destructive behaviour were also examined as symptoms that are often related to and caused by depression. Guidelines, protocols, and assessment scales were presented as checklists in need of modification individually adapted to the patient and the need for an individualistic and person-centred approach was underlined.

With its structured and holistic presentation, the training was highly appreciated and brought about a significant improvement in GPs' capacity to diagnose, treat, and monitor depressive conditions. During the three years after the training programme—the period of its maximum impact—a wide range of interrelated results connected with the training were observed. Referrals for depression to the local psychiatric institution and also the number of days of sick leave for depressive and apathetic conditions fell by more than 50% in Gotland. The amount of inpatient care at the local psychiatric clinic for depressive conditions dropped by 70% and suicides decreased significantly among females. Prescription of antidepressants rose from less than 50% of the Swedish average to more than 80%; conversely, there was a decrease of 30% in the number of sedatives, anxiolytics, and hypnotics prescribed, in relation to the Swedish average, normalizing the previous over-prescription. Three years after the training, thanks to improved diagnosis of recurrent depressive conditions, lithium prescription also rose by 30%.[1]

Another finding was that the seasonality of suicide patterns in Gotland, which was fairly marked in the 1980s, decreased significantly during the 1990s. It may confirm that the basic problem in Gotland before the training project was one of under-diagnosis and under-treatment of seasonal triggered depression, resulting in a high number of depression related suicides. This situation was improved by the training.[2]

A special cost–benefit calculation showed that the training programme, which cost roughly SEK 400,000, resulted in substantial savings for society during the three-year period of its maximum impact owing to the reductions in morbidity, suicide mortality, inpatient care, and spending on drugs.[1]

The Gotland Male Depression Scale (GMDS)

However, these changes were only temporary. By the end of the decade the suicide numbers had returned to their baseline values or slightly above, and the need for continued and updating training was apparent. New courses began in the early 1990s and follow-up refresher courses were provided at intervals of about two years until 1998.

Detailed scrutiny of the suicide-preventive effects of Gotland's training programme revealed that the positive change of reduced suicidality was found mainly in the group of female suicides; while male suicides were unaffected.[3] The male suicides were mostly violent. Moreover, a psychological autopsy of all male suicides showed that unlike the women in Gotland who committed suicide and who were mostly known to the health-care services, the great majority of men who committed suicide were known only to the police, tax authorities, or social welfare authorities that deal with alcoholics. Thus, the improvement of GP services did not reach those males.

The training, focused as it was on improving the quality of GPs' recognition and monitoring of depression, evidently had no positive impact on male suicidality in Gotland, since the men concerned committed suicide without coming into contact with health-care services. In the few cases when such contact existed, the men were diagnosed as having personality disorders, showing sociopathic behaviour or being drug abusers, and were often considered untreatable owing to their uncooperative behaviour, 'psychopathic' acting-out, aggression, or lack of compliance with and motivation for treatment. Research shows that depressive and suicidal men usually display atypical depressive symptoms. If they casually ask for help, their depression is often neither recognized nor effectively treated.

In view of the persistently high male suicide rate and from the results of our psychological autopsy of all male suicides during the 1980s, the GMDS was developed, disseminated, even in the mass media, and used in the follow-up training programmes during the 1990s that placed heavier emphasis on depressive symptoms and suicidal behaviour in males. This scale focuses on the typical 'atypical' male depressive symptoms, presenting the typical features of male depression: impaired stress tolerance, acting-out, aggression, low impulse control, irritability, indecision, abuse tendencies, temporarily 'pseudo psychopathic' or 'antisocial' behaviour, and inheritance of tendencies towards suicide, depression, and substance abuse.

This scale was based on a clinical evaluation of the male depressive picture that the psychological autopsy study had revealed and has now internationally been tested for several years as a screening instrument to detect depression in males who are in contact with primary care or other health-care or social services. The scale is even continuously being subjected to scientific evaluation and validation. Since this GMDS has been taught as a screening instrument to local primary health-care staff and presented in the Gotland mass media, a decrease in male suicides on Gotland has also been observed.

The concept of male depression and suicidality is increasingly the focus of scientific interest and is being actualized in a growing number of contexts. However, since most of the male depressives who commit suicide are not in contact with any health-care services, approaches must be developed to reach them by involving other players in society—the men's workplaces, trade unions, social networks, families and friends, as well as the mass media.[4]

International experience

Training aimed at better recognition and monitoring of depressive and depression related conditions in primary care appears to prevent suicide. Indeed, recent international data have supported the findings of the pioneering Gotland Study also showing the importance of GPs as the front line in diagnosis and treatment of depression and reducing suicide mortality. The community-intervention suicide-prevention project in Kiskunhalas region of Hungary between 2000 and 2005 also showed that education in the treatment of depression and suicidality of GPs and other health-care professionals as well as the public is an effective method of reducing suicide mortality.[5] Similarly, a recently published, randomized-controlled study from Australia demonstrated that suicidal behaviour during the two-year follow-up period was lower for old persons treated by educated GPs as compared to control GPs.[6]

Other positive results from GP education on depression and suicides according to the Gotland Model are reported from—among others— Russia, Japan, Iceland, Philippines, Iran, Slovenia, Austria, and Sweden. However, primary care education given out of context of suicide preventative measures is not sufficient to decrease suicide mortality in the long term.

The need for continuous training

Already, the original Gotland Study has demonstrated the crucial need for maintenance and booster education to counteract fading-out effects towards the baseline after 3–5 years. It showed the necessity of involving the societal support organizations male suicidants were in contact with—e.g., police, social welfare, tax authorities, labour organizations, families, and other stakeholders. Complex, permanent, and multi-level educational and organizational interventions are useful. This has been demonstrated most recently by the German Nuremberg Alliance Against Depression study and the international European Alliance Against Depression (EAAD) project—a multifaceted community-based action programme against depression and suicide. The results from these studies seem to provide further support for the effectiveness of the EAAD concept. While the majority of suicide-prevention programmes mainly affect female suicidal behaviour, these programmes seem to be beneficial for both sexes.[7,8]

As antidepressant prescription is a proxy marker of care of depressed patients, it is not surprising that a statistically significant correlation between markedly increasing antidepressant utilization and decreasing national suicide rates have been reported recently from different parts of the world, including 29 European countries.[9,10] Finally, it could be noted that the suicide-preventive effect of routine psychiatric care should be further improved by psychosocial and person-centred individualized interventions, which are proven to significantly reduce subsequent suicide mortality among suicide attempters in low- and middle-income countries.[11]

Case Study

The patient was a 52-year-old journalist, also known as an artist and writer: an intellectual, opinion moulder, entertainer, and presenter of a popular television programme. He came from an adventurous family of artists and writers. His father had been a creative teacher and heavy drinker, with long unproductive periods. Divorced many years previously, the patient was now involved with a younger woman. The relationship was functioning relatively smoothly, and the couple had one child. He was in full swing, with high public visibility, and intensely active in a wide-ranging social network.

For six months, he had been feeling increasingly uneasy, especially in the mornings. He was experiencing growing restlessness, a sense of hopelessness, and a feeling of being a fake. He had difficulty in making even minor, everyday decisions. He felt overwhelmed by everyday problems—paralysed—but, at the same time, he remained active in his work. He was talkative and sociable, but his concentration and real interest in social life were now habitually lacking.

His sleep was increasingly fragmented. Especially at night, he frequently experienced an almost irresistible, compulsive urge to take his own life, and he was becoming ever more frightened of being unable to resist this urge. He had made several nocturnal excursions to remote places with concrete plans to commit suicide by hanging, jumping, or asphyxiation in his car. He reported an inner struggle on these occasions, after which he finally managed to return home. Shocked by this experience he had sought psychiatric help, following his own research in preparation for a programme on male helplessness.

He made a pleasant, talkative, professional, easy-going, and social adequate impression. No inhibition was evident. He reported increasing consumption of alcohol—mostly wine—to 'calm down'. He stated that he was no longer able to write, since he lacked new ideas, but could manage his programme on a 'routine' basis. He had received no reactions from others—nobody had noticed his problems—but he told of his deepening despair and was horrified at his own compulsive suicidal urges.

The diagnosis was male depression, with acute suicidality. The recommended treatment was selective serotonin reuptake inhibitors combined with weekly individual psychotherapy sessions focusing on acceptance of his limitations, helplessness, weakness, and inability to cope with every demand, plus family-therapy sessions with his family to monitor his suicidality. Recovery took eight weeks, and the patient is currently receiving long-term maintenance treatment with supportive and clarifying psychotherapy and psychopharmacology.

References

1 **Rutz W**. Evaluation of an educational programme on depressive disorders given to general practitioners in Gotland. Short- and long-term effects. Dissertation. Sweden: Linköping University; 1992: 1–116.

2 Rihmer Z, Rutz W, Pihlgren H. Decreasing tendency of seasonality in suicide may indicate lowering rate of depressive suicides in the population. Psychiatry Res. 1998;**16**:233–240.

3 Rutz W, von Knorring L, Pihlgren H, Rihmer Z, Wålinder J. Prevention of male suicides: lessons from the Gotland study. Lancet. 1995;**345**:524.

4 Rutz W. Improvement of care for people suffering from depression: the need for comprehensive education. Int Clin Psychopharmacol. 1999;**14**(Suppl3):27–33.

5 Szanto K, Kalmar S, Hendin H, Rihmer Z, Mann JJ. A suicide prevention program in a region with a very high suicide rate. Arch Gen Psychiatry. 2007;**64**:914–920.

6 Almeida OP, Pirkis J, Kerse N, Sim M, Flicker I, Snowdon J, et al. A randomized trial to reduce the prevalence of depression and self-harm behaviour in older primary care patients. Ann Family Med. 2012;**10**:347–356.

7 Hegerl U, Wittmann M, Arensman E, Van Audenhove C, Bouleau J-H, Van der Feltz-Cornelis C, et al. The 'European Alliance Against Depression (EAAD)': a multifaceted, community-based action programme against depression and suicidality. W J Biol Psychiat. 2008;**9**:51–59.

8 Székely A, Konkolÿ Thege B, Mergl R, Birkás E, Rózsa S, et al. How to decrease suicide rates in both genders? An effectiveness study of a community-based intervention (EAAD). PLoS One. 2013 Sep 23;**8**(9):e75081. doi: 10.1371/journal. pone.0075081. eCollection 2013.

9 Ludwig J, Marcotte DE, Norberg K. Antidepressants and suicide. J Health Econ. 2009;**28**:659–676.

10 Gusmão R, Quintão S, McDaid D, Arensman E, Van Audenhove C, Coffey C, et al. Antidepressant utilization and suicide in Europe: an ecological multi-national study. PLoS One. 2013 Jun 19;**8**(6):e66455. Print 2013.

11 Fleischmann A, Bertolote JM, Wasserman D, Bolhari DJ, Botega NJ, de Silva D, et al. Effectiveness of brief intervention and contact for suicide attempters: a randomized controlled trial in five countries. Bull of the WHO. 2008;**86**:703–709.

Chapter 30

Collaboration between psychiatrists and other physicians

Jean-Pierre Soubrier

Suicide in different medical settings

It is well known that up to 60% of suicidal people, and in some studies even more, have consulted one or more physicians just 1–2 months before their suicidal act, regardless of whether the outcome was temporary (for attempters) or final (for those who died).[1,2] As patients, these people usually come into contact with general practitioners or specialists in various fields of somatic medicine. The setting may be a private surgery or a public outpatient clinic, and besides general practice the main specialities of the doctors concerned are internal medicine (with its various subspecialities—cardiology, gastroenterology, endocrinology), orthopaedics, neurology, gynaecology, otorhinolaryngology, and urology. The pre-suicidal phase is of the utmost importance in prevention, and medical staff who meet patients in this category therefore bear a heavy burden of responsibility.[3–5]

General practitioners, and to a lesser extent other physicians, are frequently the first and sometimes the only professional actors in the drama of suicide. What can they do, and what should they refrain from doing? What kind of help is needed? For anyone who is not a trained psychiatrist, dealing with suicidal patients is a difficult task. Psychiatrists may play a vital role in their care and treatment. However, no one should work unaided with suicidal patients and in suicide prevention. Teamwork, in which a psychiatrist plays a key role, may be a solution.

Suicide-prevention team

Every medical setting should include structures and routines whereby a psychiatrist instructs the staff concerned in how to deal with suicidal patients and their families, and also in suicide prevention. Preventing suicide is a burdensome task, and it is therefore advisable for such work to be carried out by a suicide-prevention team of several people. A psychiatrist should head the team, which should include professionals from various fields, such as a psychologist, a social worker, and a psychiatric nurse. The widespread knowledge about the team's suicide preventive activities along with a high degree of approachability is a prerequisite for the team's success.

The suicide-prevention team may be the source of knowledge and be in charge of current training in both the psychiatric clinic and the whole hospital. It may also serve as a link between health-care services and the relevant authorities in the community. Another function of the team may be to ensure continuous application of modern treatment and preventive methods within existing routines. A quality-assurance programme could be established, and this means that quality indicators need to be defined. Examples of such indicators are the percentage of suicide attempt patients examined by a psychiatrist within 24 hours of their attempt and suicidal patients' average waiting time to see a psychiatrist after referral.

Training may be provided on a regular basis to general practitioners and other doctors.[1–5]

Topics should include:

- reasons why suicidal people consult somatic doctors;
- when suicidal patients should be referred to a psychiatrist or admitted to hospital;
- how to communicate with suicidal patients' relatives; and
- follow-up after a suicide attempt.

Other important team duties include offering support to staff in emergency departments and intensive care units, and drawing up rules of conduct for the aftermath of a suicide on the ward.

Cooperation with somatic physicians

Liaison between psychiatrists, general practitioners, and other medical practitioners who treat suicidal patients has a profound impact on the course of the suicidal process at all stages. This impact is not always as positive as might be expected. A certain taboo remains, reinforced by supposed ethical considerations and respect for privacy. This may be one explanation why suicide figures are underestimated and suicide prevention is fairly difficult to implement.

Very often, suicidal patients approach the non-psychiatric physician with somatic complaints of one kind or another, and cite several examples of different symptoms without expressing any overt suicidal communication during their visit. Either these patients do not associate their suicidal tendencies with somatic symptoms, or they consider suicidal ideation a sign of weakness and are often ashamed of their suicidal thoughts or plans to take their own life. They mention their feelings of helplessness and worthlessness and their fears only in vague terms. The emotional instability and low self-esteem so characteristic of suicidal people may, instead, be compensated for by an impression of strength and competence. There is thus a marked discrepancy between patients' underlying desperation and what they express verbally during the consultation. Physicians expect suicidal patients to be depressed and may, therefore, miss suicidality unless they penetrate more deeply into the diagnosis. Symptoms of depression may be masked by physical symptoms and pain, accompanied by sleep disorders, fatigue, irritability, and anxiety.[2]

For the above reasons, it is hardly surprising if initial and also subsequent contacts between somatic doctors or general practitioners and their suicidal patients fail to prevent suicidal acts. Psychotic and alcohol or other substance abusers may present relatively surmountable problems of suicide risk assessment. If they are promptly referred to appropriate specialists who are better trained to treat such patients, their suicidal acts may be averted.

Of special importance is to train general practitioners and specialists in the careful evaluation of all patients who may be suspected of somatization or who may have psychosomatic symptoms. Clinical intuition, experience, and common sense are major tools in this context, but must be supplemented by education and training in basic suicidal assessment[6,7] (see also chapters 16 and 18).

Patient–physician relationship

All doctors should be trained in communicating with suicidal patients, to optimize diagnosis and treatment. Communication between suicidal patients and their physicians is positively or negatively affected by the physician's attitudes towards the suicide and his or her communication skills and psychological preparedness to deal with self-destructive behaviour. Suicidal patients' expectations of and attitudes towards their physicians also profoundly influence the communication and compliance with treatment recommendations.

Referral for psychiatric evaluation

Whenever there is the slightest suspicion of suicidality, patients must be referred to a psychiatrist or psychologist. Such referrals must also take place when patients present with mental disorders fail to take antidepressant medication or to comply with other treatment, or express a desire for psychological help. Patients must also be referred when they have a personal or family history of attempted suicide and lack social support.

However, seeing a psychiatrist is the dominant fear of many suicidal patients, who are apprehensive that such contact may in some way confirm relatives' opinion that they are of unsound mind. A written referral and active, urgent follow-up are, therefore, imperative.

A simple suggestion to a person to approach a psychiatrist can be directly counterproductive. Before referring patients one should inform them and, if possible, their relatives that specialist help is necessary. The referral should not be perceived by the patient as abandonment; instead, it should be a joint decision. It is helpful in this context to explain the beneficial effects of various forms of psychotherapy and drugs. The primary care or other physician should also ensure follow-up of the contact with the psychiatrist to whom the patient is referred. This is because of the need to know whether the patient has approached the psychiatrist or not. A precondition for successful referral is for the referring doctor to have well-established contacts and to be personally acquainted with private psychiatrists or public outpatient and inpatient psychiatric departments. This is all the more important if the patient is isolated and lacks social support and protective factors.

When to hospitalize a suicidal patient

In some cases, immediate hospitalization is appropriate.[3] This applies to patients with recurrent severe thoughts of suicide, serious intent to die, major depression with anxiety, and agitation or psychoses such as schizophrenia and manic–depressive disorder. It also applies to patients with borderline personalities in traumatic life situations. Admission is further required when a suicidal patient has poor family or social support. However, evaluation is no easy matter when no obvious signs of profound or severe mental disorder are present.

Emergency admission and admission to an intensive care unit

Collaboration between psychiatrists and the staff of intensive care units and emergency departments is essential for patients who have survived a suicide attempt. Confronting suicidal patients is often traumatic for all medical staff in the units concerned. Hospital staff are all too seldom trained to deal with and understand complex psychological problems. The suicidal patient constitutes a threat to staff's professional role—that of saving lives—and also evokes their own anxiety about death and threatens their personal integrity. Staff reactions are variable, and include uncertainty, fear, anxiety, uneasiness, and guilt. These feelings may result not only in distancing, escape reactions, irritation, and aggression, but also in interest and empathy. In general, medical staff are often dissatisfied with the amount of help they can give patients and their relatives, owing to the lack of knowledge and shortage of time, and also to poor collaboration with psychiatrists.[8]

Contact with relatives

The psychiatrist's most important and usual role in the emergency setting is to establish contact with the suicidal patient's relatives. It is well known that people who have attempted suicide belong to one of the major risk groups for completed suicide. Family members are often under psychological duress and need advice, psychological support, and sometimes psychiatric treatment. Last but not least, psychiatrists may help physicians to comfort relatives or close friends of patients who have died from suicide. Programmes for surviving relatives must be encouraged (see also Chapter 28).

Follow-up and treatment planning

The psychiatrist's task is to intervene in the suicidal process, to slow it, and finally to interrupt it. This can be achieved only by ensuring follow-up, with psychosocial, psychological, and medical care, with or without medication. Eventually, some patients may be referred to their general practitioner for follow-up and treatment. The general practitioner must then be in a position to plan treatment in cooperation with the patients and their families, and have easy access to a psychiatrist or suicide-prevention team for consultation whenever necessary, and to discuss cases during the follow-up period. To enhance the capacity of general practitioners to be able to support suicidal patients, they are in need of regular training programmes.[1–9]

Suicide on the ward

A dramatic situation like suicide in a hospital may induce typical post-traumatic stress disorder (PTSD) among staff. In such situations a suicide-prevention team should perform a therapeutic function by debriefing the staff and commenting on the clinical aspects of the case. In this process, cooperation with forensic physicians and forensic psychiatrists may be necessary, within a postvention programme (see also Chapter 28).

Continuous training

Collaboration between psychiatrists, psychologists, general practitioners, and other doctors should be extensive, owing to its importance in the treatment of suicidal patients and in relieving psychological tensions that may be experienced by staff. [5] Good cooperation and continuous training of physicians in primary care and other fields by their psychiatrist colleagues and the suicide-prevention team are essential elements in successful suicide prevention at every stage. The suicide-prevention team should play a key role not only in skills development but also in terms of emotional debriefing.

New developments

Finally, since society is progressing towards a de-stigmatization of various taboos towards mental disorders and suicide, new approaches are essential within a network of collaboration between physicians and psychiatrists.[10]

De-stigmatization of mental disorders[11] allows better access to healthcare and confidence in consulting a psychiatrist, allowing the suicidal person to express freely and fearlessly their own suicide ideation.[12] All these efforts supported by community-based organizations and social sector implementations are necessary to prevent suicide.[13]

References

1 **Rutz W, von Knorring L, Wallinder J**. Long-term effects of an education programme for general practitioners given by the Swedish committee for the prevention and treatment of depression. Acta Psychiatr Scand. 1992;**85**:83–88.

2 **Wolk-Wasserman D**. Contacts of suicidal neurotic and prepsychotic/psychotic patients and their significant others with public care institutions before the suicide attempt. Acta Psychiatr Scand. 1987;**75**:358–372.

3 **Litman R**. Hospital suicides: lawsuits and standards. Suicide Life Threat Behav. 1982;**12**:212–220.

4 **Soubrier JP, Debout M, Vedrinne J, Pommereau X**. *Guide de l'entretien avec un patient suicidaire*. Paris: Lundbeck-France; 1998.

5 **World Health Organization (WHO)**. Preventing suicide: a resource for general physicians. Mental behavioural disorders. Department of Mental Health, Social Change and Mental Health. Geneva; 2000.

6 **Beck AT, Brown GK, Steer RA**. Suicide ideation at its worst point: a prediction of eventual suicide in psychiatric outpatients. Suicide Life Threat Behav 1999;**29**:1–4.

7 **Jacobs DG**. Guide to suicide assessment and intervention. San Fransisco: Jossey Bass Publishers, 1999.

 8 **Wolk-Wasserman D**. The intensive care unit and the suicide attempt patient. Acta Psychiatr Scand. 1985;**71**:581–595.

 9 **Soubrier JP**. Définitions du suicide. Signification de la prévention. Ann Medicopsychol 1999;**157**:526–529.

10 **Soubrier JP**. Looking back and ahead. Suicidology and suicide prevention: do we have perspectives? World Psychiatry. 2004 Oct;**3**(3):159–160.

11 **Sartorius N, Gaebel W, Cleveland HR, Stuart H, Akiyama T, Arboleda-Flórez J, et al**. WPA Guidance on how to combat stigmatization of psychiatry and psychiatrists. World Psychiatry. 2010 Oct;**9**(3):131–144.

12 **Soubrier JP**. *Vers une dé-psychiatrisation dans l'approche de la prévention du suicide. 2èmes Assises de la FEALIPS*. Feb 2014.

13 **World Health Organization (WHO)**. Public health action for the prevention of suicide: a framework. Genève: World Health Organization, 2012.

Chapter 31

The work environment for health-care staff

Danuta Wasserman

Vulnerability of psychiatric staff

Research shows that the incidence of suicidal acts is high among health professionals,[1] and that the supportive work environment provides protection and is associated with a lower level of suicide ideation.[2] The fact that health-care workers, especially in psychiatry, are constantly confronted with issues of life and death, and with suicidal patients, raises questions relating to the improvement of work environment for psychiatric care providers and the need for regular training, supervision, and support.[3,4]

At every psychiatric clinic or department, there should be routines that allow discussions about issues of failure and feelings of inadequacy in connection with treatment of suicidal patients and a patient's suicide. The purpose is to help staff cope with their own emotional experience, take a stand on personal existential issues, and develop professionally.

Attempted suicide and suicide run directly counter not only to the instinct of self-preservation, but also to the role of health-care staff as those who provide health-care and save lives. This is why it is not unusual for suicidal people who violate this role to be given a negative reception. These negative feelings may sometimes be very strong among the staff.[5]

Sound routines keep chaos and anxiety in check

Powerful emotional reactions in the form of indifference, rejection, and antipathy should be explored fully, since they have a profound influence on suicidal patients and may even promote suicide. Constant awareness of the nocebo effect i.e., the harmful impact on patients of therapists' conduct, procedure, and treatment is necessary. Failing to admit compulsorily a patient who is at high risk of suicide and opting for a less active treatment instead or omitting, e.g. treating a patient with antidepressants may be, in certain cases, expressions of negative reactions on the staff's part, rather than of their concern for the patient.[5,6]

Negative countertransference reactions may arise even in the best-trained personnel. The suicidal conflict is, fundamentally, a highly aggressive one and it is hardly surprising that it affects staff. Bearing in mind that the behaviour of the staff may provoke or contribute to suicide should be as self-evident as awareness of the beneficial effects (placebo effects) of a trustful contact between patient and physician, especially since the reaction of the staff can have a nocebo effect and lead to the patient's suicide.

Every department in which work with suicidal persons is performed should have documented routines for diagnosis and treatment to ensure that appropriate action is taken. Good routines are particularly important in treatment of suicidal people since their care can be strongly influenced by staff's attitudes, their state of mental health and well-being, and their outlook on life, including values regarding various ethical and moral issues.

Routines and documentation relieve staffs' anxiety and uncomfortable emotions, and also promote good care, commitment, and the creativity that is released when chaos is kept in check. Conversely, unhealthy work conditions may result in 'burn-out', with apathetic, irritable, or dismissive attitudes towards patients,[7–11] as well as in depression.[12–14]

Dealing with a suicidal person is arduous work, and demands a high-level of knowledge. Staff who work with suicidal people, therefore, need regular training and support and supervision in their day-to-day work.

Case Study

A patient's suicide—an unbearable experience

Hans, aged 30 years, a hospital ward nurse and the only child of two elderly doctors, was admitted to a psychiatric ward after a two-week stay in the intensive care unit after throwing himself in front of an underground train. He was beset by problems. On the relationship front, his fiancée had broken off their engagement shortly before the wedding was due to take place; at work, major reorganizations were taking place and he was facing a demotion. His real wish was to be a doctor, but his school grades were not good enough.

The staff at the psychiatric ward thought that they had come to know Hans fairly well, and after a few weeks' care he was granted his first weekend leave. Before his departure, a doctor met him briefly. Hans appeared calm and the doctor had little time on that particular day to explore in depth his state of mind or how prepared he was for an encounter with the real-life world outside the hospital. Nor had his relatives been contacted. Hans' statement that he was going to spend the weekend with his elderly parents was simply taken on trust.

On the Monday, all the staff were shocked to receive a request to identify the body of one of their patients, brought to the hospital during the weekend. It was Hans, who had lain down on the underground track late in the evening on the same day he had left the hospital. There, invisible in the darkness, he had been run over and killed.

It was a dreadful experience for everyone on the ward. This applied not least to the doctor who had last met and talked to Hans before his leave. Even several years later, this doctor related that the event had had such a tremendous impact on him that still, every time he was reminded of it, he became agitated and his heart began to pound rapidly.

Support for staff after a suicidal act of the patient

Immediate routine measures

After a suicide or suicide attempt has taken place, the questions of how to inform the patient's relatives, who should do so, and how to protect and inform the other patients must be settled without delay. The person in charge of the ward must also decide which tasks should be cancelled for the rest of the day in order to give the personnel time for meetings and emotional working-through.

Information must also be given to the administrative head of the institution as well as to the relevant authorities. This procedure varies from country to country and is regulated by national laws.

Contacts with relatives

Relatives should be informed, without delay, face to face in their own home or asked to come to the hospital. Giving them the news by telephone is inappropriate. It is important to give relatives a chance of meeting the staff members who looked after the patient before the suicide, and also to facilitate the access to debriefing and therapy if they wish.

Immediate emotional support for staff

Being a member of the medical staff means facing suffering and death on a daily basis, and encountering emotionally trying situations. But a patient's suicide is among the most daunting experiences a psychiatrist and members of the psychiatric staff can undergo. It is, therefore, extremely important to be able to work through the feelings that are aroused.[15–18]

A suicidal act is a tragedy that affects the whole staff team and the entire clinic or department. Not only strong feelings but also irrational explanations, projections of guilt on to others, and self-reproaches are brought up. An immediate opportunity for working through the traumatic emotional aftermath of a suicidal act, individually and in a group, must be given to all the staff, as must the opportunity for everyone to relate the event from his/her own point of view. It is important for those affected to be able to speak freely about their feelings and express their anger, sorrow, and despair.

All the health-care staff involved should take part in such meeting. The people who are affected most deeply often wish to withdraw, and may take sick leave or holiday. Sometimes, one meeting is not enough and additional meetings may be necessary. Staff who react very strongly should be given the opportunity for individual therapy. It is also vital for the person who chairs such a discussion to have a structure—one that does not, however, stifle the personal emotional reactions that arise during the meeting. This discussion of the staff's emotions should be led by someone who was not involved in the event and, preferably, is employed elsewhere. Conflicts between co-workers may come to the fore in this kind of situation, and it is important for these issues to be addressed. The first impressions from the initial meeting must always be summarized by the person who heads the group.

Developing knowledge after the suicidal event

Within some 4–6 weeks after a suicide has taken place in the ward or department, a 'psychological autopsy' can be carried out. This method was developed at the Suicide Prevention Center in Los Angeles in the 1950s.[15] The purpose of such a review is to improve all the staff's skills by reconstructing the suicidal process up to the time of the suicidal act, and to go through the whole treatment process systematically.[16–18] Strong emotional reactions may also arise in this kind of retrospective review, which provides a good opportunity for these reactions to be heard and support to be provided for those in need. [16]This process should be carried out with the aim of integrating the staff's newly acquired knowledge with their previous knowledge and experience. The material from the autopsy and the police investigation can also be used. The entire review process and the final assessment should be documented in the patient's medical records.

In many clinics, a retrospective review also after a suicide attempt has been introduced as a routine, since the staff members are usually very highly motivated to reassess the actions taken in the treatment.

Training and supervision

A plan for a clinic offering regular training in suicidology—diagnostics, treatment, and preventive strategies—can be a helpful measure. Moreover, individual supervision of staff should be available. Supervision develops not only the staff's knowledge of psychiatry, but also their psychotherapeutic skills and contributes to the emotional maturity. Training is important not only for psychiatrists but also for other staff groups in psychiatric departments, as well as for somatic staff in emergency wards, and in adjacent clinics involved in the care of suicidal persons.

Enhancing the quality of suicide-preventive work

Wherever staff work with suicidal patients, there should be:

+ a plan for training courses for all the staff;
+ an individual plan for supervision of each staff member;
+ an action programme to be implemented when a suicide or suicide attempt takes place on the ward; and
+ simple epidemiological monitoring of suicide attempts and suicides.

More advanced registration of all suicidal acts that have taken place at the clinic or outpatient department can include diagnostic and treatment data, and also information on waiting times and the duration of treatment, in order to provide basic and specific local knowledge of the efficacy of treatment methods used.

References

1 Hawton K, Agerbo E, Simkin S, Platt B, Mellanby RJ. Risk of suicide in medical and related occupational groups: a national study based on Danish case population-based registers. J Affect Disord. 2011 Nov;**134**(1–3):320–326.

2 Eneroth M, Gustafsson Sendén M, Løvseth LT, Schenck-Gustafsson K, Fridner A. A comparison of risk and protective factors related to suicide ideation among residents and specialists in academic medicine. BMC Public Health. 2014 Mar **22**;14:271.

3 Ramberg IL, Wasserman D. The roles of knowledge and supervision in work with suicidal patients. Nord J Psychiatry. 2003;**57**(5):365–371.

4 Samuelsson M, Gustavsson JP, Pettersson IL, Arnetz B, Åsberg M. Suicidal feelings and work environment in psychiatric nursing personnel. Soc Psychiatry Epidemiol. 1997;**32**:391–397.

5 Wolk-Wasserman D. Some problems connected with the treatment of suicide attempt patients: transference and countertransference aspects. Crisis. 1987;**8**:69–82.

6 Maltsberger JT, Buie DH. Countertransference hate in the treatment of suicidal patients. Arch Gen Psych. 1974;**30**:625–633.

7 Kumar S. Burnout and psychiatrists: what do we know and whereto from here? Epidemiol Psychiatr Sci. 2011 Dec;**20**(4):295–301.

8 Rössler W. Stress, burnout, and job dissatisfaction in mental health workers. Eur Arch Psychiatry Clin Neurosci. 2012 Nov;262 Suppl **2**:S65–69.

9 Heponiemi T, Aalto AM, Puttonen S, Vänskä J, Elovainio M. Work-related stress, job resources, and well-being among psychiatrists and other medical specialists in Finland. Psychiatr Serv. 2014 Jun 1;**65**(6):796–801.

10 Thomas P, Billon R, Chaumier J, Barruche G, Thomas C. Psycho-social hazards for staff in geriatrics and geriatric psychiatry. O J Psych. 2014;**4**:91–98.

11 Volpe U, Luciano M, Palumbo C, Sampogna G, Del Vecchio V, Fiorillo A. Risk of burnout among early career mental health professionals. J Psychiatr Men Hlt 2014; Nov:**21**(9):774–781.

12 Kim I, Noh S, Muntaner C. Emotional demands and the risk of depression among homecare workers in the USA. Int Arch Occup Environ Health. 2013;**86**:635–664.

13 Bonde JPE. Psychosocial factors at work and risk of depression: a systematic review of the epidemiological evidence. Occup Environ Med. 2014;**5**:438–445.

14 Madathil R, Heck NC, Schuldberg D. Burnout in psychiatric nursing: examining the interplay of autonomy. Leadership style and depressive symptoms. Arch Psych Nurs. 2014;**28**:160–166.

15 **Shneidman E.** The psychological autopsy. Suicide Life Threat Behav. 1981;**11**:325–340.

16 **Fairman N, Thomas LP, Whitmore S, Meier EA, Irwin SA.** What did I miss? A qualitative assessment of the impact of patient suicide on hospice clinical staff. J Palliat Med. 2014 Jul;**17**(7):832–836.

17 **Conner KR, Beautrais AL, Brent DA, Conwell Y, Phillips MR, Schneider B.** The next generation of psychological autopsy studies. Part 1. Interview content. Suicide Life Threat Behav. 2011 Dec;**41**(6):594–613.

18 **Conner KR, Beautrais AL, Brent DA, Conwell Y, Phillips MR, Schneider B.** The next generation of psychological autopsy studies. Part 2. Interview procedures. Suicide Life Threat Behav. 2012 Feb;**42**(1):86–103.

Chapter 32

A psycho-educational perspective on family involvement in suicide prevention and postvention

Karl Andriessen and Karolina Krysinska

Although suicide is an individual act, except for relatively rare cases of a suicide pact involving two or more people, it hardly even happens in an interpersonal void. In the field of mental health-care and clinical practice there is recognition of the role of family in the everyday functioning of an individual, coping with stress, as well as in aetiology and treatment of psychopathology. Although families can play an important role in supporting the person at risk of suicide and encouraging treatment and recovery, the pathogenic function of the family seems to attract more research interest in suicidology, than its preventive potential.[1] Different lines of evidence point to the possibility of familial or genetic vulnerability for suicidal behaviour, which may be related to a genetic vulnerability for psychiatric illness, deficits in impulse control, and/or social modelling. Among life stressors frequently experienced by suicidal individuals are events related to relationships with family members, such as interpersonal conflicts, relationship breakdown, bereavement, and domestic violence. Studies on the dynamics and structure of families with a history of a suicide attempt or suicide, especially in case of suicidal children and adolescents, often reveal serious and chronic problems in the family: negative childhood experiences and traumas, damaged attachments, abuse, or neglect. There is a strong association between marital status and suicide: divorced, widowed, and separated persons have the highest suicide rates.

On the other hand, married people have lower suicide rates than unmarried individuals, and marriage and responsibility for bringing up children may serve as protective factors against suicide by reducing social isolation, providing emotional and social stability, and enhancing social integration. A number of psychosocial interventions for adolescents after a suicide attempt, which involve the family, have been developed and evaluated; often showing promising results. The multi-level involvement of the family in the care and recovery of a person who has attempted suicide, including history-taking, provision of discharge plans, interventions, and treatment, as well as increasing the knowledge regarding the impact of a suicide attempt on family members, have been recommended in mental health-care and suicide-prevention policy documents.[2]

Another important area related to family involvement in suicide is postvention; i.e., 'activities developed by, with, or for suicide survivors, in order to facilitate recovery after suicide and to prevent adverse outcomes, including suicidal behaviour'.[3] Family members can be deeply affected by the death and although many relatives of suicide victims can effectively cope with the loss, others need peer and/or professional help.

The importance of the family in the provision of care

Family members often accompany a person who made a suicide attempt to the emergency department (ED), although their encounters with the ED staff are not always positive or encouraging. A study[4] showed that 79% of adolescent suicide attempters were accompanied by their parent(s), mostly a mother or a stepmother, during their visit to the ED, and only 17% sought help alone. In another study,[5] almost half of suicide attempters were accompanied by a family member when they reached the ED. Although, in general, the patients and their families experienced appropriate and respectful treatment by the ED staff, more than half of the attempters and almost a third of their family members felt stigmatized or punished. Of interest, the experiences of family members were more positive than the experiences of the suicide attempters: the family members were more likely to feel heard by the ED staff and to receive information regarding treatment.

A number of interventions for individuals who have attempted suicide, mostly adolescents, involving their family members have been developed and evaluated. These include a compliance enhancement intervention,[6] family intervention for suicide prevention (FISP),[4] and attachment-based family therapy (ABFT).[7] A treatment modality for suicidal adults and their families originating in the attachment and family systems perspective has also been proposed.[8]

The compliance enhancement intervention aims to improve adherence to community treatment in adolescents receiving medical care in the ED or a paediatric ward after a suicide attempt.[6] This 1-hour intervention includes making a verbal contract between adolescents and their parents to attend at least four outpatient therapy sessions, to review factors which might affect treatment attendance, and an overview of expectations and misconceptions regarding treatment. The adolescents and their parents are also contacted by telephone to assess their participation in the treatment sessions. A trial looking at the effectiveness of the intervention in comparison to the standard planning group showed that at the three-month follow-up there were no significant differences between the two groups in regards to the number of sessions attended. However, after controlling for service barriers, such as insurance coverage difficulties, waiting lists, and problems with scheduling additional appointments, the adolescents in the compliance enhancement intervention group attended significantly more treatment sessions than their peers in the control group.

Another intervention for adolescent suicide attempters and their families specially designed to be delivered in the busy and fast-paced ED environment is the FISP.[4] The FISP is a 20-minute family-based cognitive behaviour therapy session aiming to mobilize family support for treatment and safety, and including a care linkage component with follow-up telephone contacts to further motivate and support linkage to outpatient treatment. The first main component of FISP is addressing the short-term risk of repeated suicidal behaviour through strengthening the coping skills of the adolescent and the family, educating the family about restricting access to potentially dangerous means of suicide, and enhancing motivation to seek follow-up treatment. Education about the importance of seeking and receiving follow-up care is the second component of the intervention. A randomized trial showed that youth in the FISP trial had significantly improved uptake of outpatient follow-up treatment, including psychotherapy and psychotherapy combined with medication, than adolescents receiving the standard ED care.

ABFT has been designed to treat adolescent depression and suicidal behaviour by addressing problem areas in the family functioning.[7] These include family disengagement, ineffective parenting, parental stress, criticism and hostility, and adolescent's negative self-concept, low treatment motivation, and engagement. The therapy involves individual and family meetings over a period of three months. A randomized controlled trial, comparing the effectiveness of ABFT for adolescents with suicidal ideation and depression and their families, and a control group receiving facilitated referral to other providers, showed promising results. Adolescents in the ABFT group had significantly lower scores of suicidal ideation at post-treatment and follow-up evaluations, and attended a significantly greater number of sessions than their peers in the control group. There was a nearly significant reduction in depressive symptoms by mid-treatment in the ABFT group; however, there were no differences regarding levels of depressive symptoms post-treatment and at follow-up.

According to the attachment and family systems perspective,[8] 'by exposing the patient to loved and internalized objects, pre-suicidal affective constriction can be decreased. By reawakening in the patient early introjects from the past, current family members can therefore play a powerful role in changing the dynamics of the pre-suicidal state and thus altering the outcome'. This treatment modality, originating in the attachment and family systems perspective, focuses on three processes: family cohesion (i.e., emotional bonding between family members), family adhesion (i.e., less close bonds in families with a history of interpersonal loss or trauma insecure attachments), and the formation of a new family (i.e., creating a network of professional and peer support for individuals bereft of a biological family due to external circumstances or due to extreme family pathology and dysfunction). Although this therapeutic framework has been thoroughly conceptualized, to-date no studies have been conducted to show its effectiveness.

Psycho-educational resources for families after a suicide attempt

In 2005, the US National Alliance on Mental Illness (NAMI) and the Suicide Prevention Resource Centre published a series of suicide prevention guides for attempt survivors, their families, and doctors. Only the resources for the attempt survivors and their families are presented here.[9,10]

1 *Taking Care of Yourself After an Attempt* (Consumer guide): This brochure discusses the availability of follow-up care and provides advice regarding recovery after a suicidal crisis and increasing the quality of life. It suggests creating a safety plan and building a support system, including involvement of family members. It provides tips to 'Learn to live again' and to effectively cope with future suicidal thoughts and crises. The resource presents also a list of mental health-care organizations and services providing professional/peer help and support.

2 *Taking Care of Yourself and Your Family After an Attempt* (Family guide): This resource material presents an overview of 'What Happens in the Emergency Department', including the goals of the ED visit, the purpose of the physical and mental health assessment, confidentiality laws and sharing of information, and the need for follow-up care, including voluntary or involuntary hospitalization. Another section provides advice for 'Reducing the Risk at Home': limiting availability to means of suicide and creating a safety plan, including getting to know the 'triggers' for suicidal ideation and behaviour, building support networks, and strengthening communication within the family. The need to maintain hope and self-care for the family members is stressed, as well as the need to get professional input whenever possible. The brochure lists mental health-care organizations and services providing professional/peer help and support.

Practical considerations for family involvement in care and treatment of at-risk individuals

On the basis of the literature a number of practical recommendations regarding involvement of the family in the care of an individual after a suicide attempt can be presented:[1,2,6,8]

1 *Overcoming stigma around suicide and opening family communication*: Talking about suicidal feelings can be difficult for the person at-risk and his/her environment, and in some cases evoke negative reactions in the family members such as anxiety, panic, feeling of helplessness, anger, guilt, or minimization of the risk. Still, being able to talk openly about one's own suicidal ideation with family or friends, might decrease the burden of psychological pain, provide a safe environment, and allow looking for professional help and alternatives for suicide.

2 *Family members can assist the history-taking after a suicide attempt*: The family can provide important information regarding the life events and changes in the living circumstances preceding the suicide attempt, family history of suicide, history of psychiatric treatment, including medication and any recent changes in the treatment arrangements.

3 *Patient's agreement to involve the family and the benefit of family involvement*: Family can be involved in the treatment or in the aftercare following a suicide attempt only after securing the agreement of the person at-risk, and only if such involvement can contribute to the effectiveness of treatment. The prerequisite for successful treatment involving the family is gathering information about the family-related events that might have triggered the suicidal crisis and taking history of earlier and current family traumas, including emotional, physical and sexual abuse or neglect, as well as the family strengths and ways of coping with stress and life events. Family involvement in treatment and care requires an agreement among all parties involved regarding the issues of boundaries, safety and confidentiality. According to clinical observations,[12] 'many suicidal patients have ambivalent relationships with family members, and they are at

risk for abuse, neglect, violence, and resentment. Clinicians should think carefully about whether involving the family poses more bene-fit than risk. Involving an angry, abusive family member can cause a suicidal patient to regress. Involving a suicidal patient in a situation that results in further losses or danger can cause additional damage, and may even worsen suicidal thoughts'.

4 *Therapeutic intervention and other follow-up care arrangements after a suicide attempt should address individual and family factors, as well as possible service barriers and ED staff attitudes:* Even the most cooperative and motivated patients/clients and their families might never engage in treatment or stop it prematurely, if they encounter negative attitudes of the ED staff and/or their access to services is hindered. The service barriers include waiting lists, delays in getting an appointment, treatment termination despite a patient's or family's desire for further sessions, or barriers related to the health insur-ance policy, such as limited coverage or inability to switch treatment providers.

After a suicide

People bereaved through suicide, experience a wide variety of grief reac-tions. Some of these might occur after all kind of deaths, such as feelings of sadness, missing and yearning for the deceased. Other feelings might be related to the unexpected or violent nature of death, such as shock, sense of unreality, trauma, and shattered illusions of personal invulner-ability, whereas anger at the deceased, and feelings of abandonment and rejection might be more typical in suicide bereavement.[11-13] Suicide also affects family relationships and dynamics. Previously existing fam-ily problems might increase, or new problems might occur due to the possible disorganizing effect of suicide on relationships.[14]

As a result, suicide survivors might enter therapy with a variety of experiences, feelings, thoughts, questions, and concerns. Approximately one-third of individuals who die by suicide (in the Western world) were in therapy before their death and survivors might seek contact with a therapist. On the other hand, surviving family members can contact a therapist irrespective of treatment of the deceased person. Therapy might be necessary for survivors who become unable to function because of the grief, in either personal or professional spheres. Therapy aims to enable the survivor to return to the pre-suicide level of functioning.[15]

An integrative, supportive, and educational approach after suicide

Psychotherapy with suicide survivors should integrate components of various theoretical and clinical models of support.[14] Systems approach focuses on family structure and interaction processes. A psycho-educational approach underscores the importance of information and learning in a supportive, therapeutic climate. Attachment theory relates to bonds within the family system, and between family members and the therapist. A narrative approach focuses on the co-creating of stories and a postvention approach aims to assist the survivors in alleviating the impact of suicide. Obviously, the balance between these complementary approaches in the provision of support in an individual case will depend on the theoretical and scholarly background of the therapist, the actual needs of the survivors, the available social support, and the context of the family. It is, however, advised that therapy would be provided in a supportive and educational climate, for individual survivors (adults and children) and families alike. An involved, humanistic, compassionate approach would be preferred to overly directive or passive approaches.[15]

Role of the therapist

1 *Assessment*: During the first contacts the clinician should assess the situation and the questions of the surviving family members. Specifically, familial relationships, factors related to the grief work, suicidal thoughts of the survivors, and the availability of a social network, should be assessed.[15,16] The assessment should clarify whether the family, sub-groups of the family, or individuals could enter therapy. A potentially difficult situation may occur when the surviving family members wish to consult the therapist of the deceased person. In this situation, a compassionate contact with the family might

be preferable over a refusal of the therapist to see the family due to fear of litigation, or a misunderstood interpretation of professional secrets.[17] A contact between the therapist surviving the suicide of the patient (the surviving therapist) and the family might be helpful for both. There is discussion in the literature whether the surviving therapist should continue therapy with the surviving family.[15,17] It might depend on the theoretical background of the therapist and the questions of the survivors. However, there might be a risk for the therapist to engage with the survivors because of own survivor feelings (of guilt, anger, etc.), and there is a risk of serious negative countertransference. As such, it is advisable to refer the surviving family members to another therapist for further treatment.

2 *Addressing grief reactions*: The therapist should assume the least psychopathology in the survivor.[15] This could allow exploring explanations for the event related to the experiences of the survivor and might diminish feelings of guilt and fear of mental illness in the surviving family members. For most survivors, bereavement through suicide is a new and 'alien' experience for which they lack any 'reference point'.[13] Therapy can provide a safe environment to acknowledge, validate, and normalize the experiences of the survivors, such as the psychological distress, guilt, shame, blaming, etc.[14] It can provide opportunities to address problem-solving skills; e.g., in dealing with familial relationships, survivor feelings (e.g., anger, hopelessness), suicidal ideation in survivors, and social or perceived stigma. Therapy can stimulate social support as an adjunct to therapy, such as via self-help (mutual aid) groups, which provide role models and might reduce feelings of stigma.[18]

3 *Demystifying suicide and the creation of a 'suicide story'*: Survivors enter therapy with many questions related to the suicide, and an important task in therapy is improving the survivor's understanding of suicide in general, as well as the suicide death they had personally experienced. Discussing the suicidal process, risk and protective factors (including a possible interaction between a biological vulnerability and environmental risk factors), the occurrence of

so-called 'warning signs', and the cultural (societal) perspective on suicide, in a warm and supportive climate, might increase insight in the suicidal mechanisms and one's own experiences. These insights might also be helpful in the creation of a personal 'suicide story',[14,15] in which the individual survivors or the surviving family formulate their own understanding of the suicidal person and the suicide they have experienced, including their own involvement with the suicidal person and the questions that remain unanswered. The performance of certain rituals, such as creating a remembrance 'place' at home (a photo or personal belongings of the deceased), eating the deceased's favourite dish at his/her birthday, visiting the grave or a favourite place of the deceased, might be a part of the process to formulate a 'suicide story'; or rituals could emerge from the 'suicide story'.[12] The story would allow integration of the suicide in one's own life and to live beyond the suicide.

4 *The need for professional education*: Survivors turn to psychotherapists in times of despair and with many questions. The therapist who is willing to work with suicide survivors should be trained in working with issues related to suicide and suicide bereavement. This include therapists' insights in own feelings and thoughts about death and suicide, and personal and professional strengths and limits. Professional back-up for therapists working with suicide survivors is necessary.[15,17]

Case Study

A woman has visited her local mental health centre. Five years ago she was in therapy after the suicide of her husband. For many years he had been struggling with problems at work, which mimicked childhood traumas of bullying at school, eventually leading to anxiety, depression, and overt suicidal thoughts. Supported by his wife and their two adolescent sons, he engaged in treatment with his GP and the psychotherapist at the mental health centre. After several months of treatment his mood seemed to stabilize and the suicidal threat seemed to have diminished. At a given moment, unexpectedly, he got fired because of ongoing problems at work. The same day, he went home and hanged himself in the garden.

During and after completion of her therapy, which included individual sessions with a psychotherapist and group sessions with the support group, she continued to go to work and to do the household, including supporting the children. However, during the recent months she has started to worry about the youngest son, now 22 years old. Though he is doing well at college and has several friends, he seems to be increasingly distressed and absent-minded. Just as his father, he does not like to talk about his feelings and thoughts. She would like to reach out to him, but she does not seem to get through, and she is afraid that he might be suicidal as well.

The psychotherapist acknowledges her feelings and worries, and together they explore the situation with the youngest son and how she could relate to him. Although her worries concerning her son could be coloured by the suicide of her husband, the son might actually be suicidal. The therapist encourages the woman to speak openly with her son and to share her concerns. Together they explore different options how she could encourage her son to tell her how he is doing in a face-to-face conversation or, if needed, in writing. They also consider involving the older son, but decide against it as it would be better to have a conversation just between the mother and the son.

A few days later, the mother opens the conversation by asking her son about his deceased father, and how much they both miss him. The son shows her a picture of the father which he has kept with him since his death. While looking at the picture they share memories, and laugh and weep together. They decide to give the picture a place in the house, and the mother gave her son a link of an online support group for people bereaved by suicide. Though she never knew whether the son contacted the group, the father's picture stayed in the place they had chosen together until after the son got married a few years later and left the house.

References

1 **Frey LM, Cerel J.** Risk for suicide and the role of family: a narrative review. J. Fam. Issues 2015;**36**(6):716–736.

2 **Suicide Prevention Australia (SPA).** Position statement: supporting suicide attempt survivors. Leichhardt, NSW: Suicide Prevention Australia; 2009.

3 **Andriessen K.** Can postvention be prevention? Crisis. 2009;**30**(1):43–47.

4 **Hughes JL, Asarnow JR.** Enhanced mental health interventions in the emergency department: suicide and suicide attempt prevention. Clin Pediatr Emerg Med. 2013;**14**(1):28–34.

5 **Cerel J, Currier GW, Conwell Y.** Consumer and family experiences in the emergency department following a suicide attempt. J Psychiatr Pract. 2006;**12**(6):341–347.

6 **Spirito A, Boergers J, Donaldson D, Bishop D, Lewander W.** An intervention trial to improve adherence to community treatment by adolescents after a suicide attempt. J Am Acad Child Adolesc Psychiatry 2002;**41**(4):435–442.

7 **Diamond GS, Wintersteen MB, Brown GK, Diamond GM, Gallop R, Shelef K, et al.** Attachment-based family therapy for adolescents with suicidal ideation: a randomized controlled trial. J Am Acad Child Adolesc Psychiatry 2010;**49**(2):122–131.

8 **Lobo Prabhu S, Molinari V, Bowers T, Lomax J**. Role of the family in suicide prevention: an attachment and family systems perspective. Bull Menninger Clin 2010;**74**(4):301–327.

9 English: (<http://www.nami.org/Content/ContentGroups/Policy/Issues_Spotlights/consumer_guide.pdf>).

10 Spanish: (<http://www.nami.org/Content/ContentGroups/Policy/Issues_Spotlights/consumer_guide_sp.pdf>).

11 **Andriessen K, Krysinska K**. Essential questions on suicide bereavement and postvention. IJERPH.2012;**9**(1):24–32.

12 **Grad O**. The sequelae of suicide. In:. O'Connor R, Platt S, Gordon J, eds. International handbook of suicide prevention. Research, policy and practice. Chichester: Wiley & Sons; 2011: 561–576.

13 **Jordan JR, McIntosh JL (eds)**. Grief after suicide: understanding the consequences and caring for the survivors. New York, NY: Routledge;2011.

14 **Kaslow NJ, Aronson SG**. Recommendations for family interventions following a suicide. Professional Psychology: Research and Practice. 2004;**35**(3):240–247.

15 **Dunne EJ**. Psychoeducational intervention strategies for survivors of suicide. Crisis. 1992;**13**(1):35–40.

16 **Kaslow NJ, Samples TC, Rhodes M, Gantt S**. A family-oriented and culturally sensitive postvention approach with suicide survivors. In: Jordan JR, McIntosh, JL, eds. Grief after suicide: understanding the consequences and caring for the survivors. New York, NY: Routledge; 2011:301–323.

17 **McGann VL, Gutin N, Jordan JR**. Guidelines for postvention care with survivor families after the suicide of a client In: Jordan JR,. McIntosh, JL, eds. Grief after suicide: understanding the consequences and caring for the survivors. New York, NY: Routledge; 2011:133–155.

18 **World Health Organisation (WHO)**. Suicide prevention: how to start a survivors' group. Geneva: International Association for Suicide Prevention—World Health Organization; 2008.

VIIIB

Public health perspective

Chapter 33

Perestroika in the former USSR: history's most effective suicide-preventive programme for men

Danuta Wasserman and Airi Värnik

Perestroika: reduced alcohol consumption and a hopeful social climate

Suicide was a prohibited topic in the USSR. Nonetheless, with the major political changes associated with *perestroika* ('restructuring') during the Gorbachev regime in the second half of the 1980s, the national archives were opened in 1989. These thus became available for research, making it possible to study, for example, how factors in society at large influence suicide rates. *Perestroika* was characterized by considerable degree of openness and freedom, as well as reform policies. Strict limits were imposed on the sale of alcohol, and a new restrictive attitude towards alcohol consumption was actively encouraged.[1]

Suicides decreased

By using previously classified material about suicide, violent death, and alcohol poisoning, we studied statistics on causes of death relating to the whole population in the 15 Soviet Socialist Republics for the years 1970–1990 and various age groups for the years 1984–1990. The highest numbers of suicides were noted in the Slav republics (Russia, Ukraine, Belorussia), Kazakhstan (with its high proportion of Slavs in the population), and the Baltic states (Lithuania, Latvia, and Estonia). In these areas the suicide rates were roughly ten times as high as in the Caucasian states (Armenia, Azerbaijan, and Georgia), where the lowest figures were reported. These wide regional variations are largely due to national and cultural differences.[2]

1984 was the last year of the period of stagnation (as it may be called) which was characterized by centralization of political and economic power, censorship, and isolation from other countries. In 1986–1988, *perestroika* was at a peak. The number of suicides for men in the USSR decreased by 40% in 1984–1986 (Fig. 33.1), against 3% in 22 European countries studied during the same period. This decline occurred in all 15 republics of the USSR. The largest falls were observed in Russia and Belorussia, where male suicides fell by 42%.[3]

The sharp decrease in suicides applied to women as well as men,[4] but of all groups in the population the largest being among men in the work-force aged between 25 and 54—possibly the age range during which one is most responsive to social changes as well as to alcohol policy. No corresponding decline for this age group was noted in any other country in the 20th century.[1–5]

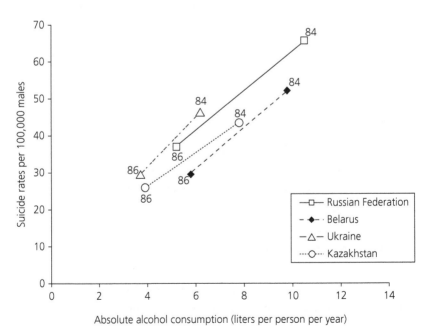

Fig. 33.1 Annual suicide rates per 100,000 males and consumption of absolute alcohol in litres per capita in Russian Federation, Belarus, Ukraine and Kazakhstan.

In Estonia, one of the former republics of the USSR, a study examining the blood alcohol concentration in suicide victims at the time of death, in a representative sample during 1981–1992 (i.e., before, during, and after the major anti-alcohol campaign), confirmed that alcohol restriction was accompanied by a decrease in suicide mortality among alcoholics of both sexes.[6] Similar results are reported in another study on suicide and alcohol consumption from Russia.[7]

These results illustrate the role of alcohol restrictions in history's most effective suicide-preventive programme for men. There is no doubt that the sudden decline in suicide rates coincided with the anti-alcohol campaign and the reform period in the former USSR known as *perestroika*. However, besides the alcohol restrictions, the role of hope of a better future and greater freedom cannot be underestimated in the reduction in mortality from violent causes, as well as from stress-related illnesses such as cardiovascular diseases.

These reductions in mortality are not due to statistical errors. Another research group has, like ourselves, shown that the reliability of mortality data was high, and no changes took place in the routines or quality of data collection during *perestroika* compared with the preceding period.[8]

Suicide rates increase when alcohol restriction ends

Unfortunately, the suicide-preventive effects observed during Gorbachev's reforms were not lasting. Unofficial alcohol production rose strikingly after 1988. Scarcity of funds ruled out a continued anti-alcohol campaign and efforts to change attitudes in the former USSR.[9] Since 1990, there has been an explosive rise in suicide rates as well as in homicide, accidents, and in overall mortality which corresponds with the collapse of the Soviet Union.[10] This development, besides high alcohol consumption, is attributed by different authors to adaptation shock anomic conditions, and modernization processes during economic, social, political, and ideological changes.[9-13]

Alcohol restrictions reduce suicides

Several 'natural experiments'—such as Prohibition in the US in 1910–1920, sharply raised alcohol prices in Denmark in 1911–1924, and restrictions on the sale of alcohol in Sweden in connection with the introduction of ration books in the first part of the 20th century—and have been proved to cause significant falls in suicide.[14–16] In the Russian Federation, in 2006 a policy regulating production and sale of ethyl alcohol and alcohol-containing products was restored, which resulted in a 9% decline in suicide mortality among Russian males.[17]

From clinical studies of suicidal people, it is well known that a sense of hopelessness is a factor that contributes strongly to suicidal thoughts and acts, and also that alcohol use disorder is an important diagnosis in this context. In light of these facts, the outcome of the vast natural experiment of *perestroika*—that both higher hopes and lower alcohol consumption in the former USSR helped to bring about the most effective suicide-prevention programme for men in our time is not surprising. Gorbachev's reforms consisted of a combination of various measures, including radical alcohol restrictions, intensive efforts to change attitudes at all levels (from the nation's top political leaders to the 'grass-roots' level), and the introduction of legal sanctions when the basic intentions of the reform were not observed. Production as well as sale of alcoholic beverages fell sharply, owing to governmental restrictions. Compliance with the law at different levels was ensured by both the imposition of various penalties for drunkenness in public or at the workplace and through effective steps to change attitudes towards the use of alcohol. At every level of Soviet society during the Gorbachev era, for example, proposing toasts in alcohol during official dinners was prohibited. Drinking no longer appeared to be an admired way of asserting one's masculinity.

Alcohol restrictions have different effects in different countries

One may wonder whether alcohol restrictions would have the same impact in other countries with different cultures. Correlations at aggregate level between alcohol consumption and suicide mortality vary from one country to another;[18] thus, the same clear associations between reduced or increased alcohol consumption and correspondingly reduced or increased suicide mortality cannot be observed in certain countries.

Obviously, it is not only the availability of alcohol but also attitudes and tolerance of the society towards alcohol use that have an impact on the number of alcoholics in the respective society. In cultures with greater acceptance of alcohol, there are more alcoholics; accordingly, these cultures promote certain forms of behaviour. It is, therefore, important to understand in depth why, in any particular nation, people drink alcohol.

Alcohol restrictions reduce suicides among alcoholics

Analyses at aggregate level are marred by great uncertainty regarding causality and associations. But a study from Denmark has shown that suicide rates among alcoholics fell when their alcohol consumption decreased as a result of sharp price rises, while the suicide rates among non-alcoholics did not change.[15,19] Studies at the individual level also clearly show the role of alcohol in mortality from suicide and provide additional arguments for interpreting results concerning reductions in suicide during *perestroika*.[6] In Russia, alcohol plays a crucial role in suicide mortality, among other reasons, due to intoxication-oriented drinking patterns.[11,20]

Treatment of psychiatric disorders should accompany diminished access to alcohol

However, when measures of suicide prevention are planned, factors other than mere restrictions on the supply of alcohol must be taken into consideration. Suicides among alcoholics are due to a range of psychiatric and psychosocial factors that cannot be influenced solely by reduced access to alcohol. Suicide-prevention measures must, therefore, include treatment of underlying psychiatric morbidity, reinforcement of social networks, and learning of adequate coping strategies to deal with difficult situations, alongside public health measures to regulate access to alcohol.

References

1 **Wasserman D, Värnik A, Dankowicz M, Eklund G.** Suicide-preventive effects of perestroika in the former USSR: the role of alcohol restriction. Acta Psychiatr Scand Suppl. 1998;**394**:1–44.

2 **Wasserman D, Värnik A, Dankowicz M.** Regional differences in the distribution of suicide in the former Soviet Union during perestroika, 1984–1990. Acta Psychiatr Scand 1998;suppl 394:5–12.

3 **Wasserman D, Värnik A, Eklund G.** Male suicides and alcohol consumption in the former USSR. Acta Psychiatr Scand. 1994;**89**: 306–313.

4 **Wasserman D, Värnik A, Eklund G.** Female suicides and alcohol consumption during perestroika in the former USSR. Acta Psychiatr Scand. 1998;suppl 394:26–33.

5 **Wasserman D, Dankowicz M, Värnik A, Olsson L.** Suicide trends in Europe, 1984–1990. In: Stefanis CN (ed.). Biopsychosocial approaches to suicide. The Netherlands: Elsevier Science; 1997.

6 **Värnik A, Kõlves K, Väli, M, Tooding LM, Wasserman D.** Do alcohol restrictions reduce suicide mortality? Addiction. 2007; **102**(2):251–256.

7 **Nemtsov A.** Suicides and alcohol consumption in Russia, 1965–1999. Drug Alcohol Depen. 2003;**71**(2):161–168.

8 **Leon D, Chenet L, Shkolnikov V, et al.** Huge variation in Russian mortality rates 1984–1994: artefact, alcohol or what? Lancet. 1997;**350**:383–388.

9 **Värnik A.** Suicide in the Baltic countries and in the former republics of the USSR. Karolinska Institute, Stockholm: Doctoral dissertation; 1997: 1–169.

10 **Värnik P, Sisask M, Värnik A, Yur'yev A, Kõlves K, Leppik L, et al.** Massive increase in injury deaths of undetermined intent in ex-USSR Baltic and Slavic countries: hidden suicides? Scand J Public Health. 2010;**38**(4):395–403.

11 **Värnik P.** Mortality from external causes, particularly suicides, in European countries: trends, socio-demographic factors and measurement issues. Tallinn University, Tallinn, Estonia: Doctoral dissertation; 2015:39–50.

12 **Pridemore WA, Chamlin MB.** A time-series analysis of the impact of heavy drinking on homicide and suicide mortality in Russia, 1956–2002. Addiction. 2006 Dec;**101**(12):1719–1729.

13 **Jukkala T, Mäkinen IH, Stickley A.** The historical development of suicide mortality in Russia, 1870–2007. Arch Suicide Res. 2015;**19**(1):117–130.

14 **Norström T.** Alcohol and suicide in Scandinavia. Br J Addict. 1988;**83**:553–559.

15 **Skog OJ.** Alcohol and suicide in Denmark 1911–1924: experiences from a 'natural experiment'. Addiction. 1993;**88**:1189–1193.

16 **Wasserman IM.** The impact of epidemic, war, prohibition and media on suicide: United States, 1910–1920. Suicide Life Threat Behav. 1992;**22**:240–254.

17 **Pridemore WA, Chamlin MB, Andreev E.** Reduction in male suicide mortality following the 2006 Russian alcohol policy: an interrupted time series analysis. Am J Public Health. 2013;**103**(11):2021–2026.

18 **Lester D.** The association between alcohol consumption and suicide and homicide rates: a study of 13 nations. Alcohol Alcohol. 1995;**30**:465–468.

19 **Skog OJ.** Alcohol and suicide: Durkheim revisited. Acta Sociol. 1991;**34**:193–206.

20 **Razvodovsky YE.** Alcohol consumption and suicide rates in Russia. Suicidology Online. 2011;**2**:67–74.

Chapter 34

Controlling the environment to prevent suicide

Annette L Beautrais

Current best evidence for preventing suicide clearly suggests that controlling the environment by restricting access to means and sites of suicide is a strategy which has strong empirical support. This evidence exists for multiple methods of suicide, at both population and individual levels, and is consistent across various countries and cultures. This chapter reviews the rationale and evidence for controlling the environment as an effective suicide-prevention strategy.

Rationale

The aetiology of suicide is complex: multiple factors contribute to all suicide attempts. However, in every attempt—two factors—the availability of means of suicide and the decision to use a specific method—are critical in determining whether an individual dies or survives. The lethality of suicide methods varies: case fatality rates (percentage who die from all those who make an attempt using a specific method) are highest for firearms (80–90%), drowning (65–80%), hanging (60–85%), car exhaust (40–60%), jumping (35–60%), charcoal burning (40–50%), and pesticide ingestion (6–75%), and lowest for medication overdose (1.5–4%).[1] If access to highly lethal methods is restricted then an attempt may be thwarted, or a less lethal method used, and the person may survive.

Many people make suicide plans which depend on using a specific method—if their preferred method is not available then they may not substitute another method. Many suicide attempts are made by people reacting impulsively to crises, with little planning. If means of suicide are not readily available, they may defer their attempt. Most people who survive near-fatal suicide attempts do not go on to make further attempts by the same—or some alternative—method. For these reasons, at an individual level, restricting access to commonly used means of suicide can defer or prevent lethal attempts.

At a population level, methods of suicide which are readily available in a particular environment tend to be those most commonly used for suicide. In Asian and Latin American countries, for example, where pesticide use in agriculture is widespread, suicide by pesticide ingestion is common. In cities with many high rise residential buildings, suicide by jumping is common. In the US where gun ownership is common and gun control is lax, almost 60% of suicides are by firearms, whereas in neighbouring Canada where population access to firearms is subject to legal restrictions, firearms account for approximately 16% of suicides.

Restricting access to means of suicide is an important prevention strategy worldwide. In 1993, the World Health Organization (WHO) promoted six suicide-prevention strategies of which five (gun possession control, detoxification of domestic gas, detoxification of car emissions, control of the availability of toxic substances (including pharmaceutical drugs), and toning down reports in the press), were well-defined efforts to control the environment.[2]

Updated recommendations are presented in the WHO Report in World Suicide Report: Preventing Suicide. A Global Imperative.[3]

Regulation of firearms

Ready access to firearms is associated with increased rates of firearm suicide.[4] The impact of legislative or policy controls of firearms on rates of firearm suicide has been observed in several countries. In Canada, enforcement of the Criminal Law Amendment Act of 1977 (Bill C-51) reduced firearm suicide, without substitution of other methods, and with most impact on youth suicides.[5] Similar reductions in firearm suicide rates following legislative restrictions on firearm ownership have been reported for Austria, Australia, Canada, Finland, New Zealand, and the UK. In the Israeli Army a policy change requiring guns to be left on base during weekend leave reduced suicides by 40%, with most of the reduction accounted for by a reduction in weekend suicides. Halving the size of the Swiss Army for economic reasons, and diminishing the number of guns kept in private homes by conscripts, was followed by a 27% reduction in the national suicide rate among men aged 18–45 (the age of those who served in the Army), with no change in control groups (women and older males).[6] Legislative controls associated with reduced firearm suicides include: restrictions on firearm registration; licensure restrictions; controls on access to automatic weapons and quantities of ammunition; extension of the waiting period for purchases; imposition of safe storage requirements; and background checks for psychiatric or violence histories deemed barriers to gun ownership.

Control of pesticides

Ingestion of pesticides accounts for one-third of all world deaths by suicide. Worldwide suicide rates could be reduced significantly if access to highly lethal pesticides was controlled. Measures that could realize this goal include sanctioning and enforcing relevant international conventions on hazardous chemicals, imposing controls on pesticide sales, reducing the toxicity of pesticides, using less toxic pesticides, promoting safe storage practices, providing public education about safe management, and improving the medical management of pesticide overdoses.[7,8] The effectiveness of such initiatives is illustrated by significant reductions in suicides in Western Samoa and Sri Lanka following introduction of legislative controls on toxic pesticides. Alternative methods were not substituted.

Control of carbon monoxide

Vehicle exhaust gas

Historically, carbon monoxide (CO) poisoning by vehicle exhaust gas was a common method of suicide in most industrialized countries. However, in the late twentieth century, many countries imposed mandatory emissions standards on vehicles for ecological, 'clean air' purposes. These standards were achieved, most commonly, by requiring the fitting of catalytic converters (which reduced the toxicity of vehicle exhaust

gases) to all new vehicles. The introduction of legislation requiring catalytic converters in new vehicles was associated with reduced suicides by
CO exhaust in both England and Australia.

Charcoal burning

Extensive media publicity introduced and ensured the adoption of a
novel method of suicide, charcoal burning, in Hong Kong, in 1998. The
method was framed by the media as a 'painless, pleasant' way to die and,
coinciding with the Asian financial crisis, appealed to a population that
had not previously been vulnerable to suicide, thereby increasing the
overall suicide rate. Hong Kong suicide researchers initiated successful prevention efforts by encouraging supermarkets to remove charcoal packs from open shelves, forcing purchasers to explicitly request
charcoal from controlled sites. Researchers also educated motel own-
ers to recognize vulnerable individuals seeking to rent accommodation
to conduct charcoal-burning suicide. Media were encouraged to mute
reporting of charcoal-burning suicides. Implementation of these measures significantly reduced charcoal-related suicide deaths, with the largest contribution to the reduction coming from purchasing restrictions
applied in stores.[9,10]

Reducing availability of medications

Self-poisoning with medications is the second or third most common
method of suicide in most European countries and contributes substantially to morbidity in many countries, accounting for the majority of
all hospital admissions for self-harm. Restricting access to drugs commonly used for self-poisoning, and especially to those with high case
fatality, can reduce morbidity, rates of hospital admission, and associated costs, as well as mortality. Drugs used in overdose suicide attempts
include prescribed psychiatric drugs as well as over-the-counter (OTC)
medications. Access to medications can be controlled in several ways:
restricting the number of prescriptions and the amount dispensed, prescribing less toxic drugs when available, wrapping individual pills in tin-
foil or in plastic blisters, recalling unused drugs, pharmacist monitoring
of large or excessive prescriptions, physicians taking precautions against

forgery, and physicians not prescribing or refilling prescriptions without seeing patients.[11] In Australia, Britain, Japan, Norway, and Sweden, the introduction of controls on prescribing of barbituates was followed by reduced suicide rates using these drugs. In a number of countries the prescription of the less toxic selective serotonin reuptake inhibitors (SSRIs) in place of tricyclic antidepressants, which are toxic in overdose, was associated with decreased suicide rates. In the UK, legislation restricting package sizes of OTC medications, including paracetamol and salicylates, was associated with lower rates of suicide and self-harm using these drugs.[12]

Hanging

Hanging is the most common means of suicide because both the means for hanging and ligature points are ubiquitously available. This ready availability makes it virtually impossible to restrict access in order to prevent suicide deaths. Virtually the only opportunity to impose controls on access to means of hanging and to ligature points is in institutional settings including psychiatric hospitals, and police and prison cells. Measures which can be taken to ensure 'safe rooms' in institutional settings include safe clothing (e.g., removing cords or laces) and eliminating or restricting access to potential ligature points such as cell window bars, doors, bed structures, light fittings, pipes, cupboards, sinks, bathroom fittings, or toilets.[13]

Barriers at jumping sites and hotspots

Most suicides by jumping occur in densely populated cities in which there are large numbers of high-rise residential buildings. However, most publicity about efforts to reduce suicides by jumping arises from a relatively small number of non-residential sites, often bridges, which have acquired notoriety, or iconic status, as places for jumping. Installation of barriers or safety nets at these popular jumping sites has reduced suicides from these sites. Less attention has been paid to preventing suicides from high-rise residential buildings, by far, the most common site for suicide deaths by jumping. Prevention measures that could be used include barriers, surveillance measures, signs, and telephone hotlines for suicidal people, mandatory safe building codes and enforcement of these standards, and muted media reporting.[3]

Controlling access to railways and subways

Suicide deaths occur on both long-distance railway tracks and in urban metro-rail systems. The incidence of railway suicides seems to be related to population density—and is particularly high in the Netherlands (10–14%) and Germany (7% of all suicides). Railway and metro sites near psychiatric hospitals often acquire reputations as suicide 'hotspots', with those who die at these sites including psychiatric patients who attend local facilities. Suicides have reduced in metro-rail systems where doors have been programmed to open directly onto the platform only when the train has stopped, and public access to tracks has been restricted. Measures to prevent suicide on open railway tracks and also in urban metro-rail systems include installation of barriers and use of patrols and television surveillance systems at favoured sites.

Media reporting

A discussion of controlling the environment to prevent suicide must go beyond issues of the means of suicide to include consideration of media influences on choice of methods and sites for suicide. The WHO, in 1993, included 'toning down media reports about suicide' as one of six major approaches to suicide prevention. A strong evidence base supports this recommendation. This evidence suggests that media reports or portrayals of suicide may influence vulnerable individuals to adopt particular methods and/or sites for suicide. Reporting practices which may encourage suicide include glamourizing or romanticizing suicide, normalizing suicide by presenting it as an understandable response to stress, gratuitously covering celebrity suicides, and providing details of specific methods of suicide, or details of suicide clusters. Media-reporting guidelines which advocate avoiding these practices are widely available.[14] The successful application of media guidelines was reported from Vienna, where, in 1978, the new underground railway system became a popular site for suicide. Mass media reported these incidents in dramatic ways. The introduction of guidelines for media to report suicides resulted in an 80% reduction in subway suicide deaths within six months, and this reduction has been sustained.[15]

Suicide clusters

Suicides which occur close together in time and/or space, beyond the rate which would be normally be expected in a community, are commonly regarded as forming a suicide 'cluster'.[16,17] Suicide clusters link two issues which are often related: (i) means of suicide; and (ii) media coverage of suicide. In suicide clusters, vulnerable individuals who either know the original decedent, or who are prompted by reports of the original death, often conveyed by mass media, may copy not only the mode of death, but also the means of suicide. Clusters are often regarded as newsworthy and seeds of social contagion are sown when clusters become the subject of dramatic and sensationalized news-reporting. Media reports commonly include details (often explicit) of the methods and sites of suicides in a given cluster, which, along with descriptions of the personal characteristics and implied motives of the person or persons who have died, provide the ingredients necessary for vulnerable people to identify with, and imitate, the victims. Reviews of clusters suggest they are more common: among young people, and in institutional settings including schools, prisons, hospital inpatient units, and the armed services; in small rural and aboriginal communities, and particularly in townships or regions which have many members who share strong family, social, cultural, or occupational relationships; within social systems that are highly enmeshed, and where structure and leadership have declined.

Knowledge of clusters has largely been informed by a relatively small number of narrative studies of single clusters.[18] However, in a population-based, case-control study, Gould and colleagues compared media coverage of youth suicide clusters with non-cluster suicides and provide the first empirical evidence that links newspaper reports about suicide to the initiation of teenage suicide clusters.[17]

Descriptions of the suicidal individual, act, and method, as well as front-page placement of the story, and the use of a headline containing the word 'suicide', all occurred more often in suicide clusters than in non-cluster suicides. These findings add weight to recommendations for muted media coverage of suicide, including method.[3]

Safe clinical practice

Despite widespread research and recommendations about the effectiveness of restricting access to lethal means of suicide, there has been a failure to translate these findings to clinical practice. Numerous studies report that many health practitioners do not routinely inquire, educate, or counsel suicidal patients or their families about restricting access to means of suicide. These failures exist across many medical settings including pediatrics, emergency departments, general practice, and mental health services. When asked the reason for not addressing means restriction, staff cite lack of time, fear of reactions, and scepticism that method restriction is effective. These responses and attitudes highlight the need for improved education of health practitioners about the effectiveness of means restrictions. The body of evidence which supports lethal means restrictions is now more than adequate to support the importance of this approach for suicide prevention; failure to routinely ask about access to means and advocate the removal of potentially lethal methods can be viewed as failure to apply best practice in care. Controlling the environment is, in fact, not foreign to practising psychiatrists. Controlling the availability of prescribed medications by providing small amounts to high-risk patients is a common practice. Controlling the environment by creating suicide-safe hospital rooms and custodial cells is standard hospital best practice.[13]

Conclusions

The research evidence about restricting access to lethal means of suicide is strong and clear. At an individual level, removing access to lethal means of suicide can thwart or defer suicide attempts. At a population level, restricting access to lethal means by imposing structural or legislative barriers can reduce suicides. Detoxifying domestic gas and vehicle exhaust gas, installing barriers at bridges, subways, and at other jumping sites, imposing legislative restrictions on access to firearms and purchasing controls on charcoal packs, are all measures which have resulted in reductions in suicide rates. Implementing media-reporting guidelines led to a striking reduction in subway suicide deaths in Vienna.

Where it is possible to restrict access to a widely available, commonly used, highly lethal method of suicide which lacks immediate substitutes, then a reduction in suicides by that method may be accompanied by a parallel reduction in overall suicide rates. Where access is restricted to methods which account for only a small fraction of total suicides, then suicides by that method may be reduced but no impact on overall suicide rates would be expected.

The extent to which restriction of one method may lead to substitution of another lethal method is difficult to anticipate or measure. At an individual level, many people who are thwarted by not gaining access to their favoured method may not switch to another method, and may not go on to make an attempt in the future. At a population level, the risk of substitution has often been used as an argument against restricting access to specific methods of suicide. However, substitution may not occur, and even if it were to occur it would take time until a new method became commonplace and many lives could be saved in the meantime. Restricting access is justified even if it would save only a small number of lives, or there is a risk of substitution. The evidence for means restriction is now so compelling that it constitutes best practice in suicide prevention. It is unethical to fail to implement effective means restriction measures capable of saving lives, in the same way it is unethical not to use best practice methods in treating suicidal patients.

At a population level, it is paradoxical that some of the most dramatic and effective suicide reductions have resulted from environmental controls which were not put in place to prevent suicides. Examples include replacing coal gas with natural gas as natural gas reserves were identified, mandating emission controls on vehicles for ecological reasons, introducing firearms controls in response to a single shooting incident, and having metro train doors open directly onto platforms to reduce costs of air-conditioning. While none of these measures were primarily introduced as public health strategies to reduce suicides they have been effective in suicide prevention as well. Indeed, when means restrictions are proposed for suicide prevention they are often met with public opposition, with the public being unwilling to tolerate some restrictions (such as bridge barriers, controls on guns, or media guidelines) in order to protect some of society's most vulnerable individuals.

In conclusion, controlling the environment is an effective approach to suicide prevention, and should be incorporated into best practice at public health and clinical levels wherever appropriate.

References

1 **Yip PS, Caine E, et al**. Means restriction for suicide prevention. Lancet. 2012;**379**(9834):2393–2399.

2 **World Health Organization (WHO)**. Guidelines for the primary prevention of mental, neurological and psychosocial disorders: suicide. Geneva: World Health Organization; 1993.

3 **World Health Organization (WHO)**. Preventing Suicide. A Global Imperative. WHO; 2014.

4 **Anglemyer A, Horvath T, Rutherford G**. The accessibility of firearms and risk for suicide and homicide victimization among household members: a systematic review and meta-analysis. Ann Intern Med. 2014;**160**(2):101–110. doi:10.7326/M13-1301.

5 **Leenaars A, Lester D**. The impact of gun control on suicide: studies from Canada. Arch Suicide Res. 1998;**4**:25–40.

6 **Reisch T, Steffen T, Habenstein A, Tschacher W**. Change in suicide rates in Switzerland before and after firearm restriction resulting from the 2003 'Army XXI' reform. Am J Psych. 2013;**170**(9):977–984. doi:10.1176/appi.ajp.2013.12091256.

7 **World Health Organization (WHO)**. Safer access to pesticides: community interventions. 2006. <www.who.int/mental_health/prevention/suicide/pesticides.pdf>.

8 **World Health Organization (WHO)**. Clinical management of acute pesticide intoxication: prevention of suicidal behaviours. 2008<http://www.who.int/mental-healthprevention/suicide/pesticides>.

9 **Kreitman N**. The coal gas story. United Kingdom suicide rates, 1960–1971. Br J Prev Soc Med. 1976;**30**:86–93.

10 **Yip PSF, Law CK, Fu KW, Law YW, Wong PW, Xu Y**. Restricting the means of suicide by charcoal burning. Br J Psychiatry. 2010;**196**:241–242.

11 **Barraclough BM, Nelson B, Bunch J, Sainsbury P**. Suicide and barbiturate prescribing. J R Coll Gen Pract 1971;**21**(112):645–653.

12 **Hawton K, Bergen H, Simkin S, Dodd S, Pocock P, Bernal W, et al**. Long-term effect of reduced pack sizes of paracetamol on poisoning deaths and liver transplant activity in England and Wales: interrupted time series analyses. BMJ. 2013;**346**:f403.

13 **Wasserman D, Rihmer Z, Rujescu D, Sarchiapone M, Sokolowski M, . . . Carli V**. European Psychiatric Association. The European Psychiatric Association (EPA) guidance on suicide treatment and prevention. Eur Psychiatry. 2012 Feb;**27**(2):129–141. doi:10.1016/j.eurpsy.2011.06.003.

14 **World Health Organization (WHO)**. Preventing suicide: a resource for media professionals. Department of Mental Health World Health Organization. Geneva; 2000. <http://www.who.int/mental_health/media/en/426.pdf>.

15 **Westerlund M, Schaller S, Schmidtke A**. The role of mass media in suicide prevention. In: Wasserman D, Wasserman C, editors. The Oxford textbook of suicidology and suicide prevention. Oxford: Oxford University Press; 2009: Ch. 69, 515–523.

16 **Haw C, et al**. Suicide clusters: a review of risk factors and mechanisms. Suicide Life Threat Behav. 2013;**43**(1):97–108.

17 **Gould M, et al**. Newspaper coverage of suicide and initiation of suicide clusters in teenagers in the USA, 1988–96: a retrospective, population-based, case-control study. Lancet Psych. 2014;**1**:34–43.

18 **Larkin G, Beautrais AL**. Geospatial mapping of suicide clusters. *Te Pou o Te Whakaaro Nui*, The National Centre of Mental Health Research, Information and Workforce Development. Auckland, New Zealand. March 2012. <http://www.tepou.co.nz/library/tepou/geospatial-mapping-of-suicide-clusters>.

Chapter 35

Suicide prevention through the Internet

Vladimir Carli

Introduction

The Internet has long since been used to reach out to large populations with information and services. In March 2011, there were 2.1 billion Internet users worldwide[1] and, in a random sample of more than 3,000 American adults, 58% of Internet users reported searching for health-related information for themselves.[2] The search for health-related information is important in spite of the fact that accessibility to the Internet differs between countries.

Many adolescents who suffer from isolation use the Internet as a way to cope with feelings of loneliness and social exclusion. Therefore, there is a unique opportunity to utilize the Internet as a means of communication, reaching vulnerable adolescents who suffer from social exclusion, mental health problems, and are undetected. The Internet also provides an opportunity to raise awareness about mental health. It has recently been shown that a school-based awareness programme called YAM (Youth Aware of Mental Health) is effective in preventing suicide attempts among young people.[3,4] The same kind of programmes could be designed to be delivered online in order to reach a wider audience of adolescents. This is important also in the context of recent findings showing that excessive Internet use is associated with mental health issues, including self-destructive behaviours[5] and that adolescents with specific behavioural patterns, which include increased media and Internet use, are at high risk of psychiatric symptoms and suicidal behaviour.[6]

Although empirical evaluation is still limited, numerous professional online suicide and mental health help sites using various approaches have been planned, launched, and evaluated with encouraging results.[7] However, the information available online can be of varying quality and some websites even encourage suicide. Thus, one important question for suicide prevention (and perhaps for health-care in general) is not only *what* these information seekers find online, but also *how* they search for information and profit from it.

The SUPREME project (suicide prevention through Internet and media-based mental health promotion)

The aim of the SUPREME project was to develop, disseminate, and evaluate an intervention website aimed at adolescent mental health promotion and suicide prevention by means of improving mental health knowledge, increasing awareness, and offering direct professional support to its users. Some sections of the website were based on the YAM programme.[4] It was optional for the participants to visit the intervention website.

Females consistently reported a higher rate of mental health problems than males. Regarding Internet use, results showed that nine out of ten subjects used the Internet at least once a day and the majority reported even more frequent use, several times a day, but for short periods. It was by far most common for the adolescents to use the Internet for social purposes, involving activities performed on social networking sites and other communicative online tools, followed by activities relating to schoolwork.

There were interesting associations between activities performed on the Internet and mental health; performing target searches (e.g., on Google) was particularly associated with depression, anxiety, and stress in both males and females, perhaps because poor well-being causes individuals to seek targeted information which relate to their mental health problem. There was also a positive correlation between the intensity of Internet use and scores on depression, anxiety, stress, and suicidal thoughts/ideation. Longitudinal analyses of the effectiveness of the intervention website showed a statistically significant decline in mental health-related outcomes, such as depression, anxiety, stress, as well as in suicidal ideation.

Youth involvement in the website development

A participatory design process is a valuable approach to help ensure that an online youth mental health promotion service meets the needs and preferences of the users.[8] The approach entails involving young people in every project stage: from the initial concept, through to the dissemination of the website. The rational behind this method is that adolescents are in the best position to understand and, therefore, to inform the design of the website, so as to ensure that it appeals to their age group.[9] Employing a youth-participation approach has been shown to be an efficient and effective way of attracting and engaging young people in different services, by enhancing usability, promoting help-seeking behaviour, and resilience in young people.

Collaborating with young people to acquire information and feedback can involve a range of different techniques. Before the Internet service is implemented it might be useful to obtain perceptions and preferences from young people through focus groups and interviews. This was implemented in the SUPREME project with the purpose of gaining a better understanding of the types of activities and information that would capture the attention of adolescents; to understand which online platforms they use and in which way the intervention website could be promoted to reach them. Tone, style, and information-dissemination techniques were discussed. In the SUPREME project, the number of participants in the focus groups was kept low to allow for an open discussion where different opinions could be accounted for. A semi-structured interview protocol with open-ended questions was used for all interviews. Online tools, such as surveys or online discussions, can also be useful for collecting a large amount of information from young people.

Online tools and content

An online youth mental health service needs to present information in an interesting format to engage users. Young people who experience distress, mood difficulties, or are seeking mental health advice are more likely to use a combination of both static (e.g., fact sheets) and interactive (e.g., forums and games) online services than those who do not experience such difficulties.[10] In order to maximize the effectiveness of the website, it might, therefore, be useful to incorporate the most popular static and interactive tools for adolescents. For example, on the SUPREME website, mental health content was presented through both static and interactive tools.

Online resources also need to adapt and adjust their service to how young people are most likely to use them, to allow the service to be more usable and efficient. Results from the SUPREME project demonstrate that adolescents use the Internet for different purposes. On average, adolescents use 23.5% of their Internet time for socializing, 18% for school or work, 16% for targeted searches, 14.5% for playing games, 14% for reading the news, 8% for visiting websites with pornographic content, and 6% for gambling. In order for a mental health-promoting website that targets young people to be effective, it is important to deliver mental health information through appropriate online activities that are popular and preferred by young people. The SUPREME results highlight that such a website needs to provide a platform for social interactions, as this was one of the main preferred online activities among the participants.

Research further suggests that personal mental ill-health experiences are highly valued, especially by young females. These can be presented through written stories or using music and video tools. To target young men, action-oriented strategies might be useful. This involves providing mental health-promoting games, video, and music formats to both present mental health information and be used as tools for users to share their own stories and thoughts relating to mental health problems.

Website design

The design of a website encompasses the look, layout, and navigation of the service provided. This is an important element that needs to be appealing and engaging for young people, especially when first entering the website. For example, it takes on average 10–20 seconds for a first-time visitor to decide whether to keep browsing or abandon the website.[11] In the SUPREME project, 44% of visitors spent on average less than 5 minutes browsing the website, while 27% of users browsed the website for more than 15 minutes on average.

The purpose and services of the website should be made clear for users when first entering it. The colour scheme, headings, fonts, location of text, labels, and navigation tools as well as the size and spacing of characters should be kept consistent throughout the website to create a professional look. To facilitate navigation throughout the site, it is recommended that the most important items should appear at the top of the page. In addition, text should be presented with a dark font on a light background to make reading easier. It is also important that information is written in a language that is familiar to adolescents, the use of jargon is avoided, and that the tone is kept professional without being patronizing. Mental health professionals and young people need to work together to ensure that the language resonates with their age group.

Website functions

A significant number of adolescents use the Internet after 11.00 p.m.[10] and a report investigating adolescents' Internet use showed that using the Internet for accessing information was predicted by late-night use (after 11.00 p.m.).[12] In the SUPREME project, 26% of young people reported that they stayed up late and lost sleep in order to use the Internet.[13] Although it is worrying that young people lose sleep to stay up and use the Internet, these results suggest that mental health professionals and trained personnel need to be able to interact with young people not only during regular opening hours (9.00–5.00 p.m.). Males, in particular, tend to use the Internet late at night.[12,14] Thus, allowing services to be responsive during the night may provide an opportunity to assist and support young men. This is especially important considering that young males, compared with their female peers, show lower help-seeking tendencies for mental health problems. Moreover, those who access the Internet during late hours have significantly higher levels of psychological distress and mood problems than adolescents who do not go online late at night.[10] This suggests that those who are perhaps most in need of support and guidance may be the ones who would benefit the most from a 24/7 open online service; however, a 24/7 service may not always be feasible. Therefore, it might be preferable to offer resources only during the hours the website is most frequented and perhaps offer an alternative option during out-of-hours contact, such as an e-mail service or links to other portals and hotlines.

Online safety and building trust with the users

In order to develop an effective website promoting mental health that engages and promotes help-seeking behaviour in young people, the site needs to be regarded as a trusted source for mental health help and advice. In addition, it needs to be a safe place for adolescents seeking support.

Knowing where mental health information comes from, who produced it, and who made the website are among the most important issues identified by young people when they seek online mental health support. Research shows that concerns about the reliability, accuracy, and quality of online mental health information are the second biggest reason for avoiding online mental health information.[15]

Nevertheless, many young people prefer to turn to the Internet for mental health support and advice. A major reason for this might be that it allows them to remain anonymous. Anonymity has, therefore, been identified as a key requirement for many people when seeking help for mental health issues. For example, in a study by Kummervold et al.,[16] 64% of people aged 18–35 who were active on a mental health discussion forum in Norway responded that they would not use the service if they had to use their real name. This was an issue also identified by the adolescents in the SUPREME project's focus groups. They generally disliked websites where they had to register their personal details and appreciated anonymity when researching information about their health on the Internet. This is an especially important issue for young men,[14] people who want to deal with mental health problems privately,[17] and people with suicidal ideation and depression.[18]

Activity in which online posts and comments from users are monitored and reviewed to avoid harmful online communication is highly beneficial. Online anonymity can sometimes empower users to post things of a more destructive nature, such as negative comments towards others or by, for example, pretending to perform self-harm activities. Therefore, it is important to have moderators that oversee conversations and remove inappropriate comments. Research suggests that chat rooms and forums that are moderated show more positive online communication compared with unmoderated ones.[19]

It is essential that an online service, in which young people can interact with trained personnel or professionals, creates a set of guidelines for staff for appropriate crisis support.[8] For example, the survey used in the SUPREME project identified that 8.5% of participants were emergency cases, where 7% were contactable for further action. Therefore, guidelines are needed to clearly outline the procedure in such emergency situations.

Promotion

In order for a youth mental health promotion website to be successful, it needs to attract the target group. Therefore, it might be useful if the site raises awareness of its presence in online places that young people visit often and promote it via search engines. However, some online activities differ between young males and females.[20] For example, among adolescents in the SUPREME project, it was more common for males to engage in online games compared with females, while females tended to use the Internet more for socializing than males. Promotion and marketing efforts should, therefore, address this in order to target both groups.

The vast majority of young people who seek mental health information on the Internet use a search engine for this purpose.[12] This was also true for the participants in the SUPREME focus groups. The Google search engine was the most commonly used engine by both healthy and inpatient focus-group participants. Among adolescents in the SUPREME project, targeted searches were also one of the main online activities. It is recommended that an online youth mental health service creates a strong presence at online websites that are frequently used by young people.

Evaluation of the website

Reviewing the website for user engagement and impact on a regular basis can be useful to ensure that it is effective and fulfils its purpose.

This stage can also be done with focus groups and interviews. However, online survey tools are especially effective for receiving feedback from a large number of users.[8]

Conclusion

The usefulness of the Internet for mental health promotion and prevention of suicide is evident. However, caution should be used when developing programmes online and guidelines, as described in this chapter, should be observed.

References

1 Internet World Stats. <http://www.internetworldstats.com/stats.htm>.

2 Atkinson NL, Saperstein SL, Pleis J. Using the internet for health-related activities: findings from a national probability sample. J Med Internet Res. 2009;11:e4.

3 Wasserman C, Hoven CW, Wasserman D, Carli V, Sarchiapone M, . . . Postuvan V. Suicide prevention for youth—a mental health awareness program: lessons learned from the Saving and Empowering Young Lives in Europe (SEYLE) intervention study. BMC Public Health. 2012;12:776.

4 Wasserman D, Hoven CW, Wasserman C, Wall M, Eisenberg R, . . . Carli V. School-based suicide prevention programmes: the SEYLE cluster-randomised, controlled trial. Lancet. 2015;385:1536–1544.

5 Kaess M, Durkee T, Brunner R, Carli V, Parzer P, . . . Wasserman D. Pathological Internet use among European adolescents: psychopathology and self-destructive behaviours. Eur Child Adolesc Psychiatry. 2014;23:1093–1102.

6 Carli V, Hoven CW, Wasserman C, Chiesa F, Guffanti G, . . . Wasserman D. A newly identified group of adolescents at "invisible" risk for psychopathology and suicidal behavior: findings from the SEYLE study. World Psychiatry. 2014;13:78–86.

7 Gilat I, Shahar G. Suicide prevention by online support groups: an action theory-based model of emotional first aid. Arch Suicide Res. 2009;13:52–63.

8 Campbell AJ, Robards F. Using technologies safely and effectively to promote young people's wellbeing: a better practice guide for services. NSW Centre for the Advancement of Adolescent Health, Westmead and the Young and Well CRC, Abbotsford. 2013.

9 Wong NT, Zimmerman MA, Parker EA. A typology of youth participation and empowerment for child and adolescent health promotion. Am J Community Psychol. 2010;46:100–114.

10 Santor DA, Poulin C, LeBlanc JC, Kusumakar V. Online health promotion, early identification of difficulties, and help seeking in young people. J Am Acad Child Adolesc Psychiatry. 2007;46:50–59.

11 **Liu C, White RW, Dumais S**. Understanding Web Browsing Behaviors through Weibull Analysis of Dwell Time. Proceeding of the 33rd International ACM SIGIR Conference on Research and Development in Information Retrieval. 2010379–2010386.

12 **Burns JM, Davenport TA, Durkin LA, Luscombe GM, Hickie IB**. The internet as a setting for mental health service utilisation by young people. Med J Aust. 2010;**192**:S22–S26.

13 **Sarchiapone M, Mandelli L, Carli V, Iosue M, Wasserman C, . . . Wasserman D**. Hours of sleep in adolescents and its association with anxiety, emotional concerns, and suicidal ideation. Sleep medicine. 2014;**15**:248–254.

14 **Ellis LA, Collin P, Davenport TA, Hurley PJ, Burns JM, Hickie IB**. Young men, mental health, and technology: implications for service design and delivery in the digital age. J Med Internet Res. 2012;**14**:e160.

15 **Horgan A, Sweeney J**. Young students' use of the Internet for mental health information and support. J Psychiatr Ment Health Nurs. 2010;**17**:117–123.

16 **Kummervold PE, Gammon D, Bergvik S, Johnsen JA, Hasvold T, Rosenvinge JH**. Social support in a wired world: use of online mental health forums in Norway. Nord J Psychiatry. 2002;**56**:59–65.

17 **Leach LS, Christensen H, Griffiths KM, Jorm AF, Mackinnon AJ**. Websites as a mode of delivering mental health information: perceptions from the Australian public. Soc Psychiatry Psychiatr Epidemiol. 2007;**42**:167–172.

18 **Ybarra ML, Eaton WW**. Internet-based mental health interventions. Ment Health Serv Res. 2005;**7**:75–87.

19 **Crutzen R, De Nooijer J**. Intervening via chat: an opportunity for adolescents' mental health promotion? Health Promot Int. 2011;**26**:238–243.

20 **Durkee T, Kaess M, Carli V, Parzer P, Wasserman C, . . . Wasserman D**. Prevalence of pathological internet use among adolescents in Europe: demographic and social factors. Addiction. 2012;**107**:2210–2222.

Chapter 36

Suicide prevention in schools

Danuta Wasserman and Véronique Narboni

Suicide prevention: the earlier, the better

School-based suicide-prevention strategies should be included in national suicide-prevention strategies as suicide in the second leading cause of death globally among young people between 15–29 years of age.[1] The choice of school-based suicide-prevention strategies reflects the convenience with which adolescents and young adults can be reached.[2]

Young people are impressionable, open to new ideas, and sometimes uncritical, all of which is part of their charm. Unfortunately, this juvenile tendency to absorb new impressions uncritically and to be easily influenced by others may sometimes have grave and harmful consequences. Adolescents are influenced by music, fashion, and youth idols—not only in terms of clothing and hairstyle, but also in their attitudes towards drugs, alcohol, and aspects of behaviour that are both desirable and undesirable.

It is not surprising that both good and bad models find imitators among teenagers. Research continues to demonstrate that vulnerable youth are susceptible to the influence of reports and portrayals of suicide in the mass media.[3]

Reports on suicide in the news media are highly influential. Several studies have found dramatic effects of televised portrayals that have led to increased rates of suicide and suicide attempts using the same methods as those displayed in the shows.

School as an arena for promotion of mental health and prevention of suicide

Children spend many hours a day at school. The school setting also affords scope for monitoring not only their physical development but also their cognitive and emotional growth, their emergent sexuality, and their social-role adjustment. The education system is a suitable arena for introducing programmes to promote mental health and prevent suicide and for establishing policies and procedures that can be adopted by the whole school system and by people working at individual schools.

A comprehensive framework for suicide prevention in schools involves a continuum of activities including mental health promotion, prevention, intervention, and postvention. Topics relating to mental health and suicide prevention may be easily woven into the school curriculum, just like teaching about reproduction, sexuality, and physical health. Instructions may also be given to school staff and parents as well, and they should have the opportunity to take part in tailored educational programmes.

Prevention of mental disorders and psychological distress early in the life cycle is extremely important, given the huge adverse repercussions of mental disorders in terms not only of suicidality, but also of children's and adolescents' scholastic performance and formation of social networks. Untreated psychiatric disorders developed during the early years of life, have serious consequences for the health of the individual throughout their entire life. Giving children and adolescents skills to cope with life stressors requires efforts, not only from parents, but also from other adults, like parents of children's friends, family friends, and school staff. This is particularly important as many children in the contemporary world come from broken families or live with parents who are incapable of giving them the support that a growing child needs (see Chapter 20: Adolescent suicide and attempted suicide).

Mental ill-health and suicidal behaviour among school pupils

Worldwide suicide is one of the leading causes of death in young people. For each adult who dies by suicide, there are approximately 27 others who have made at least one suicide attempt.[1] Suicide behaviours also have profound negative consequence on relatives and significant others.[4]

Data show that 29% of European adolescents have symptoms of subthreshold-depression and 10% were depressed, with high comorbidity.[5]

These data show that many young people are experiencing severe distress. Among school pupils, 12.5% would benefit from a qualified psychological and psychiatric treatment.[6]

Suicidal behaviour does not consist of isolated acts. Rather, it is the outcome of a process usually associated with a psychiatric disorder that, in many cases, goes undiagnosed and untreated. There is, thus, evidence that suicidal behaviour coincides with many underlying psychological and psychiatric conditions, ranging from depressive episodes, anxiety, and alcoholism, to psychotic manifestations. In addition to psychiatric illnesses, certain risk behaviours have been identified. For example, suicidal behaviours are strongly associated with various types of risk behaviour, including peer victimization, risky sexual behaviour, delinquency, substance abuse, non-suicidal self-injury (NSSI), physical inactivity, and poor nutrition.[7,8]

If these facts are not taken into account in programmes of health promotion and suicide prevention, ill-advised information campaigns may actually trigger suicide attempts or suicides among these already vulnerable young people, instead of preventing them.

Knowledge and attitudes can be influenced

The fact that psycho-educative programmes enhance awareness and boost knowledge of mental health and suicidal behaviour has been documented.

To temper untoward mental health outcomes in children and adolescents, the World Psychiatric Association's Presidential Global Child Mental Health Programme, in collaboration with the World Health Organization (WHO) and the International Association of Child and Adolescent Psychiatry and Allied Professionals, established during 2002–2005 a Child Mental Health Awareness Task Force.[9] The awareness task force designed a study which was carried out in Armenia (Yerevan), Azerbaijan (Baku), Brazil (Porto Allegre), China (Shanghai), Egypt (Alexandria), Georgia (Tbilisi and Rustavi), Israel, (North) Russia (Chernoprudsky), and Uganda (Kampala), each under the direction of a local psychiatrist. Questionnaires developed for this study aimed to determine the knowledge and attitudes of parents and teachers about child mental health treatment issues after an information campaign 75% of the teachers felt more comfortable in discussing these problems with students, or with other school personnel, and 68% reported greater comfort in discussing students' emotional problems with parents. 60% of parents also reported feeling more comfortable when talking to their children about emotional problems, while 46% felt more at ease in discussing these problems with teachers. It should be noted that the questions asked were about mental health and mental illness in general, and not about suicide treatment or prevention.

Suicidal behaviours and adolescents

Can suicidal behaviour be reduced? We know from scientific reports that ill-considered information can boost it. But is it plausible to assume that young people's development can also be influenced in a positive direction, by giving them a chance to identify with, and emulate, good models?

As yet, there have been few studies to show that programmes of suicide prevention can change suicidal behaviour (i.e., reduce the numbers of suicides and attempted suicides). In a five-year prevention and intervention programme in Dade County Public Schools (DCPS), Miami, Florida, US, a whole range of mental health problems from psychosocial to psychiatric disorder was targeted. The authors reported a reduction of the number of suicides and of suicide attempts, but unfortunately, the programme lacked controls and comparison schools.[10]

Two randomized controlled trials (RCTs) performed in the US have demonstrated a significant decrease in suicide attempts in a classroom-based intervention called 'Signs of Suicide' (SOS).[11,12] Similar findings were reported on reducing new cases of suicidal ideation and suicide attempts in an RCT in the classroom-based behavioural intervention called the 'Good Behaviour Game' (GBG).[13]

In Europe, the Saving and Empowering Young Lives in Europe (SEYLE) project[14] was developed by a consortium of 12 European countries (Austria, Estonia, France, Germany, Hungary, Ireland, Israel, Italy, Romania,

Slovakia, Spain, and Sweden) and supported with funding from Coordination Theme 1 (Health) of the European Union Seventh Framework Programme (FP7). One of SEYLE's aims was to gather information about European 15-year-old school-based adolescents' mental health, and also to test in an RCT, three different suicide-preventive interventions, evaluating the outcome of each intervention in comparison with a control group. The three prevention strategies tested were built on the concept of empowering different key actors in the school arena; namely, teachers, pupils, and other professionals working within school health.

◆ *QPR (Question, Persuade, and Refer)* is a gatekeeper programme developed in the US,[15] to train teachers and other school personnel to recognize risk of suicide behaviour in pupils and to enhance communication skills in order to motivate and help pupils in suicide crisis to seek professional care. Teachers were also given cards with local health-care contact information, to be distributed to pupils identified as being at risk. QPR targets all school staff, but it is a selective approach, since only pupils recognized as being at suicidal risk were approached by gatekeepers.

◆ *YAM (Youth Aware of Mental Health)* programme (<http://www.y-a-m.org>) is a five-hour universal intervention targeting all pupils in a school setting.[16] The programme consists of:

  • Three hours of interactive role-play sessions/workshops on themes surrounding knowledge about depression and anxiety, as well as enhancing skills to deal with adverse life events, stress and suicidal behaviours, combined with a 32-page easy-reading booklet, which pupils could take home.

  • Six educational posters displayed in every classroom with bullet points including key information from the 32-page booklet and telephone numbers to local health-care services and healthy lifestyle groups.

  • 1-hour interactive lecture about mental health at the beginning and one hour at the end of the intervention: aimed to increase mental health awareness about risk and protective factors associated with suicide.

The programme was implemented at each one of the ten SEYLE sites by instructors trained in the methodology through a detailed 32-page instruction manual.

ProfScreen (The Screening by Professionals) programme is a selective intervention based on responses to the SEYLE baseline questionnaires, which assessed risk behaviours, symptoms of psychopathology, suicidal thoughts, plans, and suicide attempts. Once pupils completed the baseline assessment, health professionals reviewed their answers and pupils who screened at or above predetermined cut-off points were invited to participate in a professional mental health clinical assessment and subsequently referred to clinical services if needed.[8]

Monitoring risk behaviours

The prevalence of risk behaviours and psychopathology among European adolescents is relatively high.[7,8] The SEYLE study explored the prevalence of alcohol use, illegal drug use, heavy smoking, reduced sleep, weight (over- and under-), sedentary behaviour, excessive use of Internet/television/videogames for reasons not related to schoolwork, and truancy.

Almost all studied risk behaviours showed an increase with age and most risk behaviours were significantly more frequent among boys. The only exceptions were sedentary behaviour and reduced sleep, which are more frequent among girls, who also have more internalizing (emotional) psychiatric symptoms, such as depression, anxiety, and suicidal ideation.

Most importantly, the SEYLE study also identified for the first time a risk group labelled as the 'invisible' risk group, which included 29% of the adolescents.[7] The 'invisible' risk group includes adolescents who spend an excessive amount of time watching television, using the Internet, or playing video games, going to sleep late in order to prolong the use of media activities and who perhaps as a direct consequence, neglect other healthy activities such as sports. The level of psychiatric symptoms found in this 'invisible' risk group was, in many cases, very similar to the high-risk group (percentage for high-risk group given in brackets): 33% (34%) suffered from subthreshold depression; 13.4% (14.7%)

were depressed; 31% (31.3%) had subthreshold anxiety; 8% (9.2%) anxiety; 42.2% (44%) had suicidal ideation; and 5.9% (10.1%) were suicide attempters.

While most parents, teachers, and clinicians would react to an adolescent using drugs or getting drunk, they may overlook adolescent from the 'invisible' risk group who engage in unconstructive behaviours such as watching too much television, not playing sports, or sleeping too little. The causality of the relationship between these risk behaviours and psychopathology remains unclear. However, common psychiatric disorders, such as depression, are known to show bidirectional relationships with reduced sleep,[17] low physical activity, and high media consumption.

Suicidal behaviours can be prevented

The results of the SEYLE RCT performed on approximately 11,000 adolescents from 168 schools in ten European countries demonstrate that a universal intervention called YAM (Youth Aware of Mental Health), targeting adolescent pupils, was significantly more effective in preventing new cases of severe suicidal ideation with plans and suicide attempts compared with the control group.[16] The YAM programme is aimed at changing adolescents' negative perceptions and improving their coping skills in the management of negative life events and stressors. The YAM school-based programme, consisting of 5-hour duration during four weeks, provided adolescents not only knowledge and training to improve coping skills, but also the opportunity to verbalize and discuss among themselves a range of issues related to mental health and suicidal behaviours.[18] The two outcomes of the SEYLE study, namely severe suicidal ideation with plans and suicide attempts, were diminished by 50% due to the YAM intervention. This effect is higher than those noted in other successful public health interventions; e.g., bullying and bully victimization (17–23%) or school-based interventions addressing smoking cessation (14%).[16]

A prevention programme like YAM promotes resilience against a range of risk behaviours and empowers adolescents to take responsibility for their lifestyles and mental health. Results from the European SEYLE study, supported by previous US studies, provide evidence and validity for the effectiveness of a universal suicide-preventive programme performed among school-based adolescents.[16]

Conclusions

Findings from the above-mentioned studies from both the US and European SEYLE study have implications for introducing evidence-based suicide-preventive programmes in schools, as well as informing and educating parents and school staff about adolescent mental health and risky lifestyles.

References

1 **World Health Organization (WHO).** World Suicide Report: Preventing suicide: a global imperative. Geneva; 2014. ISBN 978 92 4 156477 9.

2 **Gould MS, Brunstein Klomek A, Batejan K.** The roles of schools, colleges and universities in suicide prevention. In: Wasserman D, Wasserman C, eds. The Oxford textbook of suicidology and suicide prevention: a global perspective. New York, NY: Oxford University Press: 2009; 551–560.

3 **Gould MS, Kleinman M, Lake AM, Forman J, Basset Midle J.** Newspaper coverage of suicide and initiation of suicide clusters in teenagers in the USA: 1998–1996: a retrospective, population-based, case-control study. Lancet Psych. 2014;**1**(1):34–43.

4 **Andriessen K, Krysinska K.** Essential questions on suicide bereavement and postvention. Int J Environ Res Public Health. 2012 Jan;**9**(1):24–32.

5 **Balazs J, Miklosi M, Kereszteny A, Hoven CW, Carli V, Wasserman C, et al.** Adolescent subthreshold-depression and anxiety: psychopathology, functional impairment and increased suicide risk. J Child Psychol Psychiatry. 2013;**54**(6):670–677.

6 **Kaess M, Brunner R, Parzer P, Carli V, Apter A, Balazs JA, et al.** Risk-behaviour screening for identifying adolescents with mental health problems in Europe. Eur Child Adolesc Psychiatry. 2014;**23**(7):611–620

7 **Carli V, Hoven CW, Wasserman C, Chiesa F, Guffanti G, Sarchiapone M, et al.** A newly identified group of adolescents at 'invisible' risk for psychopathology and suicidal behavior: findings from the SEYLE study. World Psychiatry. 2014 Feb;**13**(1):78–86.

8 **Brunner R, Kaess M, Parzer P, Fischer G, Carli V, Hoven CW, et al.** Life-time prevalence and psychosocial correlates of adolescent direct self-injurious behavior: a comparative study of findings in 11 European countries. J Child Psychol Psychiatry. 2014;**55**(4):337–348.

9 Hoven CW, Wasserman D, Wasserman C, Mandell DJ. Awareness in nine countries: a public health approach to suicide prevention. Led Med (Tokyo). 2000;**11**(Suppl 1):S13–17.

10 Zenere FJ, Lazarus PJ. The decline of youth suicidal behavior in an urban, multi-cultural public school system following the introduction of a suicide prevention and intervention program. Suicide Life Threat Behav. 1997;**27**:387–402.

11 **Aseltine RHJ, De Martino R**. An outcome evaluation of the SOS Suicide Prevention Program. Am J Public Health. 2004;**94**:446–445.

12 **Aseltine RHJ, James A, Schilling EA, Glanovsky J**. Evaluating the SOS suicide prevention program: a replication and extension. BMC Public Health. 2007;**7**:161.

13 **Wilcox HC, Kellam SG, Brown CH, Poduska JM, Ialongo NS, Wang W, et al**. The impact of two universal randomized first- and second-grade classroom interventions on young adult suicide ideation and attempts. Drug Alcohol Depend. 2008 Jun 1;**95** (Suppl 1):S60–73.

14 **Wasserman D, Carli V, Wasserman C, Apter A, Balazs J, Bobes J, et al**. Saving and empowering young lives in Europe (SEYLE): a randomized controlled trial. BMC Public Health. 2010;**10**:192.

15 **Tompkins TL, Witt J, Abraibesh N**. Does a gatekeeper suicide prevention program work in a school setting? Evaluating training outcome and moderators of effectiveness. Suicide Life Threat Behav. 2010;**40**:506–515.

16 **Wasserman D, Hoven CW, Wasserman C, Wall M, Eisenberg R, Hadlaczky G, et al**. School-based suicide prevention programmes: the SEYLE cluster-randomised, controlled trial. Lancet 2015;**385**(9977):1536–1544.

17 **Sarchiapone M, Mandelli L, Carli V, Iosue M, Wasserman C, Hadlaczky G, et al**. Hours of sleep in adolescents and its association with anxiety, emotional concerns, and suicidal ideation. Sleep Med. 2014;**15**(2):248–254.

18 **Wasserman C, Hoven CW, Wasserman D, Carli V, Sarchiapone M, Al-Halabi S, et al**. Suicide prevention for youth—a mental health awareness program: lessons learned from the Saving and Empowering Young Lives in Europe (SEYLE) intervention study. BMC Public Health 2012;**12**:776.

Author index

Subject index